Ligament Reconstruction for Spine

Sang-Ho Lee • Sang-Ha Shin
Junseok Bae • Shin-Jae Kim
Editors

Ligament Reconstruction for Spine

Springer

Editors
Sang-Ho Lee
Wooridul Spine Hospital
Seoul, Korea (Republic of)

Sang-Ha Shin
Wooridul Spine Hospital
Seoul, Korea (Republic of)

Junseok Bae
Wooridul Spine Hospital
Seoul, Korea (Republic of)

Shin-Jae Kim
Wooridul Spine Hospital
Seoul, Korea (Republic of)

ISBN 978-981-95-3970-3 ISBN 978-981-95-3971-0 (eBook)
https://doi.org/10.1007/978-981-95-3971-0

This Springer imprint is published by the registered company Springer Nature Singapore Pte Ltd.
The registered company address is: 152 Beach Road, #21-01/04 Gateway East, Singapore 189721, Singapore

Preface

Lumbar spinal stenosis is one of the most common spinal disorders affecting the elderly. Far from being a mere manifestation of aging, it is a treatable disease with profound implications for survival and quality of life. When left untreated, spinal stenosis leads to gait disturbance, loss of independence, sarcopenia, and cardiopulmonary decline, ultimately contributing to reduced life expectancy. The burden of this condition is most evident among those over the age of 70, a rapidly growing segment of our population.

Yet paradoxically, this group has long been the most underserved. Patients in their 70s or older often present with advanced disease, multiple comorbidities, and osteoporosis, making them poor candidates for extensive procedures such as fusion surgery. Many elderly patients with multi-level stenosis are told that surgery is not possible and that they must endure their symptoms with only medication or injections. For these patients, once considered inoperable, spinal stenosis becomes not only a source of pain but also of despair, robbing them of dignity in their later years.

A new perspective is urgently needed. If we recognize lumbar spinal stenosis as primarily a disease of ligamentous hypertrophy, then decompression can substantially improve neurological symptoms. Moreover, since ligamentum flavum hypertrophy often represents a compensatory response to instability, it is essential to address stability as well. The concept of combining midline decompression technique through the removal of the interspinous ligament and the interlaminar ligament alone—preserving bone (no laminectomy, no facetectomy) and minimizing surgical trauma (no discectomy, no annulectomy)—with ligament reconstruction by two (Sagittal and Horizontal) artificial ligaments to replace the role of the interspinous and interlaminar ligaments offers an elegant and minimally invasive solution. No blood transfusion is needed, for no bone resection is necessary. Furthermore, we can decompress and stabilize five levels at the same time for multiple levels of spinal stenosis (lumbar 1, 2, 3, 4, 5 and sacrum 1), for this is a soft and flexible stabilization.

Over the past two decades, our institution has refined this technique with unwavering focus, culminating in the "SHLee Ligament." This artificial ligament, developed through successive innovations in material and design, represents the maturation of a concept that began with a simple idea: that even frail elderly patients deserve safe and effective surgical treatment. Ligament reconstruction provides shorter operative times, less blood loss, and reduced perioperative risk compared with fusion, while offering meaningful functional recovery.

For patients over 70, 80, and 90 years old who once had no hope of operative treatment, ligament reconstruction offers a new horizon. What was once considered an untreatable condition in this age group can now be addressed with safety and efficacy. Elderly patients, once told to endure, may now regain their mobility, independence, and quality of life. This is not merely a technical advancement; it is a paradigm shift that restores dignity to a population too often overlooked in modern spinal surgery.

This book is dedicated to that mission. It is intended for spine surgeons, trainees, and researchers who seek to advance care for the elderly population with spinal stenosis. Within these chapters, readers will find the theoretical foundation, surgical techniques, and clinical outcomes that define ligament reconstruction. Our hope is that this work will inspire broader adoption of the procedure and foster further innovation, particularly for the benefit of elderly patients worldwide.

We extend our gratitude to the colleagues, trainees, and patients who have supported this journey, and to the elderly patients who entrusted us with their care. Their resilience and determination have been our greatest source of motivation.

Ultimately, our aspiration reaches beyond technical refinement. Should ligament reconstruction one day be recognized at the highest level—even with the honor of a Nobel Prize—it would symbolize not personal ambition, but the fulfillment of medicine's highest calling: to alleviate suffering and to restore hope, especially for those most vulnerable. It is our sincere wish that this book contributes to that vision and to the future of spine surgery for the aging population.

Seoul, South Korea Sang-Ho Lee

Contents

Part IV Complication and Its Management of Ligament Reconstruction

About the Editors

Sang-Ho Lee is the founder of Wooridul Spine Hospital and a renowned spine specialist who has pioneered and advanced state-of-the-art minimally invasive spinal surgery for over four decades. He developed endoscopic spine surgery, successfully extending its application beyond the lumbar spine to cervical and thoracic disc diseases. He is also recognized as a pioneer in the development of advanced surgical techniques, particularly in spine ligament reconstruction.

He has published 318 SCI-indexed papers and has authored 7 medical textbooks. In 2022, his paper "Current Status and Research Hotspots in the Field of Endoscopic Spine Surgery: A Bibliometric Analysis" was published in the SCI-indexed international scientific journal "Frontiers in Surgery," which identified him as "The Most Prolific Researcher in Spinal Endoscopic Surgery."

His achievements have been recognized with the "Parviz Kambin Award" in 2015 and the "Parviz Kambin Award-Gold" in 2019. Under his leadership, Wooridul Spine Hospital was named by *Newsweek* as one of the "World's Best Smart Hospitals" in 2021, 2023, 2024, and 2025, reflecting its excellence in medical innovation and advanced clinical practice.

Sang-Ha Shin a neurosurgeon, serves as President of Wooridul Spine Hospital in Seoul, where he is devoted to clinical work, academic research, and medical education. Through numerous endoscopic and spinal stenosis surgeries, he has accumulated extensive clinical experience. In 2025, he served as President of the Spine Health Academy, contributing to the advancement of global spine care through numerous publications, conference presentations, and textbook authorship. As Director of the Wooridul International Minimally Invasive Spine Surgery Program, he is also committed to training the next generation of spine specialists and disseminating the latest surgical innovations worldwide.

Junseok Bae is Honorary President of Wooridul Spine Hospital in Seoul, where he also directs the Research Center. His clinical and academic focus is on minimally invasive and endoscopic spine surgery, and he contributes actively to education, research, and editorial work, including as Executive Editor of Neurospine. He is a member of several professional societies, including the Scoliosis Research Society (SRS), the International Society for the Study of the Lumbar Spine (ISSLS), the Society for Minimally Invasive

Spine Surgery Asia-Pacific (SMISS AP), the Korean Minimally Invasive Spine Surgery Society (KOMISS), and the Korean Society of Endoscopic Spine Surgery (KOSESS), through which he continues to support the advancement of spine care nationally and internationally.

Shin-Jae Kim is Director of the International Healthcare Center and Chair of the Social Contribution Committee at Wooridul Spine Hospital in Seoul. He earned his medical degree and Master of Medicine from Chung-Ang University, where he also completed his internship and neurosurgery residency, and he is board-certified in neurosurgery. He has also obtained international qualifications, including Fellowship of the American Board of Minimally Invasive Spine Surgery (FABMISS) and Fellowship of the Royal College of Physicians and Surgeons (FRCS). His clinical and academic focus is on minimally invasive and advanced spinal surgery, and he has been actively involved in research, publications, and education while contributing to international collaborations through lectures and conference activities. As a member of leading professional societies such as KOMISS, KOSASS, NASS, and AO Spine, he continues to play a vital role in promoting the advancement of spine surgery both in Korea and worldwide.

Part I
Introduction

1 Pathophysiology of Degenerative Lumbar Spinal Stenosis

Gene Cheh

Abstract

Degenerative lumbar spinal stenosis, which mainly affects older persons, is characterized by narrowing of the spinal canal, foramina, or lateral recesses, which causes compression of neural components. Age-related degeneration of the facet joints, ligaments, and intervertebral discs is the cause. The neural canal is narrowed by degenerative changes in the facet, including osteophyte development and hypertrophy, subchondral bone sclerosis, and cartilage degeneration. Disc dehydration, height loss, and bulging are examples of degenerative changes in the intervertebral disc that affect spinal mechanics and put more strain on nearby structures. Compression and instability are exacerbated by spondylolisthesis and ligamentum flavum thickening. Characteristic symptoms such as neurogenic claudication and radicular pain are caused by neural compression and ischemia. Age, genetic predisposition, obesity, and repetitive mechanical stress are risk factors. The intensity of symptoms might be influenced by dynamic factors, such as changes in posture. Understanding these mechanisms is essential for management.

G. Cheh (✉)
Department of Orthopedics, Cheongdam Wooridul Spine Hospital, Seoul, Korea (Republic of)
e-mail: genecheh@gmail.com

Keywords

Facet hypertrophy · Ligamentum flavum thickening · Buckled annulus · Endplate osteophyte · Neurogenic claudication

1.1 Introduction

Sciatica has afflicted humanity for centuries [1], but its true cause remained a mystery until 1934. That year, Mixter and Barr [2] identified herniated discs as the primary culprit, marking the beginning of the "disc dynasty" in spine surgery. Similarly, spinal stenosis—another major cause of radiating leg pain—was first described in 1948 by van Gelderen [3], who linked neurogenic leg symptoms to the narrowing of the lumbar spinal canal. Although surgeries for spinal stenosis were performed prior to this discovery, the condition was often misdiagnosed as an extramedullary tumor [4], much like herniated discs were mistaken for enchondromas before 1934.

Van Gelderen reported on two patients who had pain, weakness, and numbness in the leg after walking for 10–15 min. They experienced the same pain when they stood erect, and were relieved of it when they sat down. One of the men was pain-free when riding his bicycle and playing tennis. He concluded that their pain was more likely to be caused by lordotic posture than by activity.

S.-H. Lee et al. (eds.), *Ligament Reconstruction for Spine*,
https://doi.org/10.1007/978-981-95-3971-0_1

Degenerative lumbar spinal stenosis (DLSS) is a condition characterized by the narrowing of the spinal canal, neural foramina, or lateral recesses, resulting in compression of the neural elements in the lumbar spine. DLSS primarily affects older adults, often leading to back and leg pain, neurogenic claudication, and impaired mobility [5]. The etiology of this condition is multifactorial and involves degenerative changes in the facet joints and the intervertebral discs and ligaments [6].

1.2 Anatomical Changes

The lumbar spinal canal contains the cauda equina which supplies the lower limbs, pelvis, and bladder. The foramina allow for the passage of spinal nerves, while the lateral recesses provide additional space for nerve root movement. Degenerative changes in any of these structures can lead to spinal stenosis [7].

Degenerative changes in facet joints and intervertebral discs typically accompany aging, with some individuals experiencing facet arthrosis before disc degeneration, while in others, degeneration begins in the disc.

According to the Kirkaldy-Willis model, the degenerative process of the lumbar spine progresses through three stages: dysfunction, instability, and stabilization. The dysfunction stage is characterized by nuclear degeneration, annular tears, and facet arthropathy.

Following the dysfunction stage, the progression to instability or stabilization does not necessarily follow a linear sequence but can diverge into two distinct pathways: the unstable pathway, marked by abnormal spinal motion due to loosened facet joints, ligaments, decreased disc height, and increased mobility, often leading to degenerative spondylolisthesis (Fig. 1.1); and the stable pathway, where the spine undergoes advanced degeneration to restore stability. This stage is defined by osteophyte formation, enlarged facet joints, and restricted movement (Fig. 1.2). As noted by Kirkaldy-Willis, some patients initially experience instability but gradually transition to stabilization over time (Fig. 1.3).

1.2.1 Facet Joint Degeneration

Degenerative lumbar facet arthrosis plays a significant role in the etiology of spinal stenosis.

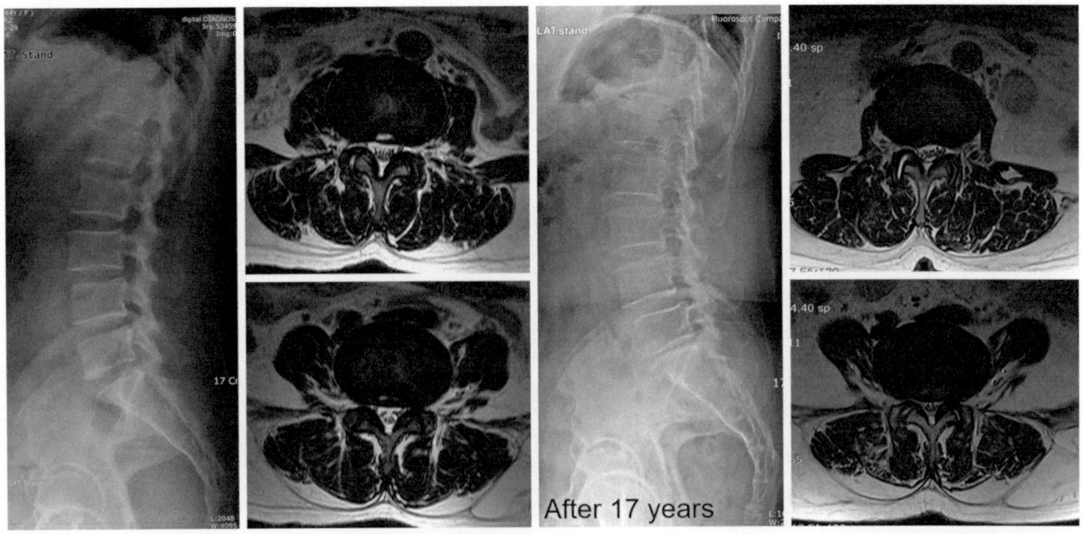

Fig. 1.1 A 61-year-old woman with low back and leg pain demonstrates facet instability that has progressed over 17 years

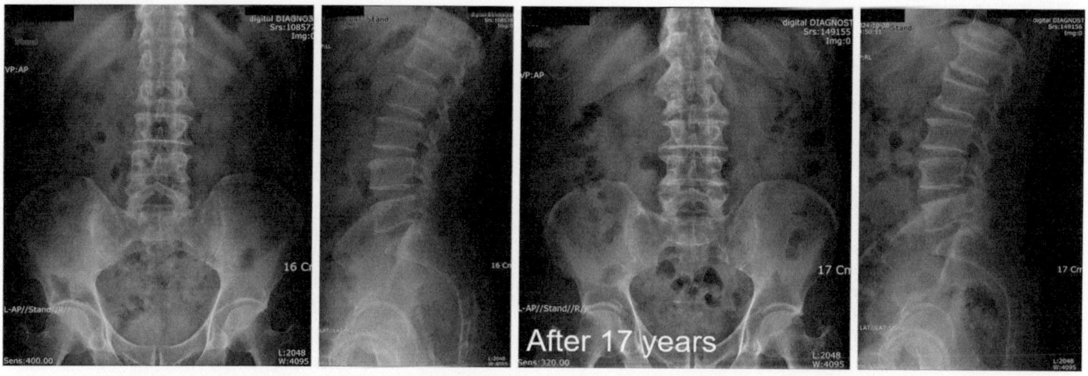

Fig. 1.2 A 74-year-old man has a claw spur stabilizing his spine compared to the radiographs from 17 years ago

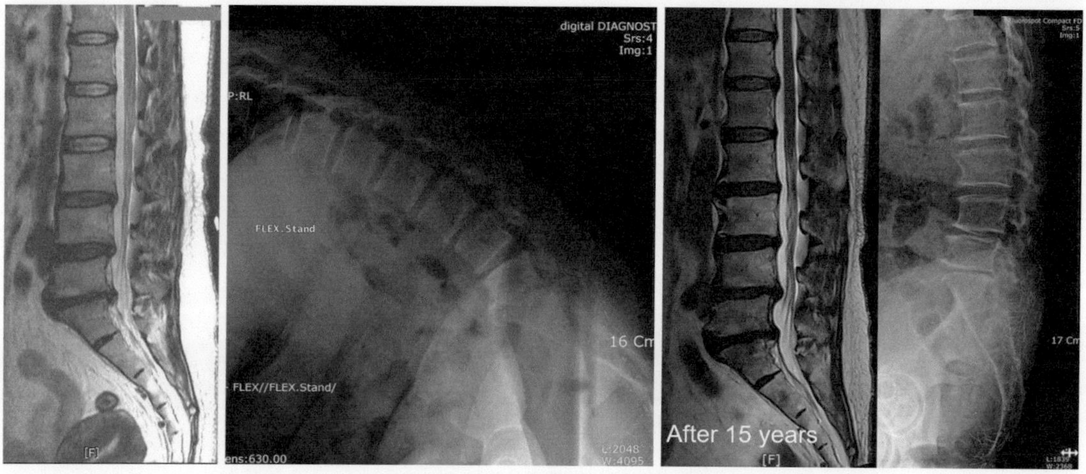

Fig. 1.3 A 62-year-old lady with previous angular instability has become stable with little stenosis on 15-year follow-up imaging

Contrary to the commonly held notion that facet arthrosis represents a mere sequela of disc degeneration [8, 9], facet degeneration precedes disc degeneration [10] (Fig. 1.4). The lumbar facet joints share the mechanical load with intervertebral discs and are essential for maintaining spinal stability while allowing for movement. The "three-joint complex" consisting of the intervertebral disc and the two facet joints function as one unit so that a pathological change in one joint will affect the other joints at that level and ultimately the adjacent spinal levels [11] (Fig. 1.5). These biomechanical roles make the lumbar facet joints prone to wear and tear, especially under conditions of repetitive stress and aging.

With degeneration, facet joints experience the breakdown of articular cartilage, joint space narrowing, osteophyte formation, and synovial inflammation. These changes result in abnormal spinal movement, pain, and instability. Hypertrophy of the facet joints, often secondary to chronic instability or mechanical stress, narrows the spinal canal, lateral recess and foramina, narrowing these spaces and compressing the exiting nerve roots [12].

Over time, mechanical stresses lead to microdamage within the cartilage, resulting in thinning, fissuring, and eventual loss of cartilage integrity especially in the area subjected to significant mechanical forces.

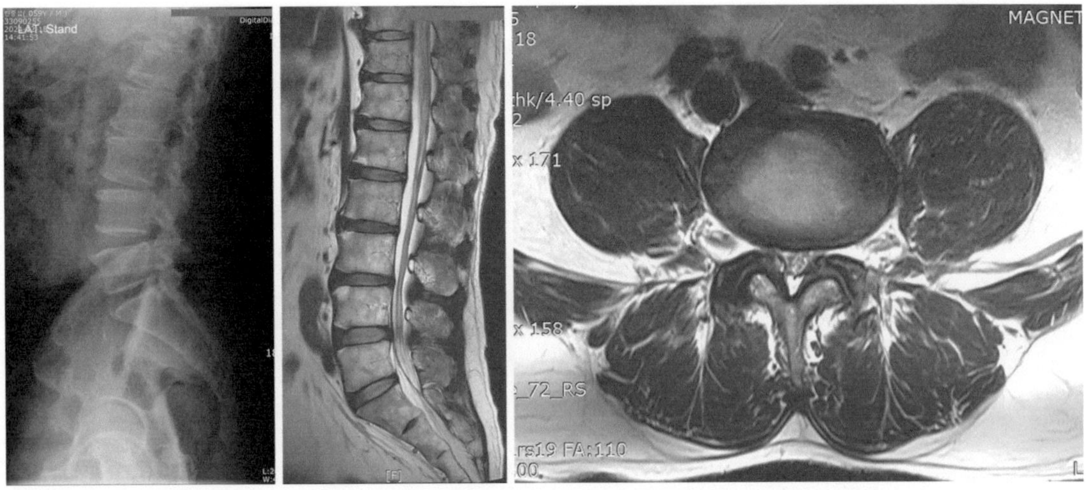

Fig. 1.4 Facet arthrosis precedes disc degeneration in this patient with spinal stenosis at L4-5

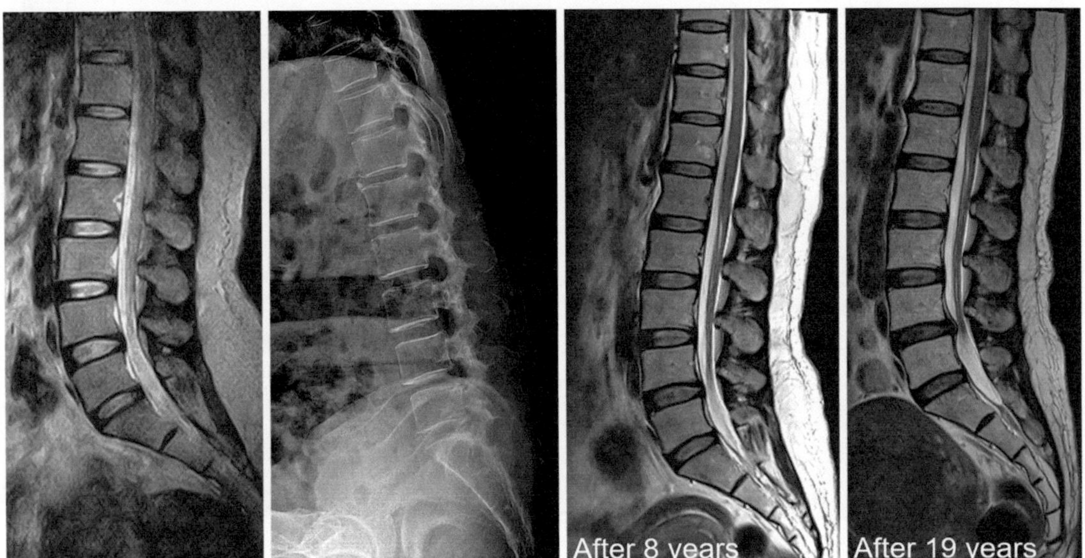

Fig. 1.5 Facet arthrosis ultimately affects disc degeneration as shown on 8-year and 19-year follow-up of a 44-year-old patient

As the protective cartilage layer erodes, the underlying subchondral bone is subjected to increased mechanical stress. In response, pathological changes such as subchondral sclerosis, microfractures, and subchondral cyst occur.

Subchondral sclerosis is an adaptation to the increased load. Although this compensatory mechanism initially stabilizes the joint, it leads to a loss of bone elasticity, making the joint more prone to further degeneration.

Repeated mechanical stress on the subchondral bone can result in microfractures, which can also lead to changes in joint congruence, further destabilizing the joint.

Degenerative changes in the subchondral bone can result in the formation of subchondral cysts, fluid-filled cavities within the bone (Fig. 1.6).

As the joint becomes increasingly unstable, the body attempts to compensate by producing osteophytes along the edges of the joint. These

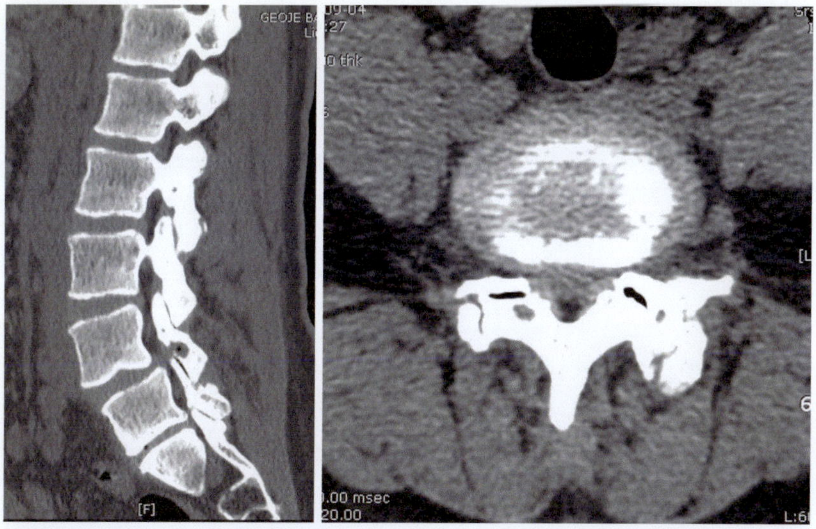

Fig. 1.6 Subchondral cyst

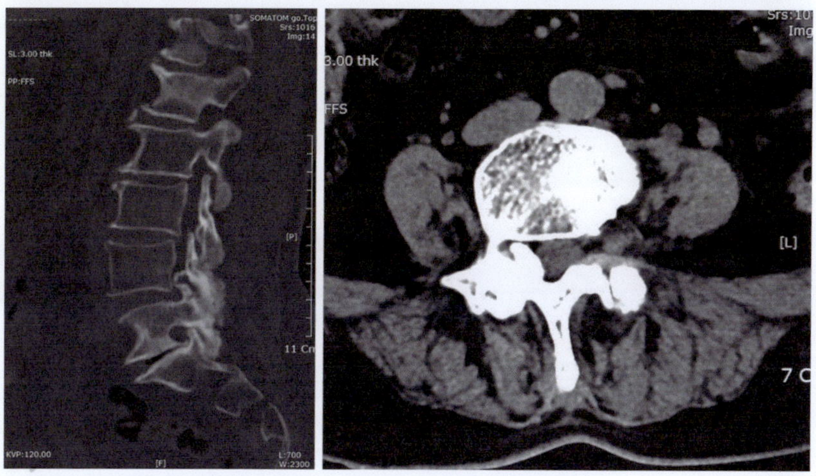

Fig. 1.7 Foraminal stenosis by ossification of the ligamentum flavum

osteophytes develop as part of a maladaptive bone remodeling process aimed at stabilizing the joint. However, osteophytes limit the joint motion and contribute to stiffness. Osteophytes can impinge on nearby neural structures (Fig. 1.7).

Facet arthrosis is associated with chronic inflammation of the synovial membrane. Synovitis leads to an increase in synovial fluid production, causing joint effusion. This swelling can stretch the joint capsule and form facet cyst (Fig. 1.8).

1.2.2 Thickening of the Ligamentum Flavum

The ligament flavum arises from the lower half of the anterior surface of the lamina above and attaches to the posterior surface and upper border of the lamina below. The ligamentum flavum's high elasticity plays a vital role in maintaining an upright posture and enabling the spine to return to its original shape after flexion. Its elasticity facilitates smooth, controlled spinal movements

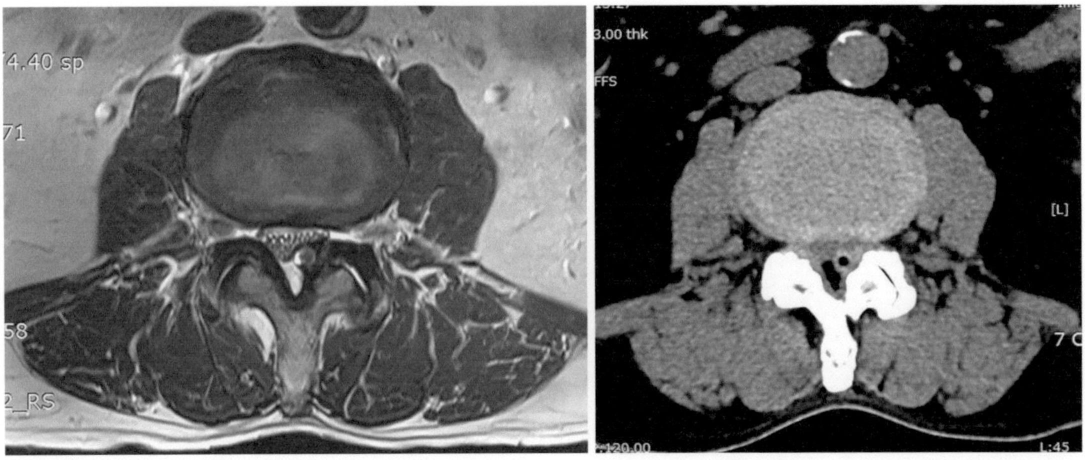

Fig. 1.8 Facet cyst

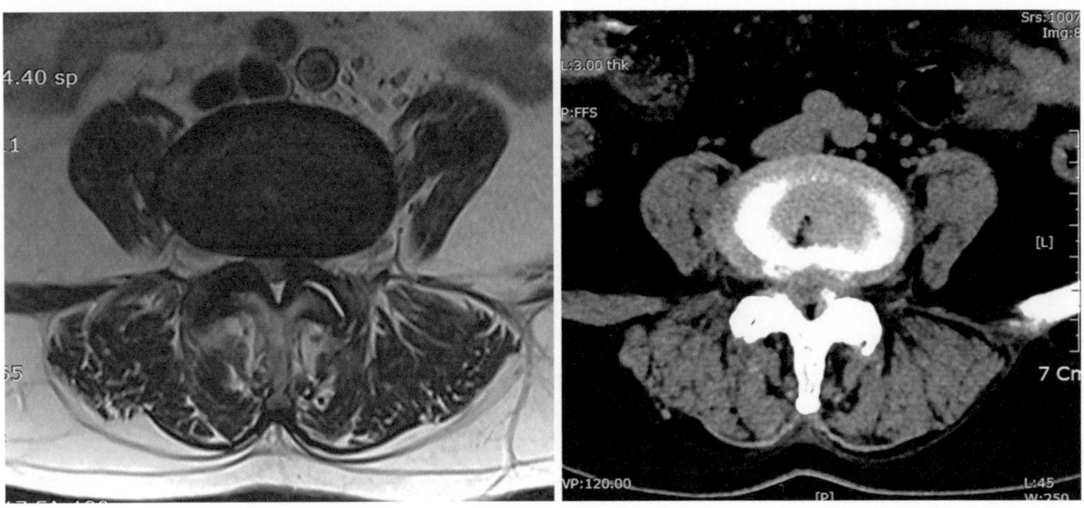

Fig. 1.9 Facet effusion and calcified ligamentum flavum

and minimizes the energy required to return the spine to a neutral posture, promoting efficient motion. The ligamentum flavum resists excessive separation of adjacent vertebral laminae and prevents the ligament from buckling into the spinal canal during extension, thereby avoiding canal compression.

However, repetitive mechanical stress can lead to a loss of elasticity in the ligamentum flavum, resulting in increased collagen fiber thickness and calcium deposition within the ligament (Fig. 1.9). These degenerative changes cause thickening of ligamentum flavum, which can narrow the spinal canal and compress the cauda equina and nerve roots.

1.2.3 Intervertebral Disc Degeneration

In some individuals, degenerative changes in the discs may precede facet arthrosis (Fig. 1.10). The intervertebral discs are fibrocartilaginous structures that provide cushioning and flexibility between vertebrae. With age or genetic predisposition, the discs undergo degenerative changes

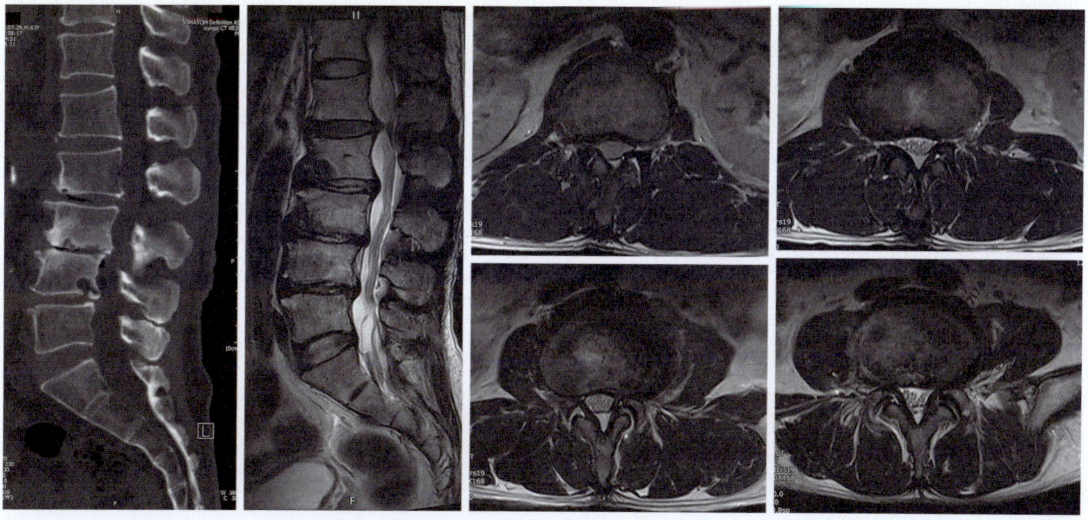

Fig. 1.10 Predominant discopathy with minimal stenosis

that include loss of water content, reduced disc height, and bulging. These changes reduce the disc's ability to absorb mechanical forces, causing abnormal load distribution across the vertebral bodies and facet joints. Bulging discs can directly encroach on the spinal canal and foramina, leading to compression of neural elements.

The progressive deterioration of the intervertebral discs can lead to a cascade of anatomical and physiological changes. The disc dehydration and shrinkage cause a decrease in intervertebral disc height, leading to reduced space between vertebrae and increased stress on surrounding spinal structures.

With weakening of the annulus fibrosus, tears can occur, particularly in the posterior regions of the disc where stress is greatest. In some cases, the nucleus pulposus may protrude through these tears, causing a herniated disc that can compress spinal nerves and cause radicular pain.

As disc height decreases, the buckled annulus narrows the spinal canal and foramen. The load on the facet joints increases leading to facet joint osteoarthritis, which further contributes to disc degeneration.

Osteophytes form along the edges of the vertebral endplate as a response to chronic mechanical stress or disc degeneration. While this process initially serves to stabilize the spinal column, excessive osteophyte formation can protrude into the spinal canal or foramina, further narrowing these spaces and compressing neural structures.

Subchondral sclerosis and cyst form in response to mechanical stress on the denuded cartilage endplate [13].

1.3 Spondylolisthesis and Scoliosis

The facet joint capsule may become lax as the joint degenerates, further contributing to joint instability. Capsular laxity allows for excessive motion between vertebrae, increasing the risk of spondylolisthesis and further joint damage.

As the facet joints lose their ability to effectively stabilize the spine, the mechanical load shifts to the intervertebral discs. This compensatory mechanism accelerates disc degeneration, leading to a vicious cycle of spinal degeneration.

When the two vertebrae are misaligned, the pathways through them are also narrowed. Degenerative spondylolisthesis, where forward slippage of the vertebral body occurs, the spinal canal narrows but the foramen widens. Foraminal stenosis is rare in the degenerative spondylolisthesis, though not impossible.

Scoliosis can alter the distribution of mechanical forces in the lumbar spine, placing increased stress on the facet joints and accelerating the degenerative process. Both central canal and foraminal stenosis can occur in the degenerative scoliosis. Canal stenosis is caused by rotatory encroachment of the Inferior articular process on the concave side (Fig. 1.11). If there is a fixed tilt with an asymmetrical collapse of the disc, a foraminal stenosis that results in nerve compression between the endplate osteophyte and superior articular process is common (Fig. 1.12).

Open subluxations, characterized by the disc being wedged open on the convex side where the vertebra above is slipping, predominantly result in contralateral lateral recess and foraminal stenosis. Closed dislocations, where the disc is wedged closed on the convex side as the vertebra above slips, exhibit an ipsilateral pattern of stenosis [14] (Fig. 1.13).

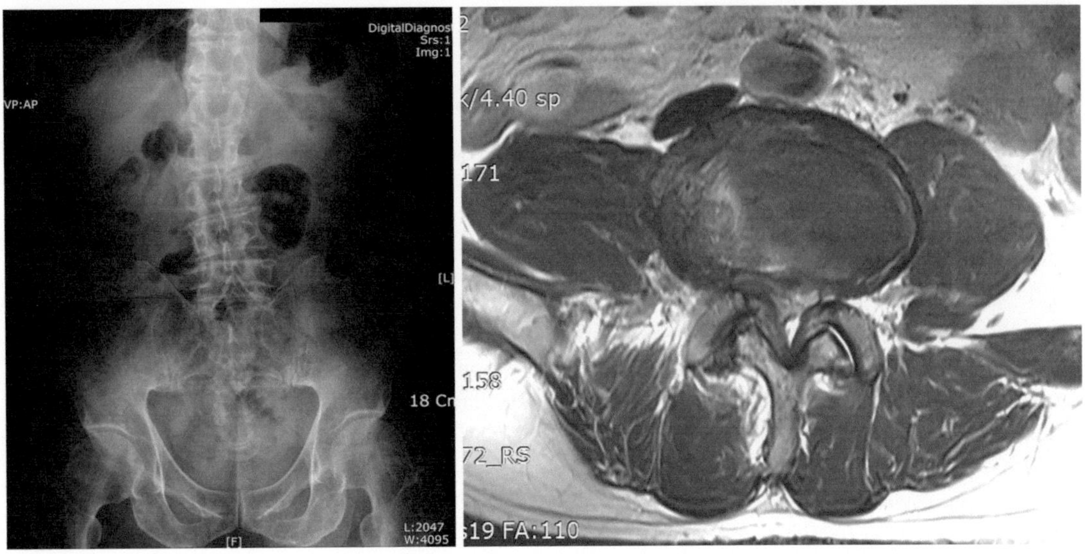

Fig. 1.11 Canal stenosis at the concavity of the scoliosis

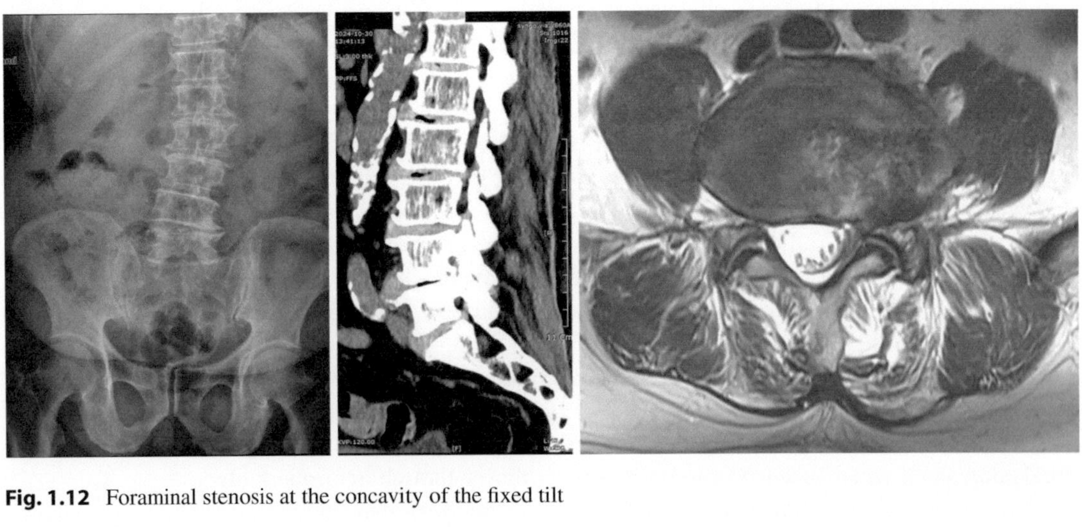

Fig. 1.12 Foraminal stenosis at the concavity of the fixed tilt

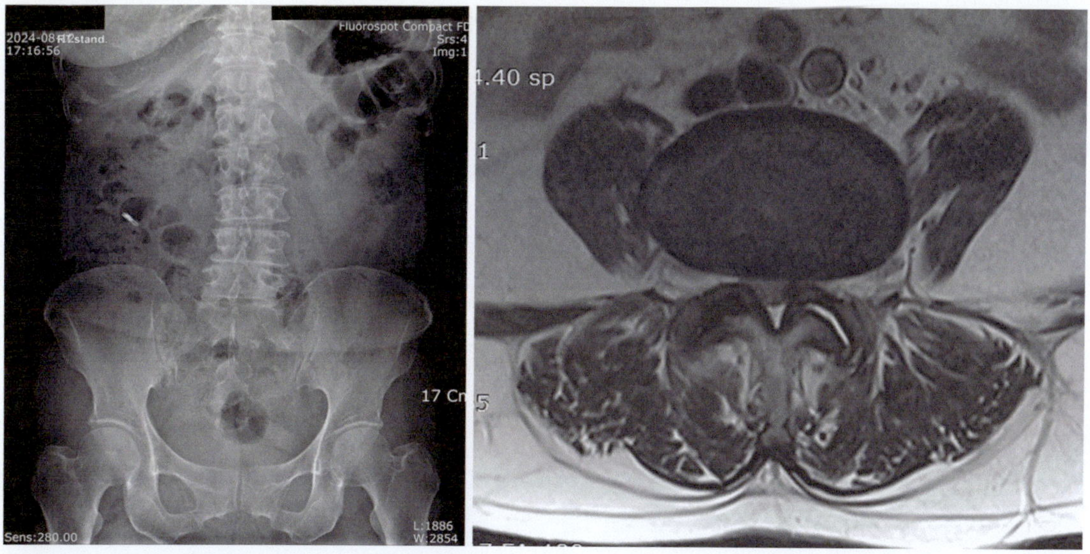

Fig. 1.13 Canal stenosis at the convexity of the scoliosis

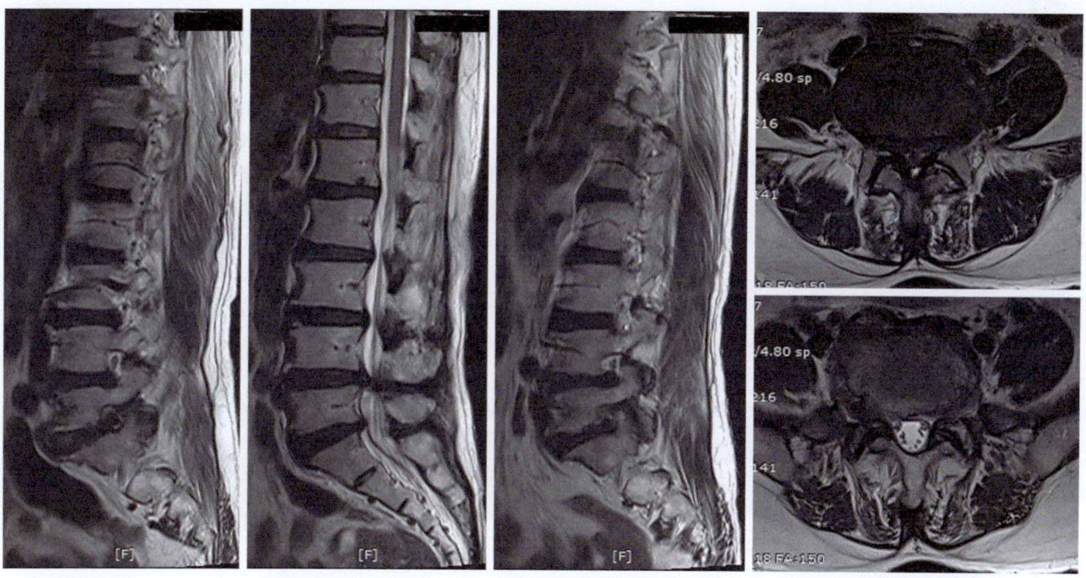

Fig. 1.14 Foraminal stenosis at L5-S1 and canal stenosis at L4-5

1.4 L5-S1

The lumbosacral junction is a transitional spinal segment that accounts for half of the lumbar lordosis and plays a critical role in transferring upper body loads to the pelvis. The L5-S1 intervertebral disc endures significant mechanical stress, making it particularly prone to degeneration, with discopathy being more common than facet joint arthritis at this level. The coronally oriented facet joints at L5-S1 resist spondylolisthesis by providing a mechanical block. However, disc height loss can cause the superior articular process to slide downward, leading to retrolisthesis, which contributes to central canal stenosis being rare but foraminal stenosis common at L5-S1 (Fig. 1.14).

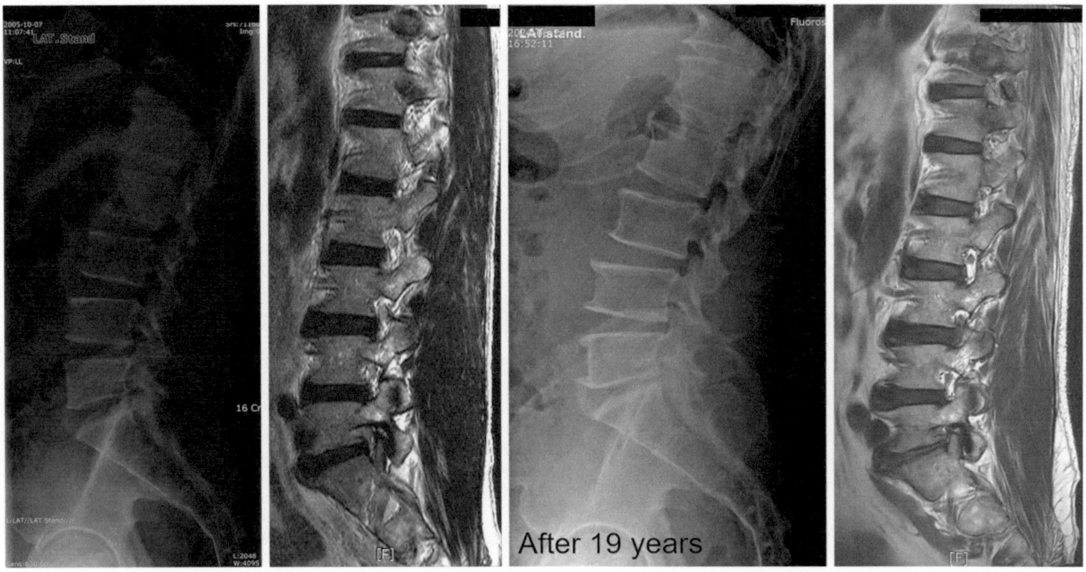

Fig. 1.15 Changes in the L5-S1 foramen over 19 years

Key contributors to foraminal stenosis include a buckled annulus from disc collapse, endplate osteophytes, a hypertrophied superior articular process, buckled ligamentum flavum, and retrolisthesis (Fig. 1.15). L5-S1 is a frequent site of dynamic foraminal stenosis, exacerbated by the trapezoidal shape of the L5 vertebral body and the anterior thickness of the L5-S1 disc, which contribute to narrow foramina. Extension further worsens foraminal stenosis by causing anterior displacement of the superior articular process. This dynamic nature of foraminal stenosis can be challenging to detect on MRIs.

1.5 Dynamic Nature of Spinal Stenosis

Because spinal stenosis is a dynamic illness, posture frequently affects its symptoms, especially those of central canal stenosis. The ligamentum flavum stretches when the lower back is in flexion, increasing the amount of space in the spinal canal and relieving pressure on the spinal nerves. On the other hand, the ligamentum flavum buckles inward when the spine is extended or standing erect, squeezing the spinal nerves against the disc bulge.

When standing for long periods of time or climbing downhill, where the extension of the spine is more noticeable, the back pain or leg discomfort appears rapidly. By creating more room in the spinal canal and neural foramina, sitting or bending forward reduces symptoms.

Supine MRI demonstrates static stenosis, but it may underestimate the degree of canal and foraminal narrowing. Standing MRIs are not commonly accessible and may cause discomfort for patients in a loaded position, despite the fact that they may offer deeper insights into this dynamic problem. The clinical diagnosis of radicular pain may be enhanced by methods to imaging the spine under loading conditions or to establish criteria for identifying patients at risk for occult stenosis during loading of the spine [15].

1.6 Pathophysiological Mechanisms

The hallmark symptoms of DLSS, including neurogenic claudication and radicular pain, are primarily a result of neural compression. The narrowing of the spinal canal or foramina creates direct mechanical pressure on the nerve roots and cauda equina.

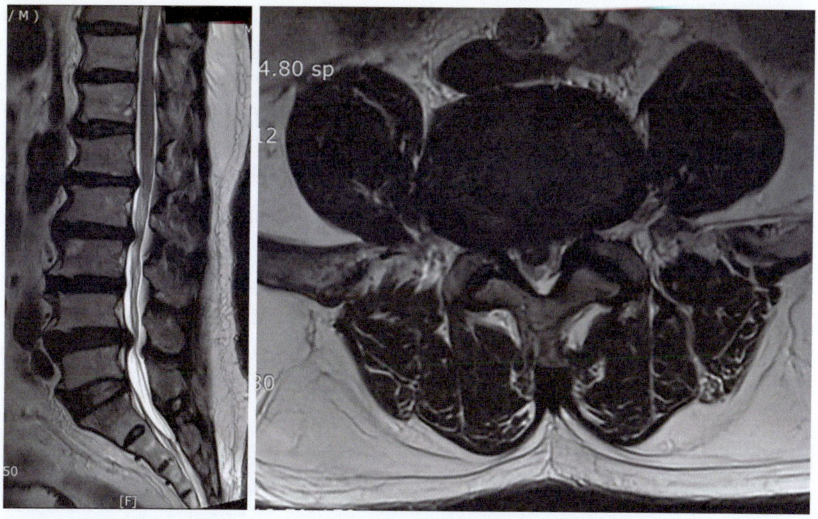

Fig. 1.16 A herniated lumbar disc can cause neurogenic claudication when it compresses the cauda equina

Neurogenic claudication is characterized by leg pain, weakness, or numbness exacerbated by walking or prolonged standing and relieved by sitting or leaning forward [16]. The classic "shopping cart sign" is commonly observed in patients, where leaning forward while pushing a cart relieves the pain by increasing the spinal canal diameter. The lordotic posture, rather than exercise causes neurogenic claudication [17].

Neurogenic claudication is typically linked to stenosis involving at least two levels [18]. The proposed mechanism involves two-level venous compression, leading to venous pooling around one or more nerve roots, which contributes to the pathophysiology of the condition. Neurogenic claudication is frequently caused by compression of the cauda equina or ganglion at the foramen (Fig. 1.16).

Radicular pain is the pain radiating along the distribution of the compressed nerve roots. In DLSS, this often manifests as sciatica, where pain radiates from the lumbar spine into the buttocks, thighs, and legs.

Chronic nerve compression rarely causes motor weakness, but sensory changes, such as numbness, tingling, or burning sensations, are common.

Compression of neural elements in DLSS reduces arterial blood flow to the cauda equina and nerve roots. The nerve roots and cauda equina rely on an intricate network of microvasculature for oxygen and nutrients. Stenosis can impede this blood supply, leading to ischemia, which exacerbates nerve dysfunction and contributes ischemic pain and weakness. Alternatively, blood pooling in the veins causes insufficient oxygenation in the capillary bed, a buildup of metabolites in the cauda equina, and consequent pain and claudication [19]. Additionally, walking may make symptoms worse because the spinal nerve roots' increased oxygen demand may be greater than the blood flow that is available.

1.7 Risk Factors Contributing to Spinal Stenosis

Several risk factors are implicated in the development and progression of lumbar spinal stenosis.

The most significant risk factor is aging. As individuals age, the cumulative effects of mechanical stress and biological changes in cartilage and bone contribute to spinal stenosis. Age-related changes such as disc dehydration, ligamentous laxity, and osteoarthritis are key contributors to the onset of DLSS. Additionally, age-related microvascular changes may further impair blood flow to the nerve roots, exacerbating ischemic damage.

Although age is the primary risk factor, genetic and environmental influences also play a role in the development of DLSS. Genetic predisposition to disc degeneration or osteoarthritis can accelerate the onset of spinal stenosis. Excess body weight increases the mechanical load on the lumbar spine, accelerating the wear and tear on the facet joints. Individuals who engage in activities that involve repetitive bending, twisting, or heavy lifting are at increased risk due to the excessive mechanical stress placed on the joints.

The alignment of the spine influences the development of stenosis. Less lumbar lordosis results in disc loading and discopathy, while more lumbar lordosis or repeated extension stress results in facet arthritis.

Roussouly [20] identified four types of lumbar spine, with type 4 lordosis being the most prone to spinal stenosis. In type 4 lordosis, the increased number of vertebrae in a lordotic orientation and a state of segmental hyperextension exists. Roussouly Type 1 creates a long thoracolumbar kyphosis, transitioning abruptly into a straighter lumbar spine. The reduced number of vertebrae forming lumbar lordosis and limited shock-absorbing capacity leads to mechanical overload, accelerated joint degeneration, and a high risk of arthritic changes in the facet joints.

Excessive stress on the facet joints occurs when compensatory hyperlordosis develops to counteract thoracolumbar kyphosis, leading to stenosis in the lower lumbar region (Fig. 1.17).

Spinal fusion or ankylosed spine, stress is concentrated in the adjacent segment, causing facet overload and accelerating degeneration (Fig. 1.18).

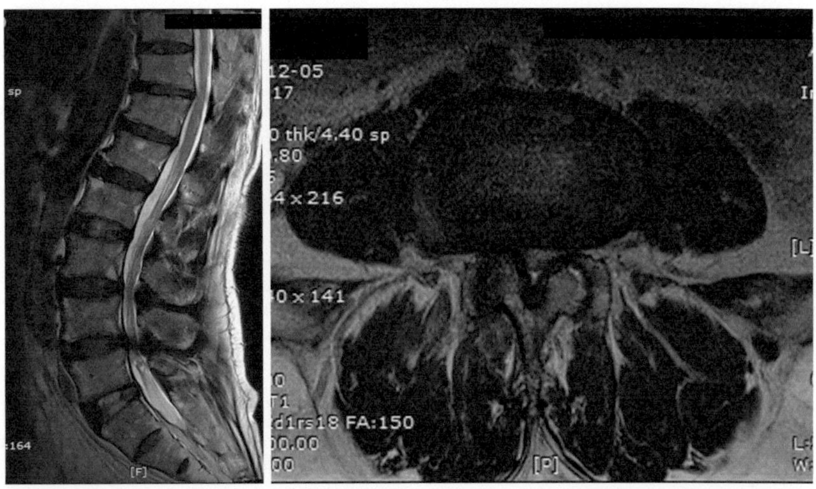

Fig. 1.17 Spinal stenosis due to compensatory lumbar lordosis in a patient with TL kyphosis

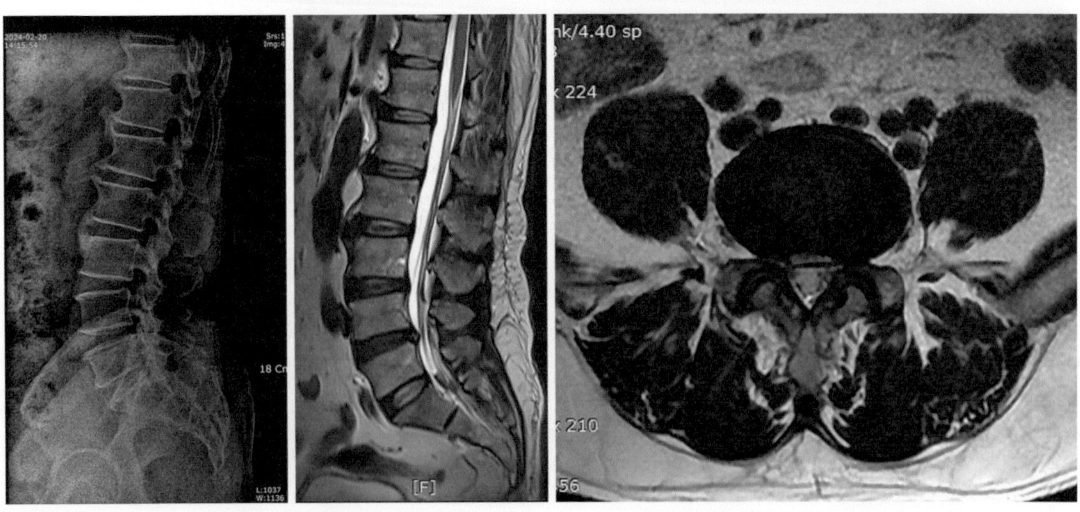

Fig. 1.18 Spinal stenosis adjacent to the ankylosing segment

The presence of transitional vertebrae and the number of lumbar vertebrae can contribute to excessive loading on the facet joint which in turn promotes degenerative changes.

1.8 Summary

Degenerative lumbar spinal stenosis is caused by a confluence of age-related, mechanical, and maybe hereditary variables. The combination of osteoarthritis in the facet joints, disc degeneration, ligamentous hypertrophy, and spondylolisthesis narrows the spinal canal and foramina, compressing the nerves and resulting in the hallmark symptoms of neurogenic claudication or radiculopathy.

References

1. Truumees E. A history of lumbar disc herniation from Hippocrates to the 1990s. Clin Orthop Relat Res. 2015;473:1885–95.
2. Mixter WJ, Barr JS. Rupture of the intervertebral disc with involvement of the spinal canal. N Engl J Med. 1934;211:210–5.
3. Van Gelderen C. Ein orthotisches (lordotisches) Kaudasyndrom. Acta Psychiatr Neurol. 1948;23:57–68.
4. Bailey P, Casamajor L. Osteoarthritis of the spine as a cause of compression of the spinal cord and its root: with report of five cases. J Nerv Ment Dis. 1911;38:588–609.
5. Genevay S, Atlas SJ. Lumbar spinal stenosis. Best Pract Res Clin Rheumatol. 2010;24(2):253–65.
6. Rauschning W. Pathoanatomy of lumbar disc degeneration and stenosis. Acta Orthop Scand. 1993;64(Suppl 251):3–12.
7. Szpalski M, Gunzburg R. Lumbar spinal stenosis in the elderly: an overview. Eur Spine J. 2003;12(Suppl 2):S170–5.
8. Butler D, Trafimow JH, Andersson GBJ, McNeill TW, Huckman MS. Discs degenerate before facets. Spine. 1990;15:111–3.
9. Deer T, Sayed D, et al. A review of lumbar spinal stenosis with intermittent neurogenic claudication: disease and diagnosis. Pain Med. 2019;20(Suppl 2):S32–44.
10. Eubanks JD, Lee MJ, Cassinelli E, Ahn NU. Does lumbar facet arthrosis precede disc degeneration? Clin Orthop Relat Res. 2007;464:184–9.
11. Kirkaldy-Willis WH, Wedge JH, Yong-Hing K, Reilly J. Pathology and pathogenesis of lumbar spondylosis and stenosis. Spine. 1978;3(4):319–28.
12. Botwin KP, Gruber RD. Lumbar spinal stenosis: anatomy and pathogenesis. Phys Med Rehabil Clin N Am. 2003;14:1–15.
13. Rauschning W. New perspectives in spinal anatomy. Spine. 2016;41(7 Suppl):S4–5.
14. Gardner ROE, Torrie PAG, et al. A radiological evaluation of lateral vertebral subluxation associated with spinal stenosis in the lumbar spine in degenerative scoliosis. Spine Deform. 2013;1:365–70.
15. Nowicki BH, Yu S, Reinartz J, Pintar FA, Yoganandan N, Haughton V. Occult lumbar lateral spinal stenosis in neural foramina subjected to physiologic loading. Am J Neuroradiol. 1996;17(9):1605–14.
16. Verbiest H. A radicular syndrome from developmental narrowing of the lumbar vertebral canal. J Bone Joint Surg Br. 1954;36(2):230–7.
17. Dyck P, Doyle JB. "Bicycle test" of van Gelderen in diagnosis of intermittent cauda equina compression syndrome. J Neurosurg. 1977;46:667–70.
18. Porter RW, Ward D. Cauda equina dysfunction: the significance of two-level pathology. Spine. 1992;17:9–15.
19. Rydevik B, Brown MD, Lundborg G. Pathoanatomy and pathophysiology of nerve root compression. Spine. 1984;9(1):7–15.
20. Roussouly P, Gollogly S, Berthonnaud E, Dimnet J. Classification of the normal variation in the sagittal alignment of the human lumbar spine and pelvis in the standing position. Spine. 2005;30:346–53.

Clinical Presentation of Lumbar Spinal Stenosis

2

Wonsok Chang

Abstract

Lumbar spinal stenosis (LSS), a disease that mainly affects people over 50 years old, may have a dramatic presentation with pain, difficulty in walking, and changes in urinary functions in addition to root symptoms, such as numbness, burning, and feeling of heaviness in the legs.

Keywords

Lumbar spinal stenosis · Neurogenic claudication · Vascular claudication · Sciatica · Low back pain

Patients with lumbar spinal stenosis generally seek for care when the disease affects their capability to work, walk distances, or participate in other occupational activities.

Despite a clinical definition that often relies on anatomic findings, the clinical diagnosis and the assessment of the severity of lumbar spinal stenosis depends primarily on the patient's description of their symptoms and on the physical examination (Table 2.1).

Table 2.1 Symptoms of spinal stenosis

Pain	Typically in the lower back or neck, radiating to the arms or legs
Numbness or tingling	Often felt in the extremities, such as arms, hands, legs, or feet
Weakness	Muscular weakness may occur in the affected area, leading to difficulty in lifting or gripping objects
Cramping	Muscle cramps or spasms, especially during physical activity or prolonged standing
Sciatica	Compression of the nerves can lead to sciatic nerve pain, causing shooting pain down the leg

When interventions are being considered, correlation with imaging findings is also essential.

Extension may be more limited than flexion [1]. Hamstring tightness is often described. The neurologic examination typically is normal, and findings when present are usually mild motor weakness or sensory changes.

Patients typically present with discomfort in the lower back, buttocks, and thighs, sometimes extending to the lower legs and feet.

The lower leg pain may be unilateral or bilateral and sometimes may be accompanied by tingling sensation and paresthesia of the feet and lower legs, reflecting compression of sensory nerve fibers. If compression of nerve becomes serious, patients would feel worsening of balance and a wide-based gait reflecting compression of the posterior column medial lemniscus fibers that

W. Chang (✉)
Department of Anesthesiology, Cheongdam Wooridul Spine Hospital, Seoul, Korea (Republic of)

S.-H. Lee et al. (eds.), *Ligament Reconstruction for Spine*,
https://doi.org/10.1007/978-981-95-3971-0_2

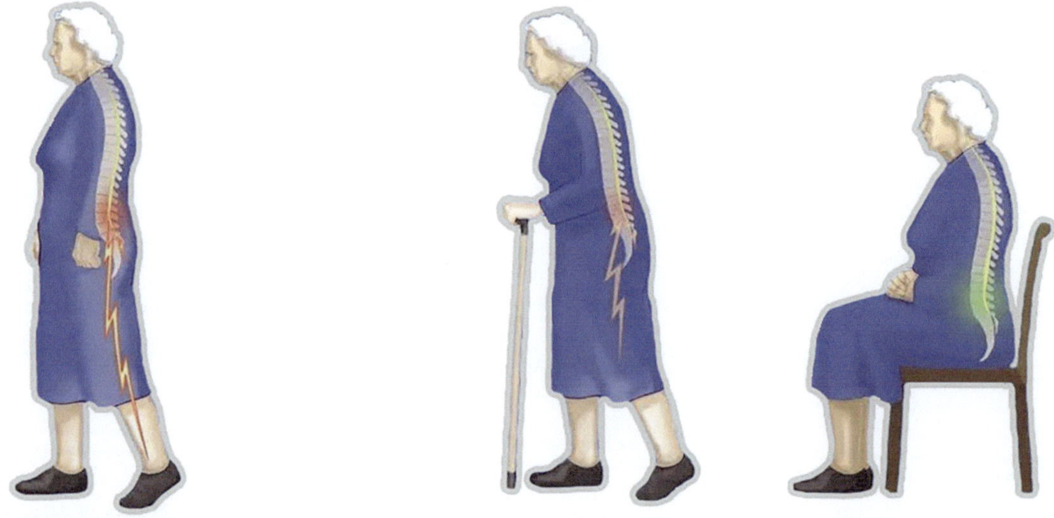

Fig. 2.1 Symptoms of spinal stenosis

provide awareness of position. The condition is more common in older individuals and often improves with sitting or forward bending (Fig. 2.1). Patients with lumbar stenosis also can report nocturnal leg cramps [2] and neurogenic bladder symptoms [3].

In the classical situation, patients are described as complaining of neurogenic claudication, also referred to as pseudoclaudication. Neurogenic claudication refers to leg symptoms encompassing the buttock, groin, and anterior thigh, as well as radiation down the posterior part of the leg to the feet. Patients feel pain, weakness, heaviness, or tiredness in the legs after standing erect or walking a variable distance. Relief comes from sitting or flexing the lumbar spine, in contrast to ischemic claudication of the legs, which resolves on standing still. Patients with neurogenic claudication report that lying on back is often associated with less relief while lying on the side is more comfortable.

Chronic low back pain may exist before limb symptoms by several years. The described symptoms are largely based on patients seen at orthopedic or neurosurgical clinics, the majority of whom have had surgical decompression. Other series have been limited to patients with sciatica or low back pain. Accordingly, the clinical description has focused on patients with more advanced disease and "classical" symptoms and signs. But, patients with lumbar spinal stenosis may present without neurogenic claudication and provoke a range of differential diagnoses.

Unlike neurogenic claudication that is more commonly bilateral and associated with central canal stenosis, radicular symptoms due to spinal stenosis are more often unilateral and related to stenosis of the lateral recess or the foraminal canal. Patients tend to be younger and often have pain at rest and at night which is increased by the Valsalva maneuver [4]. Leg pain is often described as severe and radicular in distribution, and may be exacerbated with lumbar extension to the painful side. Examination findings may include a limited lumbar range of motion especially in extension, focal motor weakness in a specific root distribution, variable straight-leg tension signs, and diminished subjective sensation and reflexes in specific root distributions.

References

1. Johnsson KE, Rosen I, Uden A. The natural course of lumbar spinal stenosis. Acta Orthop Scand Suppl. 1993;251:67–8.
2. Matsumoto M, Watanabe K, Tsuji T, Ishii K, Takaishi H, Nakamura M, et al. Nocturnal leg cramps: a common complaint in patients with lumbar spinal canal stenosis. Spine. 2009;34(5):E189–94.
3. Inui Y, Doita M, Ouchi K, Tsukuda M, Fujita N, Kurosaka M. Clinical and radiologic features of lumbar spinal stenosis and disc herniation with neuropathic bladder. Spine. 2004;29(8):869–73.
4. Jenis LG, An HS. Spine update. Lumbar foraminal stenosis. Spine. 2000;25(3):389–94.

Radiologic Evaluation of Lumbar Spinal Stenosis

3

Pratyush Shahi and Sang-Ha Shin

Abstract

Lumbar spinal stenosis causes compression of the nerve roots leading to symptoms such as pain, claudication, and weakness. Plain radiographs, computerised tomography (CT), and magnetic resonance imaging (MRI) are the main imaging modalities utilised in the assessment of spinal stenosis. Plain radiographs help in the assessment of spondylolisthesis, instability, disc height, and sagittal and coronal alignment. CT helps to determine if the spinal stenosis is bony or due to soft tissues. It also helps to identify facet arthropathy, calcified disc, pars defect, ossified ligamentum flavum, and osteophytes. MRI is the most important imaging tool in evaluation of spinal stenosis as it provides optimal visualisation of soft tissues. It helps in the identification of disc herniation, ligamentum flavum hypertrophy, facet cyst and effusion, and abutment/compression of dural sac and nerve roots. Stenosis can involve the central canal, lateral recess, neural foramen, or a combination of these. Localisation and grading of lumbar spinal stenosis along with clinical correlation are vital for treatment success.

Keywords

Spinal stenosis · X-ray · CT · MRI · Grading

3.1 Introduction

Spinal stenosis is a common pathological condition seen in the lumbar spine. It causes compression of the dural sac and nerve roots leading to symptoms such as pain, claudication, tingling, numbness, weakness, and urinary retention. Stenosis can be congenital or acquired. Congenital spinal stenosis can be due to short pedicles, achondroplasia, spinal dysraphism, and mucopolysaccharidoses. Acquired spinal stenosis, however, is more common and can have degenerative, traumatic, and iatrogenic etiologies. Radiological evaluation and its clinical corroboration are vital in formulating the treatment plan for patients with spinal stenosis. This chapter will discuss the radiological assessment of lumbar spinal stenosis secondary to degenerative conditions.

P. Shahi
Department of Orthopedics, Cheongdam Wooridul Spine Hospital, Seoul, Korea (Republic of)

S.-H. Shin (✉)
Department of Neurosurgery, Cheongdam Wooridul Spine Hospital, Seoul, Korea (Republic of)
e-mail: burrhoer@wooridul.co.kr

S.-H. Lee et al. (eds.), *Ligament Reconstruction for Spine*,
https://doi.org/10.1007/978-981-95-3971-0_3

3.2 Radiological Modalities

Plain radiographs, computerised tomography (CT), and magnetic resonance imaging (MRI) are usually utilised for the assessment of spinal stenosis.

3.2.1 Plain Radiographs

Various X-rays provide essential information on important parameters related to lumbar spinal stenosis. Lateral radiograph of the lumbar spine helps in the assessment of lumbar lordosis, spondylolisthesis, disc height, endplate changes, and foraminal height (Fig. 3.1a). Anteroposterior (AP) X-ray helps to evaluate any asymmetric loss of disc space and presence of lumbar scoliosis (Fig. 3.1b). Dynamic flexion-extension X-rays are done to check for translational and angular motion suggesting instability in cases of spondylolisthesis (Fig. 3.1c, d). Full length radiographs help in the assessment of sagittal and coronal alignment and calculation of various deformity parameters (Fig. 3.2).

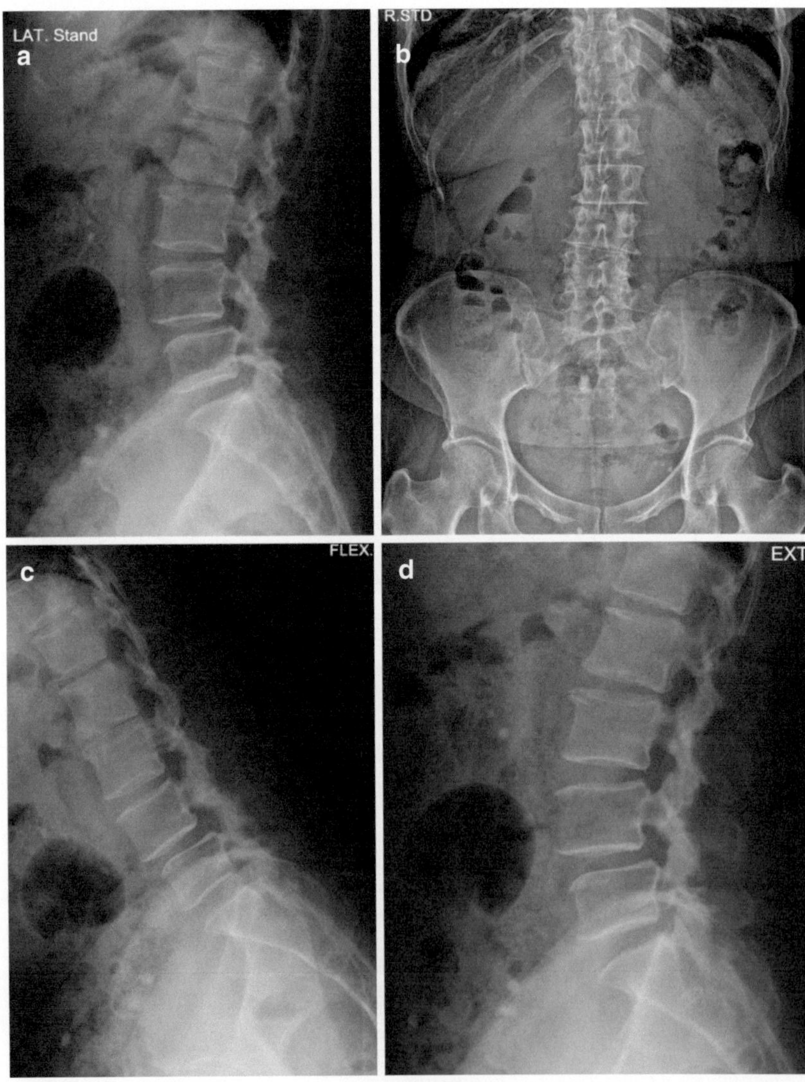

Fig. 3.1 Plain radiograph of lumbar spine. (**a**) Lateral view showing spondylolisthesis at L4–5; (**b**) Anteroposterior view showing mild adult degenerative scoliosis; (**c**, **d**) Dynamic X-rays showing unstable spondylolisthesis at L4-5

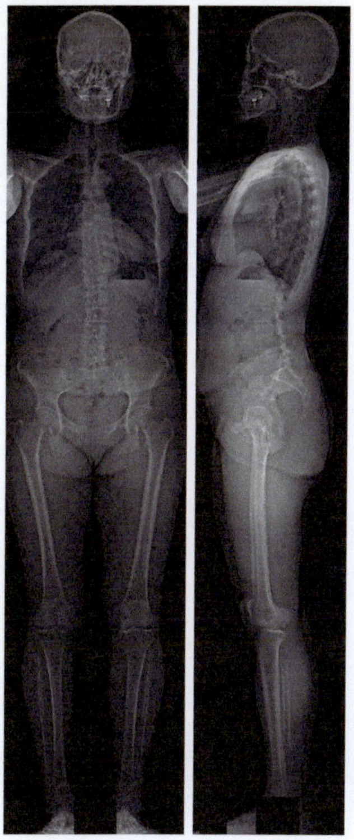

Fig. 3.2 Full length radiographs for assessment of sagittal and coronal alignment

3.2.2 CT

CT scan is a valuable radiological tool in cases with lumbar spinal stenosis. It helps in the delineation of spinal stenosis being bony or due to soft tissues and the identification of facet arthropathy, calcified or hard disc, pars defect, ossified ligamentum flavum, posterior vertebral and juxtafacetal osteophytes, and ankylosis (Fig. 3.3). Postoperatively, CT is used in the assessment of implant loosening, implant migration, fusion status, and heterotopic bone growth (Fig. 3.3). Quantitative CT (qCT) is now also being used to determine the bone mineral density of the lumbar spine utilising Hounsefield units.

3.2.3 MRI

MRI is the most important imaging modality in the assessment and quantification of lumbar spinal stenosis. It allows for the best visualisation of soft tissues, and hence is optimal for the identification of disc herniation, ligamentum flavum

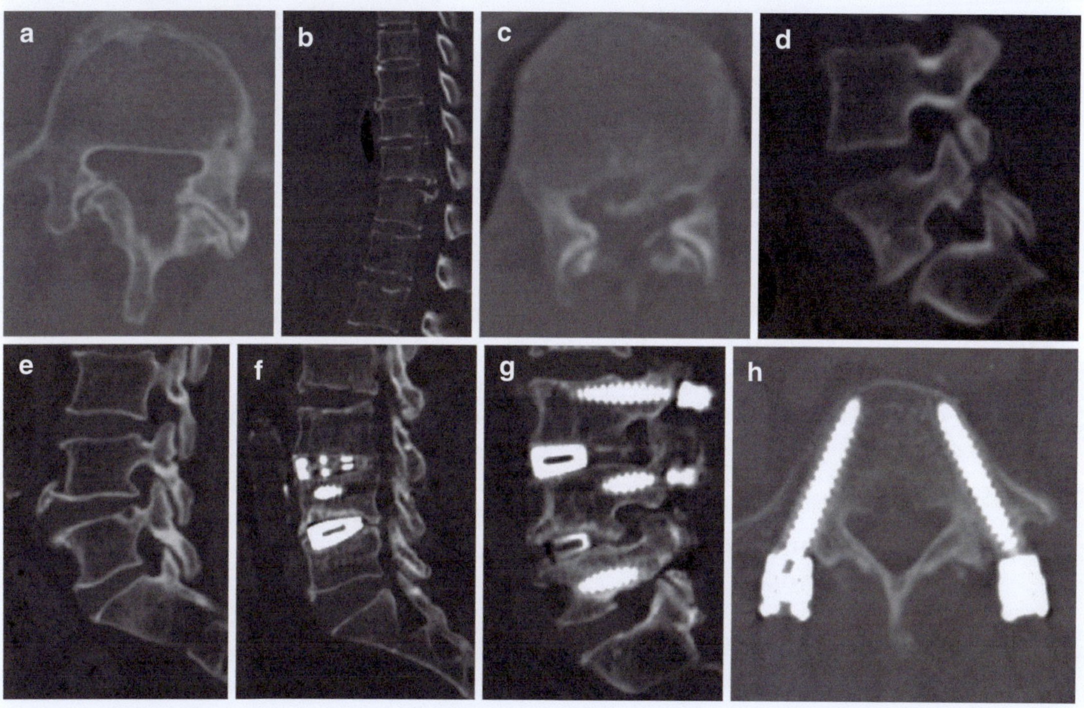

Fig. 3.3 Computerised tomography (CT) showing facet arthropathy (**a**), hard disc herniation (**b**, **c**), pars defect (**d**), and posterior vertebral osteophyte at L4–5 (**e**). Postoperative CT is helpful in assessment of implant and fusion status (**f**–**h**)

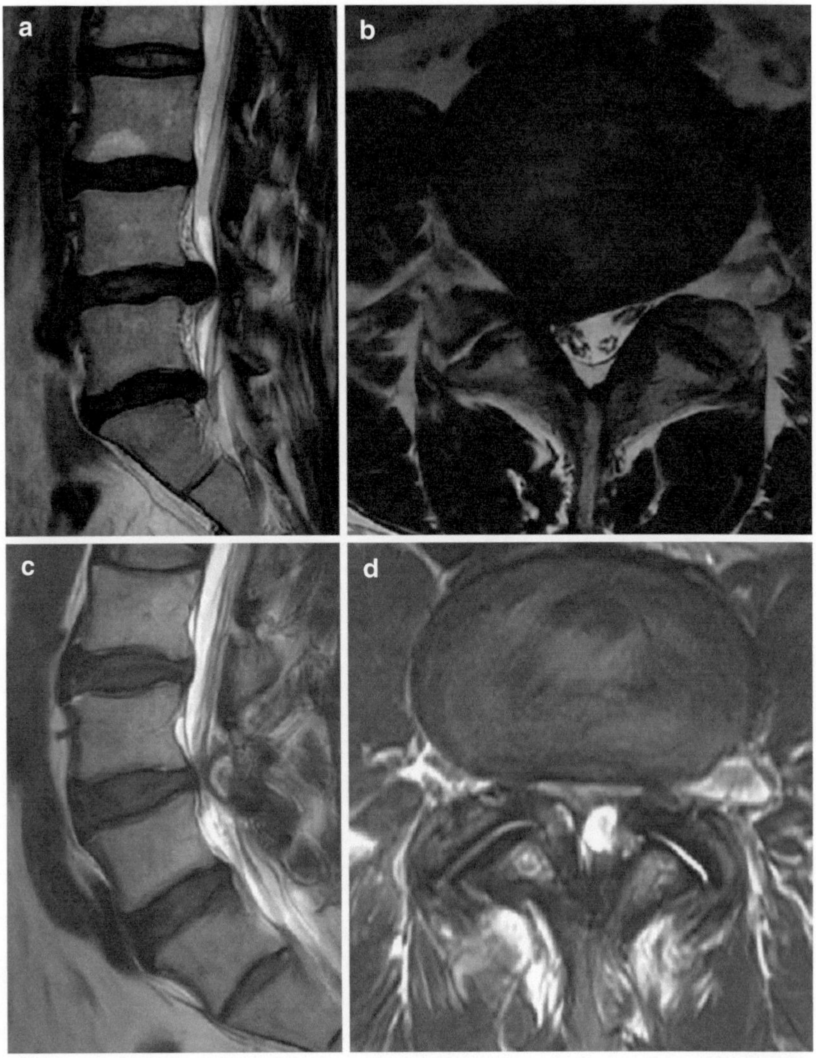

Fig. 3.4 Magnetic resonance imaging (MRI) showing right paracentral disc herniation at L4–5 (**a**, **b**) and left paracentral cyst at L4–5 (**c**, **d**)

hypertrophy, facet cyst and effusion, and abutment/compression of dural sac and nerve roots (Fig. 3.4). MRI helps in the assessment of the site and severity of spinal stenosis and the grading of facetal hypertrophy.

3.3 Localisation and Grading of Spinal Stenosis

Stenosis can involve the central canal, lateral recess, neural foramen, or a combination of these.

3.3.1 Central Stenosis

Central stenosis can be due to hypertrophied ligamentum flavum, disc herniation, or epidural lipomatosis. It classically leads to neurogenic claudication where the walking distance of the patient gets reduced. Grading of central stenosis is done on axial T2 MRI. Various grading systems have been proposed in the literature. The Schizas classification [1] (Fig. 3.5) based on the CSF/rootlet ratio is described here:

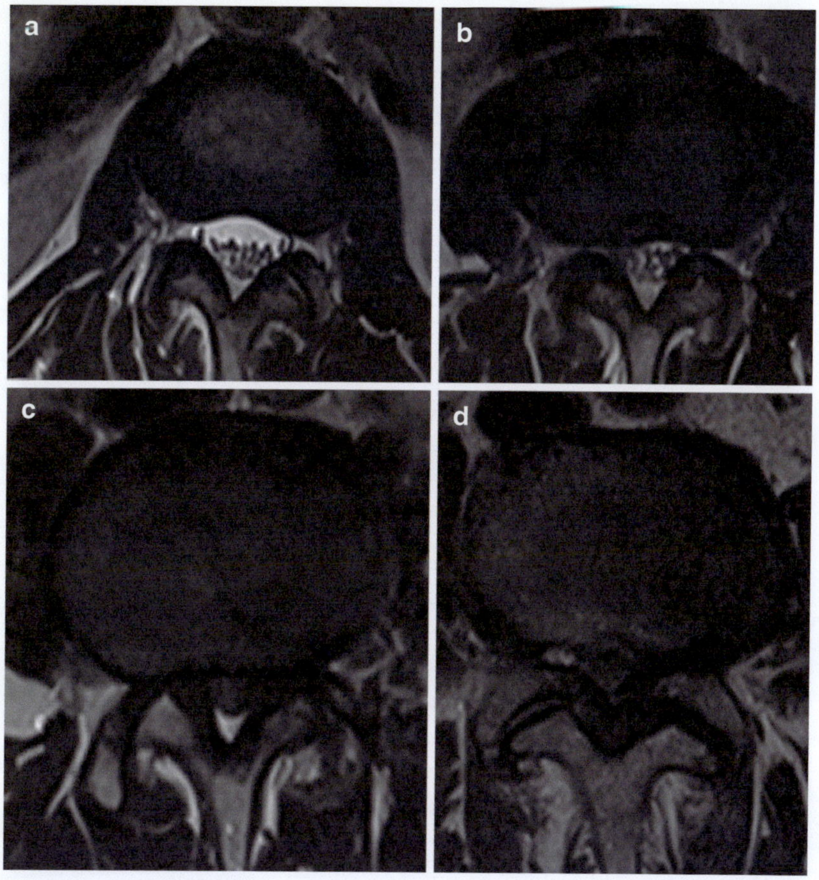

Fig. 3.5 Schizas grading of central spinal stenosis. (**a**) grade A: no or minor stenosis, (**b**) grade B: moderate stenosis, (**c**) grade C: severe stenosis, and (**d**) grade D: extreme stenosis

- Grade A: no or minor stenosis—clear CSF visible inside the dural sac but its distribution is inhomogeneous.
  - A1: rootlets lie dorsally and occupy less than half of the dural sac area.
  - A2: rootlets lie dorsally in contact with the dura but in a horseshoe configuration.
  - A3: rootlets lie dorsally and occupy more than half of the dural sac area.

    A4: rootlets lie centrally and occupy majority of the dural sac area.
- Grade B: moderate stenosis—rootlets occupy whole of the dural sac but can still be individualised, some CSF signal still present.
- Grade C: severe stenosis—no recognisable rootlets, dural sac shows homogeneous grey signal, no CSF signal visible, epidural fat present posteriorly.
- Grade D: extreme stenosis—no epidural fat posteriorly in addition to no recognisable rootlets.

3.3.2 Lateral Recess Stenosis

Lateral recess stenosis results from disc herniation, hypertrophy of the ligamentum flavum, facet hypertrophy, or facet cyst. It causes compression of the traversing nerve root leading to radiculopathy. It is best assessed on axial T2 images and can be classified as normal, abutment of traversing root, and compression of traversing root [2] (Fig. 3.6).

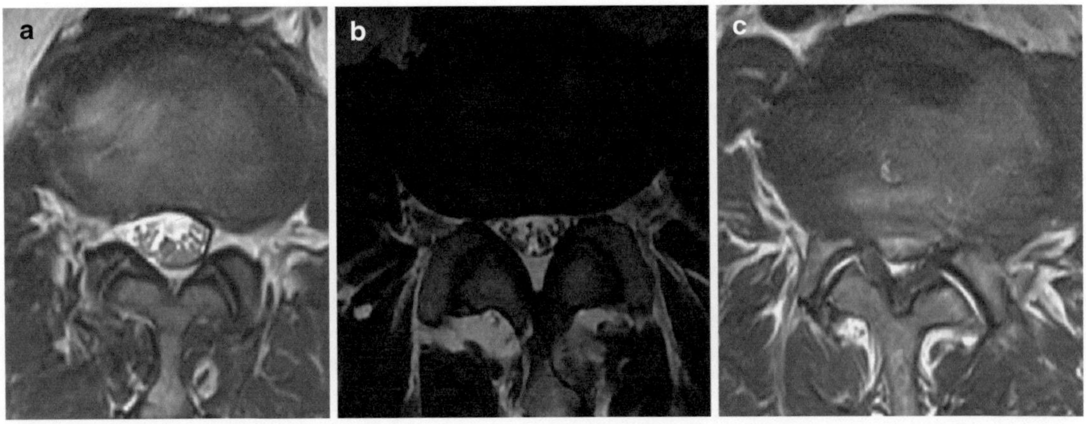

Fig. 3.6 Grading of lateral recess stenosis. (**a**) normal, (**b**) abutment of traversing root, and (**c**) compression of traversing root

3.3.3 Neural Foraminal Stenosis

Foraminal stenosis can be due to disc herniation, vertebral osteophyte, facetal hypertrophy/subluxation, disc space collapse, or ligamentum flavum hypertrophy. It leads to compression of the exiting nerve root causing radiculopathy. It is best assessed on sagittal T1 images. Lee classification [3] (Fig. 3.7) is widely used to grade foraminal stenosis and is described below:

- Grade 0: normal—nerve root is surrounded by fat circumferentially.
- Grade 1: mild—perineural fat is not seen in one dimension, either anteroposterior or superoinferior.
- Grade 2: moderate—perineural fat is not seen circumferentially but nerve root is not compressed.
- Grade 3: severe—absence of perineural fat visualisation with compression (morphologic change) of the nerve root.

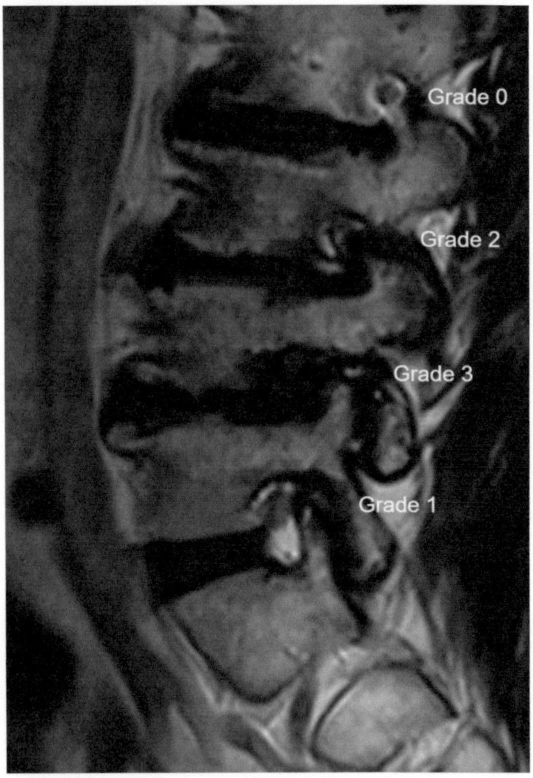

Fig. 3.7 Lee classification of foraminal stenosis

3.3.4 Facet Arthropathy

It is important to assess and grade facet arthropathy as it can lead to central, lateral recess, or foraminal stenosis. The Weishaupt grading system of facet arthropathy [4] (Fig. 3.8) is used in CT or MRI and is described below:

- Grade 0: normal facet joint space (width 2–4 mm).
- Grade 1: facet joint space narrowed (<2 mm) and/or small osteophytes and/or mild articular process hypertrophy.

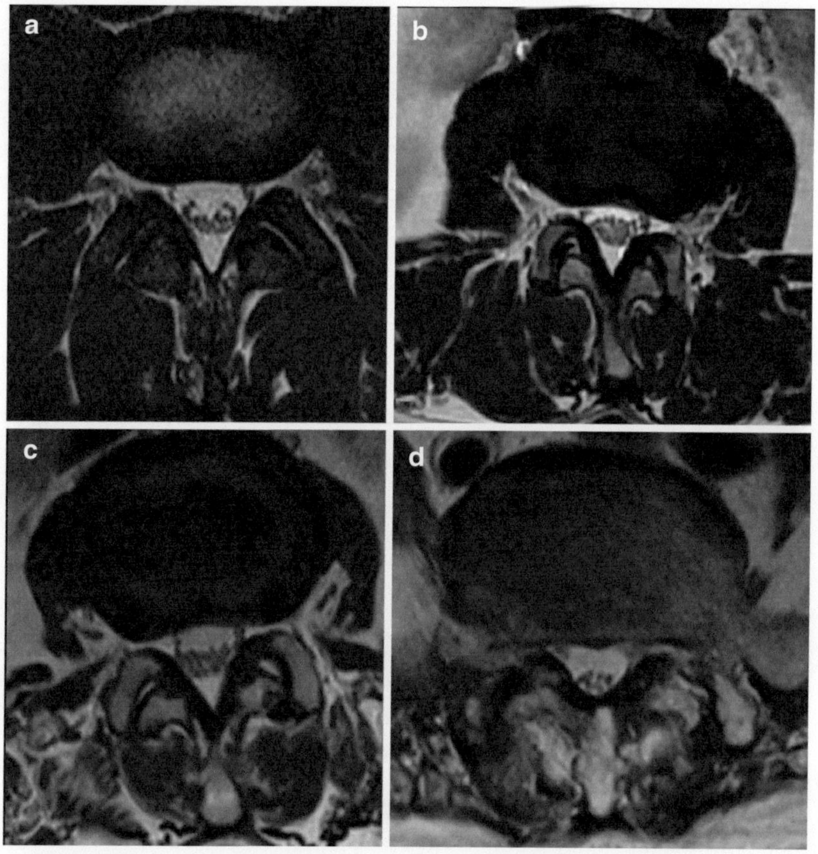

Fig. 3.8 Weishaupt grading system of facet arthropathy. (**a**) grade 0, (**b**) grade 1, (**c**) grade 2, and (**d**) grade 3

- Grade 2: facet joint space narrowed and/or moderate osteophytes and/or moderate articular process hypertrophy and/or mild subarticular bone erosions.
- Grade 3: facet joint space narrowed and/or large osteophytes and/or severe articular process hypertrophy and/or severe subarticular bone erosions and/or subchondral cysts.

3.4 Clinical Correlation of Radiological Spinal Stenosis

Several studies have analysed whether the severity of radiological lumbar spinal stenosis and clinical symptoms are correlated. Andrasinova et al. conducted an observational cross-sectional study of 84 patients who had neurogenic claudication secondary to degenerative central stenosis of the lumbar spine [5]. They found a significant correlation between neurological impairment in lower limbs and severity of stenosis on Schizas grading. However, no association was found between the degree of stenosis and pain, disability, or walking capacity. Lohman et al. studied 117 patients and 351 intervertebral levels and concluded that there was no correlation between severity of clinical symptoms and dural sac cross-sectional area [6]. A prospective study of 123 patients conducted by Athiviraham et al. demonstrated that the degree of radiological lumbar spinal stenosis did not correlate with clinical symptoms, even after standardisation of vertebral body size [7]. Fushimi et al. conducted a cross-sectional study of 239 volunteers and found that only the most severe lumbar stenosis was associated with typical clinical symptoms [8]. However, not all cases with typical symptoms were found to have severe spinal stenosis. It is clear, therefore, that the current evidence supports poor or no correlation between clinical symptoms and degree of spinal stenosis on radiological assessment. As such, it is pertinent for the physician to not be over-reliant on what is seen on imaging but rather be more cognizant about clinical and radiological corroboration before devising a treatment plan. Identifying the correct target spinal level and site with the help of localising symptoms/signs, radiological correlation, and diagnostic injections when needed is a prerequisite for good surgical outcomes.

3.5 Summary

Lumbar spinal stenosis is a common condition that leads to symptoms such as pain, claudication, and weakness as a result of the compression of nerve roots. MRI is the most valuable imaging modality in the assessment of spinal stenosis, although plain radiograph and CT also provide vital information. Stenosis can involve the central canal, lateral recess, or neural foramen. Localisation and grading of stenosis along with clinical corroboration are essential for treatment success.

References

1. Schizas C, Theumann N, Burn A, Tansey R, Wardlaw D, Smith FW, Kulik G. Qualitative grading of severity of lumbar spinal stenosis based on the morphology of the dural sac on magnetic resonance images. Spine (Phila Pa 1976). 2010;35(21):1919–24. https://doi.org/10.1097/BRS.0b013e3181d359bd. PMID: 20671589.
2. Deng F, Mishra S, Miskin N, Sun EX, Huang RY, Mandell J. Spine imaging. In: Sun EX, Shi J, Mandell JC, editors. Core radiology: a visual approach to diagnostic imaging. 2nd ed. Cambridge: Cambridge University Press; 2021. p. 860–907.
3. Lee S, Lee JW, Yeom JS, Kim KJ, Kim HJ, Chung SK, Kang HS. A practical MRI grading system for lumbar foraminal stenosis. AJR Am J Roentgenol. 2010;194(4):1095–8. https://doi.org/10.2214/AJR.09.2772. PMID: 20308517.
4. Weishaupt D, Zanetti M, Boos N, Hodler J. MR imaging and CT in osteoarthritis of the lumbar facet joints. Skeletal Radiol. 1999;28(4):215–9. https://doi.org/10.1007/s002560050503. PMID: 10384992.
5. Andrasinova T, Adamova B, Buskova J, Kerkovsky M, Jarkovsky J, Bednarik J. Is there a correlation between degree of radiologic lumbar spinal stenosis and its clinical manifestation? Clin Spine Surg. 2018;31(8):E403–8. https://doi.org/10.1097/BSD.0000000000000681. PMID: 29939845.
6. Lohman CM, Tallroth K, Kettunen JA, Lindgren KA. Comparison of radiologic signs and clinical symptoms of spinal stenosis. Spine (Phila Pa 1976). 2006;31(16):1834–40. https://doi.org/10.1097/01.brs.0000227370.65573.ac. PMID: 16845360.
7. Athiviraham A, Yen D, Scott C, Soboleski D. Clinical correlation of radiological spinal stenosis after standardization for vertebral body size. Clin Radiol. 2007;62(8):776–80. https://doi.org/10.1016/j.crad.2007.02.011. Epub 2007 May 7. PMID: 17604767.
8. Fushimi Y, Otani K, Tominaga R, Nakamura M, Sekiguchi M, Konno SI. The association between clinical symptoms of lumbar spinal stenosis and MRI axial imaging findings. Fukushima J Med Sci. 2021;67(3):150–60. https://doi.org/10.5387/fms.2021-22. Epub 2021 Dec 11. PMID: 34897162; PMCID: PMC8784199.

4 Anatomical Considerations of the Lumbar Spine for Ligament Reconstruction

Ji Young Cho

Abstract

Lumbar spinal stenosis (LSS) is a prevalent condition characterized by the narrowing of the spinal canal in the lower back, affecting millions worldwide. This study examines the anatomical considerations crucial for ligament reconstruction in LSS patients. We focus on the morphology and biomechanical properties of key ligamentous structures, particularly the ligamentum flavum (LF) and interspinous ligament. The LF exhibits significant variations across lumbar levels, with thickness increasing caudally. Its unique attachments and elastic properties play a vital role in spinal stability. The interspinous ligament, connecting adjacent spinous processes, is noteworthy for its potential as a pain generator. Our analysis reveals that precise understanding of these ligamentous structures is essential for successful surgical interventions. We discuss the implications of ligament anatomy on interspinous surgical approaches, including ligamentectomy and ligament reconstruction. The study highlights the importance of preserving spinal stability while addressing pathological changes in ligamentous structures.

Keywords

Lumbar spinal stenosis · Ligamentum flavum Supraspinous ligament · Ligamentectomy Ligament reconsruction

4.1 Introduction

In this chapter, we will discuss the anatomy of ligamentum flavum, supraspinous ligament and nerve roots.

4.2 Ligamentum Flavum (LF)

The ligamentum flavum is a significant anatomical structure in the spine, extending from the second cervical vertebra to the first sacral vertebra. It is a short, thick ligament that connects the laminae of adjacent vertebrae. The ligament's name, "flavum," derives from its distinctive yellow color, which is due to its high elastin content. Anatomically, the ligamentum flavum is composed of approximately 80% elastin fibers and 20% collagen fibers, giving it unique elastic properties.

J. Y. Cho (✉)
Department of Neurosurgery, Gangbuk Woori Spine Hospital, Gangbuk, Korea (Republic of)
e-mail: nscjy@naver.com

S.-H. Lee et al. (eds.), *Ligament Reconstruction for Spine*,
https://doi.org/10.1007/978-981-95-3971-0_4

4.2.1 Morphology

This ligament attaches to the anterior surface of the lamina above and the posterior surface and upper margin of the lamina below. Its dimensions vary along the spine, with a height ranging from 14 to 22 mm, a width of 11–23 mm at its lower part, and a thickness of 3.5–6 mm. The ligamentum flavum exhibits regional variations, being thinnest in the cervical region and progressively thickening in the thoracic and lumbar regions, with the greatest thickness observed in the lower lumbar levels [1].

Morphologically, the ligamentum flavum (LF) shows notable variations across lumbar levels. At L1-L2 and L2-L3, it is relatively thin and rounded, while at L3-L4, it takes on a triangular shape. By L4-L5 and L5-S1, the LF becomes thicker and develops a trefoil shape due to increased mechanical stress (Fig. 4.1). These morphological changes are crucial for surgical planning, as hypertrophy or calcification of the LF can narrow the spinal canal, requiring precise decompression techniques. The attachments of the LF also vary by level. It originates from the lower half of the anterior surface of the lamina above and attaches to the posterior surface and upper margin of the lamina below, creating a cup-like grasp on the upper border of the lower lamina (Fig. 4.2).

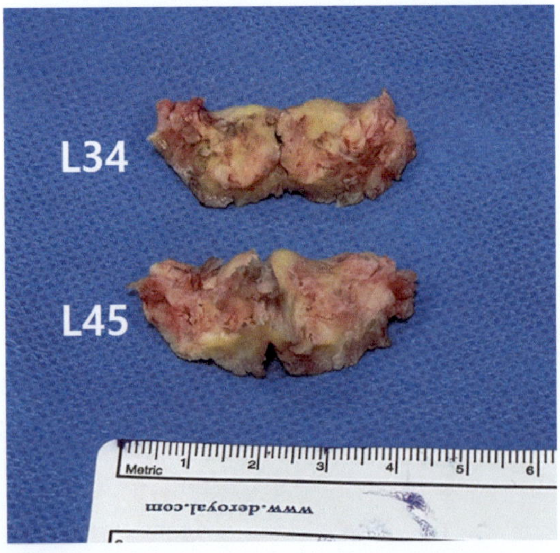

Fig. 4.1 En-block removed ligamentum flavum (LF). The LF is a butterfly shape. The LF at the lower level is larger and thicker

Microscopically, the ligamentum flavum consists primarily of longitudinally arranged elastic fibers interspersed with thin bundles of collagen fibers. Spindle-shaped fibroblasts are sparsely distributed throughout the ligament. The tissue contains a limited number of capillaries and small thin-walled blood vessels, but notably lacks nerve trunks or endings [2, 3].

Functionally, the ligamentum flavum maintains a state of pretension even in the neutral position of the spine, which prevents buckling of the ligament into the spinal canal. In the lumbar vertebrae, this pretension is further enhanced by traction and tension forces from surrounding structures. The unique anatomical properties of the ligamentum flavum contribute significantly to spinal stability and flexibility, making it a crucial consideration in various spinal conditions and surgical interventions [4, 5].

The ligamentum flavum (LF) in the lumbar spine exhibits notable differences in the arrangement and composition of its fibers across different levels, influenced by mechanical stress, aging, and degenerative changes.

4.2.2 Degenerative Changes

The ligamentum flavum (LF) in the lumbar spine exhibits significant differences in fiber composition and arrangement across various levels, primarily influenced by mechanical stress, aging, and degeneration [6]. Elastic fibers, which constitute approximately 80% of the ligament, provide elasticity essential for spinal stability and flexibility. However, their proportion decreases with age and degenerative changes, particularly at lower lumbar levels such as L4-L5 and L5-S1 [7]. These levels experience a significant reduction in elastic fiber density compared to upper lumbar segments like L2-L3 due to chronic mechanical strain. As elastic fibers diminish, they are replaced by collagen fibers, leading to fibrosis, reduced elasticity, and ligament thickening (Fig. 4.3). This shift is more pronounced in the lower lumbar spine, where the elastic-to-collagen

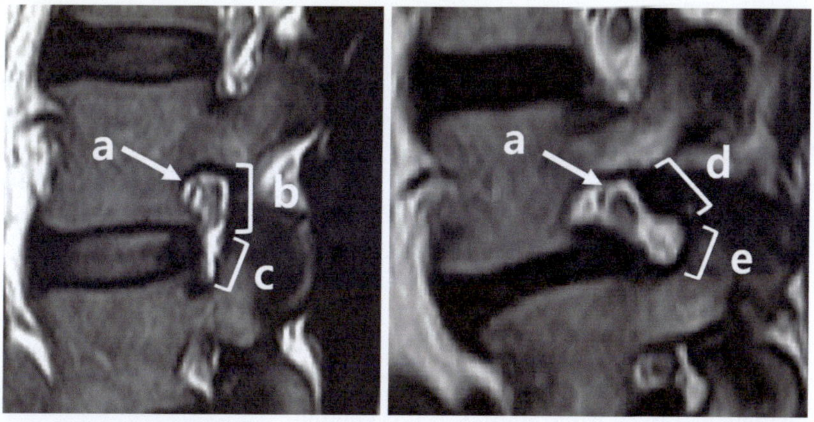

Fig. 4.2 Sagittal view of foramen at MR images. Exiting nerve root (**a**), ligamentum flavum (**b**, **d**), and empty zone (**c**, **e**). Empty zone was defined as caudal area uncovered with ligamentum flavum. This empty zone was preserved although degenerative listhesis

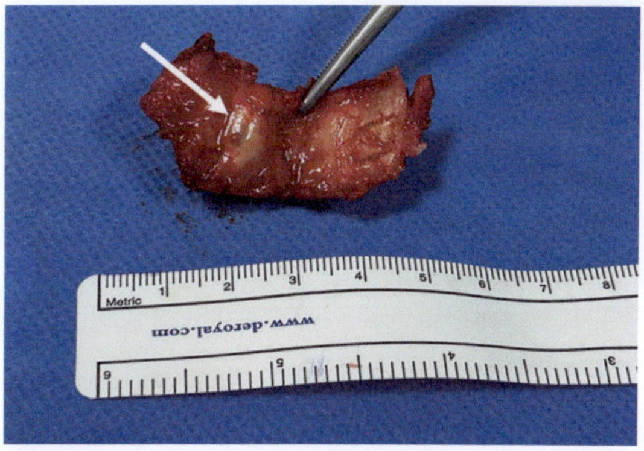

Fig. 4.3 A piece of ligamentum flavum was removed. A cyst of the ligamentum flavum, found due to degeneration

ratio is notably lower, contributing to stiffness and potential bulging into the spinal canal [8].

Structurally, the LF consists of two layers: the superficial layer, which contains oblique fibers oriented medially and upwards, and the deep layer, which has craniocaudal fibers aligned with vertical stress. Degeneration is typically more severe in the superficial layer than in the deep layer at lower lumbar levels. Additionally, the dorsal (posterior) side of the ligament experiences greater mechanical stress than the ventral (anterior) side. Degenerative changes such as elastic fiber fragmentation and collagen proliferation are more prominent dorsally due to repetitive loading [9].

Among lumbar levels, L4-L5 and L5-S1 are most affected by degenerative changes because they bear the greatest load and have high mobility. These segments show advanced elastic fiber degeneration, increased collagen content, fibrosis, calcification, and even chondrometaplasia. These changes result in ligament thickening and are strongly associated with conditions like lumbar spinal stenosis (LSS). In contrast, upper lumbar levels such as L2-L3 and L3-L4 exhibit less degeneration, with relatively preserved elastic fibers that maintain better elasticity and function [5, 10].

The progressive replacement of elastic fibers with collagen at lower lumbar levels leads to ligament hypertrophy, reduced flexibility, and narrowing of the spinal canal. These changes are key contributors to conditions like lumbar spinal stenosis or nerve compression caused by herniation. Understanding these histological differences is critical for guiding surgical interventions such as decompression or laminectomy at severely affected levels like L4-L5. In summary, the ligamentum flavum's fiber composition varies significantly across lumbar spine levels, with lower segments being more vulnerable to degenerative changes due to increased mechanical stress.

4.3 Supraspinous Ligament

The supraspinous ligament is a robust fibrous cord that extends along the tips of the spinous processes of the vertebral column, spanning from the seventh cervical vertebra (C7) to the sacrum, typically terminating at L3 or L4. This ligament exhibits a complex structure composed of three distinct layers: a superficial layer with the longest fibers extending over 3–4 vertebrae, an intermediate layer spanning 2–3 vertebrae, and a deep layer connecting adjacent vertebrae that is continuous with the interspinous ligaments [9, 11].

Anatomically, the supraspinous ligament is primarily composed of collagen and elastin fibers, which contribute to its yellowish appearance. The ligament demonstrates regional variations along the spine, being thicker and broader in the lumbar region compared to the thoracic region. In the lumbar area, it merges with the thoracolumbar fascia, while above C7, it is continuous with the nuchal ligament.

The dimensions of the supraspinous ligament vary, with heights ranging from 14 to 22 mm, widths of 11–23 mm in the lower part, and thicknesses between 3.5 and 6 mm. Microscopically, the ligament consists mainly of longitudinally arranged elastic fibers interspersed with thin bundles of collagen fibers and sparse fibroblasts. It has a limited blood supply, containing few capillaries and small thin-walled vessels.

The unique anatomical properties of the supraspinous ligament, including its layered structure and composition, contribute significantly to its crucial role in maintaining spinal stability and flexibility. Particularly, it plays a vital part in limiting flexion of the vertebral column, thus protecting the spine from excessive forward bending movements [12].

4.4 Interspinous Ligament

The interspinous ligament is a fibrous structure that connects the spinous processes of adjacent vertebrae, extending from the cervical region (C1) to the sacrum (S1). It is primarily composed of collagen fibers, with some elastic fibers concentrated in its anterior portion. The anatomy of the interspinous ligament varies depending on the spinal region. In the cervical spine, it is thin and underdeveloped, often blending with the nuchal ligament. In the thoracic spine, it is narrow and elongated, while in the lumbar spine, it becomes broader, thicker, and quadrilateral in shape. The fibers of the lumbar interspinous ligament are arranged in an oblique or S-shaped pattern.

Functionally, the interspinous ligament plays a key role in stabilizing the spine by limiting excessive flexion and preventing excessive separation of adjacent spinous processes. It also contributes to resisting compressive forces during spinal extension and provides graded resistance during lumbar flexion. Additionally, it works in conjunction with other spinal ligaments, such as the supraspinous ligament and ligamentum flavum, to maintain overall spinal integrity and mobility [9].

4.5 Traversing and Exiting Nerve Roots

The lumbar spine contains two distinct types of nerve roots: traversing and exiting nerve roots, each with unique anatomical characteristics and clinical significance. Exiting nerve roots leave the spine directly at their corresponding vertebral level, passing through the neural foramen lateral to the pedicle. For instance, the L4 nerve root exits at the L4-L5 level. These roots are particularly vulnerable to far lateral disc herniations and foraminal stenosis due to their lateral position [13].

In contrast, traversing nerve roots cross the intervertebral disc level before exiting at the level below, occupying a more central position within the lateral recess of the spinal canal. The L5 nerve root, for example, traverses the L4-L5 level before exiting. These roots are more susceptible to central or posterolateral disc herniations. Traversing roots follow an oblique course downwards and laterally towards the intervertebral foramen, passing across the disc space and beneath the pedicles of the inferior segment.

At each disc level, two nerve roots are present: one traversing and one exiting. The upper lumbar nerve roots tend to orient more at a right angle to the dural sac compared to the distal nerve roots. Understanding this complex anatomy is crucial for accurate diagnosis of radiculopathy, interpretation of imaging studies, and planning of surgical interventions [14, 15].

4.6 Summary

Understanding ligament anatomy is crucial for interspinous surgical approaches, such as ligementectomy and ligament reconstruction. These procedures often involve reconstucting ligamentous structures like the interspinous ligament to decompress the spinal canal or stabilize the spine, especially in conditions like lumbar spinal stenosis. Accurate anatomical knowledge ensures precise intervention, reducing complications and improving outcomes in ligament-related surgeries.

References

1. Javid A, Hidetomi T, Mohammad SR, Koli T, Akinobu S, et al. Anatomical analysis of the relation between human ligamntum flavum and posterior spinal bony prominence. J Orthop Sci. 2017;22(2):260–5.
2. Nakamura T, Matsumoto T, Takahashi K, Nishida K, Nishida Y, Chiba K, et al. Osteoclastic activity of human intervertebral disc cells in response to tumor necrosis factor-alpha: a possible mechanism of intervertebral disc resorption. J Orthop Res. 2014;32(3):358–64.
3. Sakamaki T, Sairyo K, Katoh S, Higashino K, Sakai T, Yasui N. Bilateral radiculopathy secondary to foraminal stenosis at L5-S1: a case report and review of the literature. Spine. 2009;34(25):2691–7.
4. Panjabi MM, White AA III. Biomechanics in the musculoskeletal system. New York: Churchill Livingstone; 2001.
5. Schrcoder P, Grob D, Rahn BA. Morphologic and histologic studies of the ligamentum flavum in the lumbar spine: a contribution to its physiologic and pathologic anatomy in view of microsurgical operations on herniated lumbar discs (microdiscectomy). Spine (Phila Pa 1976). 1999;24(3):326–9.
6. Sairyo K, Biyani A, Goel V, Leaman D, Booth R, Thomas J, et al. Pathomechanism of ligamentum flavum hypertrophy: a multidisciplinary investigation based on clinical, biomechanical, histologic, and biologic assessments. Spine. 2005;30(23):2649–56.
7. Hansson T, Suzuki N, Hebelka H, Gaulitz A. The narrowing of the lumbar spinal canal during loaded MRI: the effects of the disc and ligamentum flavum. Spine. 2009;34(12):1316–25.
8. Scapinelli R. Morphological changes in the lumbar spine in relation to age and its clinical significance. Surg Radiol Anat. 2006;28(3):209–13.
9. Solomonow M. Ligaments: a source of musculoskeletal disorders. J Electromyogr Kinesiol. 2006;16(6):549–67.
10. Postacchini F, Gumina S. Ligamenta flava in lumbar disc herniation and spinal stenosis: light and electron microscopic morphology in humans and experimental animals (dogs). Spine (Phila Pa 1976). 1998;23(5):525–30.
11. Willard FH, Vleeming A, Schuenke MD, Danneels L, Schleip R. The thoracolumbar fascia: anatomy, function and clinical considerations. J Anat. 2012;221(6):507–36.
12. Tandring S, editor. Gray's anatomy: the anatomical basis of clinical practice. 42nd ed. London: Elsevier; 2020.
13. Jenis LG, An HS. Spine update: lumbar foraminal stenosis. Spine. 2000;25(3):386–91.
14. Takahashi Y, Nakagawa H, Hashizume Y, Nishikawa Y, Ohtani K, Ogata T, et al. The relationship between radiographic findings and morphological changes in the ligamentum flavum: a study using cadavers and clinical cases with myelography and computed tomography-myelography correlations. AJNR Am J Neuroradiol. 2008;29(1):104–9.
15. Chhabra A, Thakkar RS, Clerx M, Carrino JA. Magnetic resonance neurography: current perspectives and literature review. Radiographics. 2016;36(6):1792–810.

Historical Considerations of Soft Lumbar Stabilization

5

Sang-Ho Lee and Jeong woo Kwun

Abstract

The evolution of soft lumbar stabilization has revolutionized spinal care, addressing pathologies while preserving motion and reducing fusion-related risks. Early rigid stabilization methods faced challenges like adjacent segment degeneration. The advent of dynamic stabilization systems, such as pedicle screw-based and interspinous spacer devices, offered motion preservation and reduced stress on adjacent segments, forming the foundation of soft stabilization. Advances in biomaterials, biomechanics, and minimally invasive techniques further enhanced outcomes. Combining decompression with dynamic stabilization has proven effective for managing lumbar pathologies. Modern technologies like imaging and robotics continue to refine these approaches, providing safer, motion-preserving solutions and improving patient quality of life.

Keyword

Soft stabilization · Dynamic stabilization
Interspinous spacer based system · Pedicle screw-based system · Artificial ligament

S.-H. Lee (✉) · J. w. Kwun
Department of Neurosurgery, Cheongdam Wooridul Spine Hospital, Seoul, Korea (Republic of)
e-mail: sh500909@wooridul.co.kr

5.1 Introduction

The evolution of soft lumbar stabilization represents a remarkable progression in medical history, driven by the need to address spinal pathologies while preserving motion and reducing the risks associated with traditional fusion techniques. From its conceptual roots to modern advancements, this approach has undergone significant transformation, shaped by clinical insights and technological innovations.

5.2 Historical Considerations of Soft Lumbar Stabilization

5.2.1 Early Approaches to Spinal Stabilization

Spinal pathologies, particularly degenerative disc diseases, spinal stenosis, herniations, and spinal instability, have long posed significant challenges. Historically, spinal fusion was the primary treatment for these conditions. Techniques dating back to the early twentieth century focused on achieving rigid stabilization through bone grafting and metallic implants.

The first recorded attempts at spinal stabilization involved bone grafts harvested from the iliac crest, a method popularized by surgeons such as Albee and Hibbs in the 1910s [1, 2]. These techniques aimed to eliminate pain by immobilizing

S.-H. Lee et al. (eds.), *Ligament Reconstruction for Spine*,
https://doi.org/10.1007/978-981-95-3971-0_5

affected segments, but they often resulted in loss of motion, adjacent segment degeneration, and prolonged recovery periods.

5.2.2 The Advent of Motion Preservation Concepts

By the mid-twentieth century, the limitations of spinal fusion became increasingly evident. Rigid stabilization often led to biomechanical stress on adjacent segments, accelerating degeneration and creating new clinical challenges. This prompted a paradigm shift toward motion preservation.

Initial efforts to develop non-fusion technologies began with interspinous spacers and flexible rods. The goal was to maintain spinal stability while allowing limited motion, thereby reducing stress on adjacent segments. Early devices were rudimentary and faced challenges in biomechanical performance and durability.

5.2.3 Emergence of Dynamic Stabilization Systems

The 1980s and 1990s saw the emergence of true dynamic stabilization systems. These systems can be broadly classified into *pedicle screw-based systems* and *interspinous spacer-based systems*, each addressing specific clinical needs while preserving motion and reducing stress on adjacent segments.

- *Pedicle Screw-Based Systems*: Pedicle screw-based systems anchor devices directly to the spine using screws inserted into the pedicles. These systems provide stability by controlling segmental motion while allowing some degree of flexibility.
  - *Graf Ligament System*: Introduced in the late 1980s, the Graf ligament system used pedicle screws connected by elastic bands or polyester cords. It reduced abnormal motion without fully immobilizing the spinal segments, making it an early example of motion-preserving technology [3–5].
  - *Dynesys System*: Developed in the 1990s, the Dynesys system utilized pedicle screws along with polyethylene-terephthalate cords and polycarbonate urethane spacers. It aimed to maintain spinal alignment and motion while stabilizing hypermobile segments. Although effective in many cases, outcomes were mixed, with some studies reporting persistent pain and reoperation rates [6, 7].
- *Interspinous Spacer-Based Systems*: Interspinous spacer systems are designed to stabilize the spine by inserting a device between adjacent spinous processes, reducing excessive flexion-extension motion while preserving overall spinal mobility.
  - *Wallis System*: The Wallis system, developed by Senegas in 1986, was one of the first interspinous spacers. It provided stabilization by buffering the spinous processes, reducing hypermobility and restoring alignment while preserving motion. The Wallis system laid the groundwork for subsequent interspinous devices and remains a landmark innovation in dynamic stabilization [3, 8].

This distinction between pedicle screw-based and interspinous spacer-based systems highlights the evolution of dynamic stabilization devices. While pedicle screw-based systems offer robust stabilization for severe instability, interspinous spacers are well-suited for early degenerative conditions and mild instability.

5.2.4 Evolution of Biomaterials and Biomechanics

Biomechanical studies have demonstrated the effectiveness of dynamic stabilization in reducing stress on adjacent segments. Systems like Dynesys have been shown to significantly reduce motion in targeted segments while preserving some degree of flexibility, thus minimizing the risk of adjacent segment disease [9]. Additionally, research has indicated that Dynesys could offer stability while mitigating load transfer issues to adjacent levels.

5.2.5 Clinical Challenges and Adaptations

Despite early successes, dynamic stabilization faced criticism regarding its long-term efficacy and complication rates. Challenges such as screw loosening, implant failure, and inadequate pain relief underscored the need for continued innovation.

The combination of decompression and dynamic stabilization has been highlighted in several studies as an effective approach for managing lumbar stenosis and degenerative spondylolisthesis [10]. These approaches, when carefully applied to appropriate cases, have shown favorable outcomes in improving patient mobility and reducing pain.

5.2.6 Integration with Modern Technologies

The twenty-first century has witnessed the integration of advanced imaging, computer modeling, and robotics into spinal surgery. These technologies have enhanced the precision of device placement, personalized treatment planning, and real-time intraoperative adjustments.

Additionally, the advent of minimally invasive techniques has complemented dynamic stabilization by reducing surgical trauma and improving recovery times. Interspinous dynamic stabilization systems have been proposed as safe and effective alternatives, offering well-defined indications and clinical guidance [11].

5.3 Historical Consideration of Soft Lumbar Stabilization at Wooridul Hospital

Wooridul Hospital in South Korea has been a pioneer in advancing spinal care through dynamic stabilization techniques, particularly focusing on ligament reconstruction as a transformative approach. This historical overview highlights the evolution of devices and methods in dynamic stabilization.

5.3.1 Early Adoption and Development of Dynamic Stabilization Devices

- *Conceptual Beginnings*: Inspired by Senegas (1988), Wooridul Hospital initially adopted dynamic stabilization principles to address degenerative lumbar spinal stenosis (DLSS) and mild segmental instability.
- *Locker as an Interspinous Spacer*: In its early stages, Wooridul Hospital adopted the Locker system, which served as an interspinous spacer designed to provide spinal stability. The Locker device was structurally simple and easy to implement, making it a practical initial choice for dynamic stabilization [12, 13] (Fig. 5.1).
- *Interspinous Artificial Ligament*: To address the shortcomings of the Locker system, Wooridul transitioned to using an artificial ligament with a tension band system to provide stability. This approach marked a significant step in the development of soft

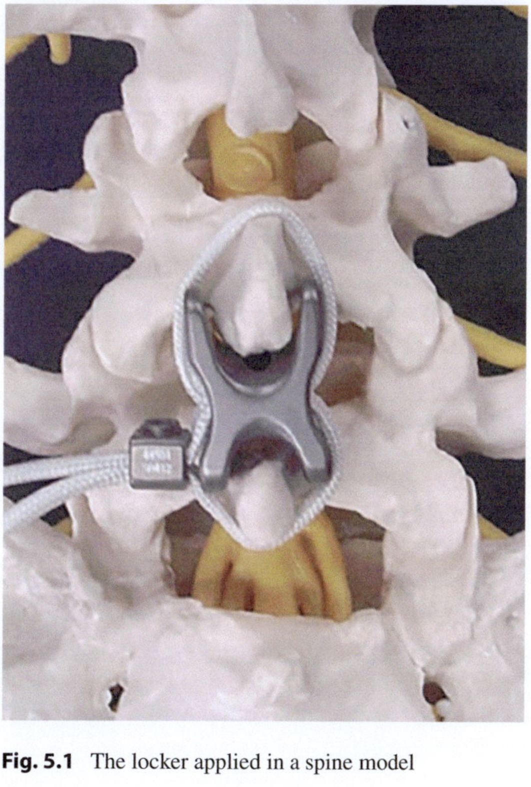

Fig. 5.1 The locker applied in a spine model

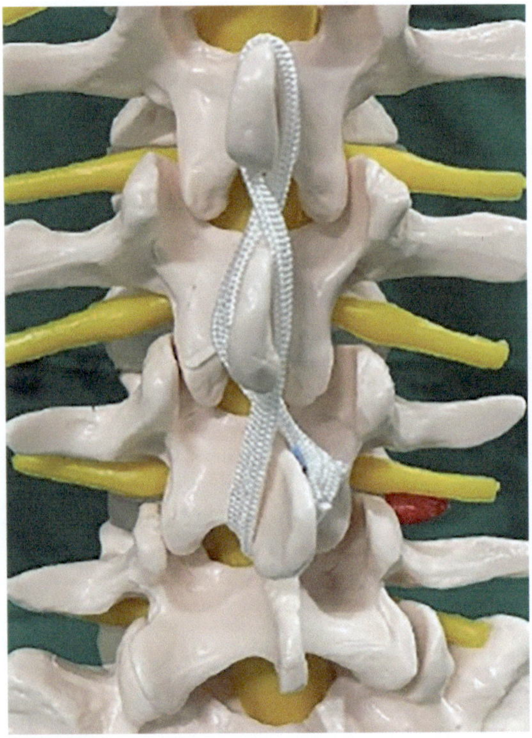

Fig. 5.2 The artificial ligament applied in a spine model

stabilization techniques, as the artificial ligament allowed for both stabilization and motion preservation, aligning with the principles of dynamic and less rigid spinal treatments. Despite its effectiveness, certain challenges remained in achieving optimal outcomes for all patient groups [14–18] (Fig. 5.2).

5.3.2 Transition to SHLee Ligament

- *Development of SHLee Ligament*: Building on the experiences with interspinous artificial ligament, Wooridul Hospital developed the SHLee ligament, which offered superior biomechanical stability and adaptability. The SHLee ligament was designed to meet the diverse needs of patients while addressing the limitations observed in earlier devices (Fig. 5.3).
- *Clinical Excellence*: The SHLee ligament maximized spinal stability while preserving motion, significantly reducing the risk of adjacent segment disease. It became a cornerstone of Wooridul Hospital's soft stabilization strategy.

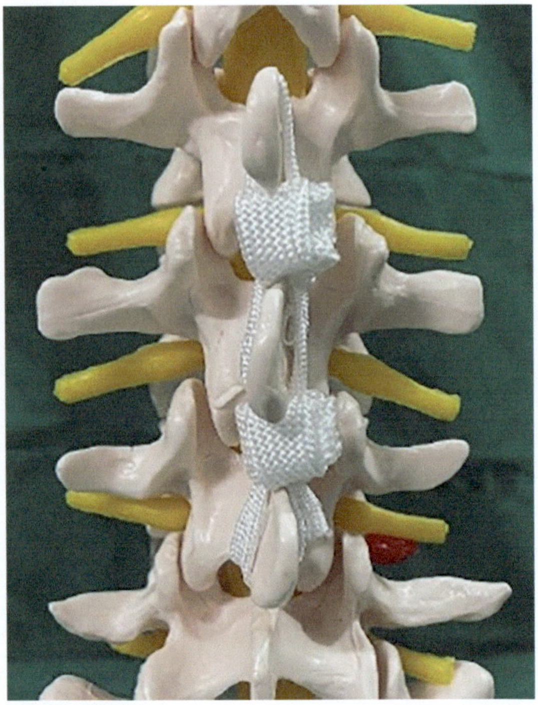

Fig. 5.3 SH Lee ligament applied in a spine model

5.3.3 Clinical Applications and Expansion of Techniques

- *Integration of OMD + Ligament reconstruction*: The combination of Open Midline Decompression (OMD) and Ligament reconstruction emerged as a key treatment method for managing spinal stenosis, neural compression, and segmental instability. This approach preserved the integrity of facet joints and lamina, maintaining spinal structure [19].
- *Expanded Applications*: The SHLee ligament proved effective for patients with mild instability, osteoporosis, or complex medical conditions, demonstrating its adaptability and safety.

5.4 Summary

Wooridul Hospital has contributed significantly to this evolution by developing the SHLee ligament, a groundbreaking advancement in ligament reconstruction. The hospital's dedication to innovation and patient-centered care ensures continued progress in motion-preserving spinal treatments, setting new standards for global excellence. The historical development of spinal dynamic stabilization reflects a relentless pursuit of better outcomes for patients suffering from spinal pathologies. From the early days of rigid fusion to the sophisticated motion-preserving systems of today, this journey highlights the importance of balancing innovation with clinical rigor. As research and technology advance, dynamic stabilization is likely to remain at the forefront of spinal surgery, offering hope to millions worldwide.

References

1. Albee FH. Transplantation of a portion of the tibia into the spine for Pott's disease: a preliminary report. JAMA. 1911;57(885):14–6. https://doi.org/10.1097/BLO.0b013e3180686a0f.
2. Hibbs RA. An operation for progressive spinal deformities: a preliminary report of three cases from the service of the Orthopaedic hospital. N Y Med J. 1911;93(1013):17–20. https://doi.org/10.1097/BLO.0b013e3180686b30.
3. Gomleksiz C, Sasani M, Oktenoglu T, Ozer AF. A short history of posterior dynamic stabilization. Adv Orthop. 2012;2012:Article 629698, 1–12. https://doi.org/10.1155/2012/629698.
4. Hadlow SV, Fagan AB, Hillier TM, Fraser RD. The Graf ligamentoplasty procedure: comparison with posterolateral fusion in the management of low back pain. Spine. 1998;23(10):1172–9. https://doi.org/10.1097/00007632-199805150-00020.
5. Kanayama M, et al. A minimum 10-year follow-up of posterior dynamic stabilization using the Graf artificial ligament. Spine. 2007;32(18):1992–6. https://doi.org/10.1097/BRS.0b013e318133faae.
6. Stoll TM, Dubois G, Schwarzenbach O. The dynamic neutralization system for the spine: a multi-center study of a novel non-fusion system. Eur Spine J. 2002; https://doi.org/10.1007/s00586-002-0438-2.
7. Grob D. et al. Clinical experience with Dynesys semirigid fixation system for lumbar spine: outcomes in 50 cases. 2005; https://doi.org/10.1097/01.brs.0000152564.24843.20.
8. Sénégas J. Mechanical supplementation by non-rigid fixation in degenerative intervertebral lumbar segments: the Wallis system. Eur Spine J. 2002;11(Suppl. 2):S164–9. https://doi.org/10.1007/s00586-002-0423-9.
9. Putzier M, et al. The surgical treatment of the lumbar disc prolapse: Nucleotomy with additional Transpedicular dynamic stabilization versus Nucleotomy alone. Spine. 2005;30(5):E109–14. https://doi.org/10.1097/01.brs.0000152564.24843.20.
10. Schaeren S, et al. Minimum four-year follow-up of spinal stenosis with degenerative spondylolisthesis treated with decompression and dynamic stabilization. Spine (Phila Pa 1976). 2008; https://doi.org/10.1097/BRS.0b013e31817ebfbf.
11. Lee SH, et al. A systematic review of interspinous dynamic stabilization. Clin Orthop Surg. 2015; https://doi.org/10.4055/cios.2015.7.3.323.
12. Lee DY, Lee SH, Shim CS, Lee HY. Decompression and interspinous dynamic stabilization using the locker for lumbar canal stenosis associated with low-grade degenerative spondylolisthesis. Minim Invasive Neurosurg. 2010;53(2):117–21. https://doi.org/10.1055/s-0030-1249704.
13. Shim CS, Park SW, Lee SH, Lim TJ, Chun K, Kim DH. Biomechanical evaluation of an interspinous stabilizing device, Locker. Spine. 2008;33(22):E820–7. https://doi.org/10.1097/BRS.0b013e31818fb0b9.
14. Lee SH, Enes M, Hoogland T. Soft stabilization with interspinous artificial ligament for mildly unstable lumbar spinal stenosis: a multicenter comparison. Arch Orthop Trauma Surg. 2009;130(8):1–10. https://doi.org/10.1007/s00402-009-1031-5.
15. Lee SH, Lee JH, Hong SW, Chung SE, Yoo SH, Lee HY. Spinopelvic alignment after interspinous soft stabilization with a tension band system in grade 1 degenerative lumbar spondylolisthesis. Spine. 2010;35(15):E691–701. https://doi.org/10.1097/BRS.0b013e3181d2607e.
16. Hong SW, Lee HY, Kim KH, Lee SH. Interspinous ligamentoplasty in the treatment of degenerative spondylolisthesis: midterm clinical results. J Neurosurg Spine. 2010;13(1):27–35. https://doi.org/10.3171/2010.3.SPINE0957.
17. Lee SH, Lee JH, Hong SW, Shim CS, Chung SE, Yoo SH, Lee HY. Factors affecting clinical outcomes in treating patients with grade 1 degenerative spondylolisthesis using interspinous soft stabilization with a tension band system: a minimum 5-year follow-up. Spine. 2012;37(7):563–72. https://doi.org/10.1097/BRS.0b013e31821c0b97.
18. Lee SH, Lee HY, Baek OK, Bae JS, Yoo SH, Lee JH. Clinical significance of achieving a flexion limitation with a tension band system in grade 1 degenerative spondylolisthesis: a minimum 5-year follow-up. Spine. 2015;40(6):E349–58. https://doi.org/10.1097/BRS.0000000000000766.
19. Lee DY, Lee SH, Shim CS, Lee HY. Decompression and interspinous dynamic stabilization using the Locker for lumbar canal stenosis associated with low-grade degenerative spondylolisthesis. Minim Invasive Neurosurg. 2010;53(2):117–21. https://doi.org/10.1055/s-0030-1249704.

6 Biomechanical Evaluation of Soft Lumbar Stabilization

Dae Jin Kim

Abstract

Interspinous soft stabilization (ISS) is a dynamic approach to managing lumbar degenerative disorders, focusing on preserving motion while providing segmental stability. Utilizing artificial ligaments to mimic the biomechanical properties of the posterior ligament complex (PLC), ISS addresses limitations of rigid spinal fusion, such as increased stress on adjacent segments and loss of mobility. Biomechanical studies have demonstrated that ISS effectively restores over 80% of native spinal stiffness and reduces adjacent segment stress by 20–30%. These findings highlight its potential to provide stability without compromising the natural kinematics of the lumbar spine. ISS achieves critical biomechanical goals, including motion preservation, load redistribution, and the maintenance of sagittal alignment. By reducing excessive flexion and extension instability, ISS stabilizes the spine while maintaining dynamic load-sharing mechanisms. Furthermore, ISS minimizes stress concentrations on intervertebral discs and facet joints, promoting balanced load distribution across treated and adjacent segments. Experimental evidence demonstrates ISS's effectiveness in maintaining rotational and flexion–extension stability under various physiological loads. These biomechanical properties underscore the value of ISS as a motion-preserving alternative to rigid fusion, offering a scientifically grounded solution to lumbar instability. By addressing key biomechanical challenges, ISS optimizes stabilization while minimizing the risk of adjacent segment degeneration.

Keywords

Interspinous Soft Stabilization (ISS) · Biomechanical evaluation · Posterior Ligament Complex (PLC) · Motion preservation · Lumbar stability

6.1 Introduction

The management of lumbar degenerative disorders has evolved significantly with the advent of soft stabilization techniques. Among these, the use of interspinous artificial ligaments for soft stabilization provides a less invasive alternative to rigid spinal fusion, aiming to preserve motion while maintaining segmental stability. This approach addresses the limitations of traditional fusion surgeries, such as adjacent segment disease and loss of lumbar lordosis [1]. By allowing controlled movement and reducing abnormal load transmission, interspinous artificial ligaments

D. J. Kim (✉)
Department of Neurosurgery, Busan Wooridul Spine Hospital, Busan, Korea (Republic of)

S.-H. Lee et al. (eds.), *Ligament Reconstruction for Spine*,
https://doi.org/10.1007/978-981-95-3971-0_6

have emerged as a promising intervention for treating conditions like grade 1 degenerative spondylolisthesis and lumbar stenosis [15]. Interspinous stabilization techniques are particularly advantageous in patients who are poor candidates for fusion due to advanced age, comorbidities, or other factors. These techniques have demonstrated clinical efficacy in reducing pain, improving function, and maintaining spinal alignment [2]. This chapter explores the biomechanics underlying the use of interspinous artificial ligaments, focusing on their design, testing methodologies, and biomechanical implications in stabilizing the lumbar spine. The integration of this technique into clinical practice has the potential to redefine surgical strategies for spine stabilization while preserving physiological motion [5].

6.2 Testing Protocols for Biomechanical Evaluation of Lumbar Posterior Ligament Complex in Laboratory Setting

Biomechanical testing of the lumbar posterior ligament complex (PLC) is a cornerstone in understanding its critical role in spinal stability and in evaluating the efficacy of surgical interventions. The PLC, composed of the ligamentum flavum, interspinous ligament, and supraspinous ligament, serves as a primary stabilizer, particularly in flexion and extension. Laboratory-based biomechanical evaluations provide a controlled environment to systematically analyze the mechanical behavior and functional contributions of these structures under various loading conditions [13].

6.2.1 Standardized Testing Protocols: Rationale and Components

The development and implementation of standardized testing protocols are essential for ensuring reproducibility and comparability across studies. These protocols typically address key aspects such as specimen preparation, loading modalities, and measurement parameters.

- *Specimen Preparation*: Multisegmental specimens, including two or more functional spinal units (FSUs), are often preferred, as they better replicate the in vivo biomechanical environment by capturing the interactions between adjacent segments. Careful dissection and preservation of the ligamentous structures are critical to maintaining specimen integrity [7].
- *Loading Modalities*: Dynamic, quasistatic, and pure moment loading approaches are widely utilized. Pure moment loading, for example, allows for the isolation of angular motion while minimizing shear forces, making it ideal for evaluating the mechanical properties of individual ligaments [8].
- *Preconditioning*: To account for viscoelastic properties, preconditioning cycles are applied, where the specimen undergoes repeated loading and unloading to stabilize its mechanical response. This ensures that subsequent data collection is not influenced by the transient effects of initial loading [10].

6.2.2 Common Biomechanical Testing Approaches

Several testing protocols have been established to evaluate the PLC's contribution to spinal mechanics:

1. *Flexibility Testing*:
    - This protocol involves applying pure moments to assess the load-displacement behavior and range of motion (ROM) of the spinal segment. It is particularly effective in characterizing the stiffness and flexibility of the PLC in different planes of motion, including flexion, extension, and lateral bending [8].
2. *Hybrid Testing*:
    - A combination of flexibility and stiffness testing, this approach adjusts the applied moments to simulate in vivo conditions. It

is designed to capture both the dynamic and static stabilization roles of the PLC [7].

3. *Stiffness Testing*:
   - This displacement-controlled method measures the force response of the PLC during incremental loading. It is particularly useful for quantifying the structural rigidity and load-bearing capacity of individual ligamentous components [11].

6.2.3 Loading Parameters and Advanced Techniques

Advanced loading techniques, such as follower loads and compressive preloads, have been developed to replicate physiological conditions more accurately. The follower load technique applies compressive forces along the natural curvature of the spine, mimicking the stabilizing effects of surrounding musculature. Preloads simulate baseline forces acting on the spine in a neutral posture, providing a realistic starting point for dynamic assessments [9, 10]. Furthermore, high-resolution imaging and motion capture systems are increasingly integrated into biomechanical studies to provide real-time data on ligament deformation, strain distribution, and joint kinematics. These advancements enable a more comprehensive understanding of the PLC's biomechanical behavior [12].

6.2.4 Challenges and Future Directions

While standardized protocols have advanced the field, inconsistencies in specimen preparation and testing equipment persist. Future research should aim to establish universal guidelines and integrate computational modeling for more predictive and individualized assessments [16].

6.3 Biomechanical Properties of Lumbar Posterior Ligament Complex

The lumbar posterior ligament complex (PLC) plays a vital role in maintaining spinal stability and facilitating biomechanical function. Comprised of the ligamentum flavum, interspinous ligament, and supraspinous ligament, the PLC provides significant resistance to flexion and contributes to overall spinal integrity. This chapter delves into the structural and functional characteristics of the PLC, its response to mechanical loads, and the importance of surgical strategies that address its degeneration through artificial ligament replacement.

6.3.1 Structural and Functional Characteristics of the PLC

The ligamentum flavum, with its high elastin content, is uniquely adapted to provide elastic recoil and resistance to deformation during flexion–extension movements. It contributes approximately 22% to the total resistance to flexion forces in the lumbar spine [17]. Meanwhile, the interspinous and supraspinous ligaments are primarily composed of collagen, providing tensile strength and limiting hyperflexion. Together, these structures resist around 6% of flexion forces, underscoring their combined contribution to spinal stability [19]. The PLC exhibits nonlinear load-displacement behavior, with stiffness increasing as the ligaments approach their physiological limits. This property is crucial for preventing excessive motion and ensuring that spinal movements remain within safe ranges. Additionally, the PLC plays a role in proprioception, aiding in the coordination of spinal motion [18].

6.3.2 Biomechanical Response to Loading

Under normal physiological loads, the PLC contributes approximately 30–40% of passive stability in the lumbar spine. During flexion, the ligamentum flavum undergoes elongation, absorbing tensile forces and reducing stress on adjacent structures. The interspinous and supraspinous ligaments, in turn, distribute tensile loads across multiple vertebral levels, mitigating localized strain [17, 18]. Pathological changes, such as hypertrophy and degeneration, alter the mechanical properties of the PLC. For instance, ligamentum flavum hypertrophy increases its mechanical stiffness, which can lead to malalignment and an increased risk of spinal canal stenosis. Similarly, degeneration of the interspinous and supraspinous ligaments compromises their tensile strength, resulting in abnormal load distribution and potential segmental instability [19, 20].

6.3.3 Replacing Degenerated PLC with Artificial Ligaments

Degeneration of the PLC often necessitates surgical intervention to restore stability and functionality to the lumbar spine. Artificial ligament systems have emerged as a promising solution, providing mechanical support that mimics the native properties of the PLC. These systems are designed to replicate the tensile strength and elastic properties of healthy ligaments, enabling controlled motion while reducing abnormal stress transmission [15]. Dynamic stabilization devices, which incorporate artificial ligaments, offer an effective alternative to rigid spinal fusion by preserving segmental motion. Such systems have demonstrated biomechanical efficacy in redistributing loads and maintaining spinal alignment. Additionally, their use minimizes the risk of adjacent segment disease (ASD), a common complication of traditional fusion surgeries [14].

6.3.4 Importance of Facet Joint Preservation

In addition to addressing PLC degeneration, maintaining the integrity of the facet joints during surgery is critical for spinal stability. Facet joints bear axial loads and resist shear forces, making their preservation essential in artificial ligament implantation procedures. Techniques that prioritize facet joint preservation ensure optimal load sharing across the spinal column and reduce the risk of accelerated degeneration at adjacent levels. Facet-sparing approaches, as referenced in minimally invasive procedures, involve limited resection or targeted decompression to maintain joint integrity [4]. These methods not only enhance postoperative stability but also align with the mechanical principles of artificial ligament systems, which depend on a balanced distribution of forces across spinal structures. By integrating facet joint preservation with artificial ligament replacement, surgical outcomes can be significantly improved, offering patients restored functionality and reduced complication rates [14].

6.4 Biomechanics of Interspinous Soft Stabilization

Interspinous soft stabilization (ISS) has emerged as an innovative approach in spinal surgery, providing dynamic stabilization while maintaining motion. This technique utilizes artificial ligaments positioned between the spinous processes to stabilize the spine, reduce stress on adjacent segments, and restore lumbar functionality. By replicating the biomechanical properties of the posterior ligament complex (PLC), ISS addresses significant limitations of rigid spinal fusion, such as adjacent segment disease (ASD) and loss of motion.

6.4.1 Biomechanical Principles of Interspinous Soft Stabilization

Interspinous soft stabilization (ISS) is designed to mimic the biomechanical behavior of the posterior ligament complex (PLC) while preserving physiological motion in the lumbar spine. The artificial ligaments used in ISS are made from elastic and tension-resisting materials such as polyester and polyethylene terephthalate. These materials replicate the natural mechanical properties of spinal ligaments, providing both tensile strength and flexibility. The ligaments are anchored to the spinous processes in a configuration that limits excessive flexion while permitting controlled extension, facilitating dynamic load sharing between stabilized and adjacent spinal segments [3, 14].

Key Biomechanical Objectives

- *Preservation of Segmental Motion*: ISS enables controlled motion within the treated segment, unlike rigid fusion techniques that eliminate mobility. By maintaining physiological flexion–extension motion, ISS reduces the transfer of abnormal mechanical forces to adjacent segments, minimizing the risk of adjacent segment disease (ASD). Biomechanical tests have demonstrated that ISS retains over 80% of the native stiffness of the spine [1, 3].
- *Restoration of Sagittal Alignment*: Through tension band mechanics, ISS enhances segmental lumbar lordosis, ensuring proper sagittal alignment. Maintaining this alignment is critical for preserving spinopelvic balance and reducing compensatory pelvic tilt. This effect is particularly beneficial in patients with spondylolisthesis or lumbar spinal stenosis [14].
- *Dynamic Stabilization*: ISS reduces the neutral zone, which represents the range of motion under minimal force, without completely eliminating motion. This stabilization prevents excessive instability while allowing the spine to retain its dynamic properties. Such stabilization is particularly effective in mild to moderate spondylolisthesis [15].

6.4.2 Biomechanical Mechanisms

The biomechanics of ISS are influenced by its ability to distribute loads and maintain stability under various physiological conditions:

- *Flexion and Extension*: During flexion, ISS limits excessive movement by distributing tensile forces across the tension band. This mechanism prevents overstretching of the posterior elements while maintaining sufficient flexibility for physiological motion. In extension, the elastic properties of the artificial ligament allow controlled elongation, avoiding abrupt restriction and ensuring smooth motion [1, 3].
- *Axial Rotation*: In cases of torsional stress, ISS provides rotational stability by restricting excessive axial motion. Cadaveric studies have shown that ISS maintains rotational stiffness at levels comparable to the intact spine [4].
- *Load Distribution*: The anchoring of ISS at the spinous processes ensures even distribution of compressive and tensile forces across both the treated and adjacent segments. This mechanism reduces localized stress on intervertebral discs and facet joints, preserving their structural integrity and reducing degeneration [1, 3].
- *Stress Reduction on Adjacent Segments*: Unlike rigid fusion, which increases stress on adjacent segments, ISS mitigates this risk by preserving natural motion and allowing dynamic adaptation to mechanical loads. Studies have demonstrated that ISS reduces adjacent segment stress by approximately 28%, significantly lowering the likelihood of ASD [3, 6].

By achieving these objectives, ISS offers a biomechanically favorable alternative to traditional fusion techniques, improving outcomes for patients requiring spinal stabilization.

6.4.3 Experimental Evidence Supporting Interspinous Soft Stabilization

The application of interspinous soft stabilization using artificial ligaments has been rigorously investigated through biomechanical and clinical studies. These efforts collectively underscore its potential to address lumbar spinal instability while preserving motion, offering a less invasive alternative to spinal fusion.

Voydeville et al. [1] conducted a pivotal biomechanical study to evaluate the efficacy of artificial ligaments in stabilizing lumbar spine segments following induced instability. Using six fresh L4/L5 cadaveric specimens, the researchers simulated instability by performing partial arthrectomies and fenestrations between the spinous processes, creating conditions that significantly increased motion in flexion–extension, lateral bending, and axial rotation. To restore stability, an artificial ligament system composed of polyester material and integrated with a wedge design was applied. This setup mimicked the function of natural ligaments while preserving some degree of motion. The experimental protocol involved mounting each specimen on a custom-designed test rig equipped with a multi-axis motion analysis system. Controlled loads ranging from −7 Nm to +7 Nm were incrementally applied across flexion–extension, lateral bending, and axial rotation. The angular displacements and translational motions of the spinal unit were recorded under three conditions: intact, destabilized, and stabilized with the artificial ligament. Results showed that the artificial ligament effectively restored stability to levels comparable to the intact state across all axes of motion ($p < 0.05$). In addition to reducing excessive motion, the ligament system redistributed loads uniformly, mitigating stress concentrations on the spinous processes. The inclusion of a wedge component improved biomechanical performance by maintaining optimal ligament tension and preventing impingement between the spinous processes. These findings established that artificial ligaments provide an effective and less invasive alternative to traditional rigid fixation techniques. By rigorously demonstrating the biomechanical viability of artificial ligaments, this study laid the foundation for their clinical application in managing lumbar instability, bridging the gap between decompression and fusion surgery.

Caserta and colleagues [3] conducted a biomechanical evaluation of elastic stabilization systems. Their study revealed that elastic stabilization reduced stress on adjacent segments by up to 28% during flexion, highlighting its ability to prevent adjacent segment degeneration while addressing instability. These findings supported the use of soft stabilization as a motion-preserving alternative to rigid fusion.

Mulholland and Sengupta [21] provided a comprehensive evaluation of soft stabilization systems, focusing on their biomechanical principles and clinical applications. Their findings emphasized that soft stabilization reduces abnormal load transmission across intervertebral discs while maintaining sagittal balance, making it a viable option for patients with mechanical back pain.

Shim and colleagues [15] compared the clinical outcomes of soft stabilization with those of PLIF in patients with grade I degenerative spondylolisthesis. Their results demonstrated similar improvements in functional scores but with significantly reduced operative times and blood loss in the soft stabilization group, further validating its efficacy and safety.

Sang-Ho Lee and his team have extensively evaluated interspinous soft stabilization through multiple studies. Their 2010 multicenter study [2] involving 556 patients with mildly unstable degenerative lumbar spinal stenosis demonstrated an 80.4% clinical success rate, as measured by MacNab criteria. This study highlighted the reproducibility and safety of the technique in preventing post-decompression instability. In another 2010 study [14], Lee and colleagues investigated spinopelvic alignment following interspinous soft stabilization with a tension band system in grade I degenerative spondylolisthesis. They found that the technique maintained lumbar lordosis and sagittal balance, achieving clinical outcomes comparable to posterior lumbar interbody fusion (PLIF) but with fewer complications and shorter recovery times. Expanding on this, their 2012 research [5] identified radiological factors influencing clinical outcomes in patients treated with soft stabilization. They reported that improvements in segmental lumbar lordosis were strongly correlated with reduced back pain and enhanced functional outcomes, further substantiating the biomechanical benefits of this approach.

6.4.4 Clinical Implications

Interspinous soft stabilization (ISS) offers distinct advantages over traditional fusion surgeries by addressing spinal instability biomechanics while preserving natural motion. Unlike rigid fusion, which increases stress on adjacent segments and often leads to adjacent segment degeneration, ISS redistributes mechanical loads and maintains sagittal alignment [21]. This approach minimizes complications such as pseudarthrosis and donor-site morbidity while reducing operative time, blood loss, and recovery duration. The preservation of segmental motion prevents accelerated degeneration of adjacent levels, a frequent complication in fusion surgeries. Clinical studies report reduced revision rates and improved patient satisfaction with ISS compared to rigid fusion. For patients with mild instability or low-grade spondylolisthesis, ISS has demonstrated equivalent or superior outcomes in pain relief and functional improvement [5]. Future developments in ISS technology focus on enhancing material properties and device designs. Innovations such as bioadaptive materials and patient-specific implants aim to improve compatibility and clinical outcomes, paving the way for more personalized and effective spinal treatments [17]. These advancements, coupled with minimally invasive techniques, hold the potential to expand the application of ISS and further optimize patient outcomes.

6.5 Summary

This chapter delves into the biomechanics of interspinous soft stabilization (ISS), emphasizing its innovative approach to addressing lumbar instability while preserving natural motion. By exploring the biomechanical principles of the posterior ligament complex (PLC), the chapter highlights how ISS balances load distribution, maintains sagittal alignment, and supports dynamic stability. Through advanced biomechanical evaluations and experimental evidence, ISS emerges as a motion-preserving alternative to traditional fusion surgery. This approach minimizes stress on adjacent segments, mitigates degeneration, and optimizes spinal stability, presenting a transformative paradigm in lumbar spine stabilization techniques.

References

1. Voydeville G, et al. Experimental lumbar instability and artificial ligament. Eur J Orthop Surg Traumatol. 2000;10:167–76.
2. Lee SH, et al. Soft stabilization with interspinous artificial ligament for mildly unstable lumbar spinal stenosis. Arch Orthop Trauma Surg. 2010;130:1335–41.
3. Caserta S, et al. Elastic stabilization alone or combined with rigid fusion in spinal surgery: a biomechanical study. Eur Spine J. 2002;11(Suppl. 2):S192–7.
4. Hamasaki T, et al. Biomechanical assessment of minimally invasive decompression for lumbar spinal canal stenosis. J Spinal Disord Tech. 2009;22:486–91.
5. Lee SH, et al. Factors affecting clinical outcomes in treating patients with grade 1 degenerative spondylolisthesis using interspinous soft stabilization with a tension band system. Spine. 2012;37:563–72.
6. Gonzalez-Blohm SA, et al. Current testing protocols for biomechanical evaluation of lumbar spinal implants in laboratory setting: a review of the literature. Biomed Res Int. 2015; https://doi.org/10.1155/2015/506181.
7. Panjabi MM. Biomechanical evaluation of spinal fixation devices. Spine. 1976; https://doi.org/10.1097/00007632-198810000-00013.
8. Wilke HJ, et al. Is it possible to simulate physiologic loading conditions by applying pure moments? A comparison of in vivo and in vitro load components in an internal fixator. Spine. 2001;
9. Patwardhan AG, et al. A follower load increases the load-carrying capacity of

the lumbar spine. Spine. 2003; https://doi.org/10.1097/00007632-199905150-00014.
10. Costi JJ, Ledet EH, O'Connell GD. Spine biomechanical testing methodologies: The controversy of consensus vs scientific evidence. JOR Spine. 2021;
11. Dickey JP, Kerr DJ. Effect of specimen length: are the mechanics of individual motion segments comparable in functional spinal units and multisegment specimens? Med Eng Phys. 2003;
12. Cripton PA, et al. The role of testing apparatus in spine biomechanics. J Biomech. 2000;
13. Anderson B, Shahidi B. The impact of spine pathology on posterior ligamentous complex structure and function. Curr Rev Musculoskelet Med. 2023;16:616–26.
14. Lee SH, et al. Spinopelvic alignment after interspinous soft stabilization with a tension band system in grade 1 degenerative lumbar spondylolisthesis. Spine. 2010;35:E691–701.
15. Shim CS, et al. Soft stabilization with an artificial intervertebral ligament in grade I degenerative spondylolisthesis. SAS J. 2007;1:118–24.
16. Han KS, et al. Spinal muscles can create compressive follower loads in the lumbar spine in a neutral standing posture. Med Eng Phys. 2011;33(4):472–8.
17. Widmer J, et al. Biomechanical contribution of spinal structures to stability of the lumbar spine—novel biomechanical insights. Spine J. 2020;20:1705–16.
18. Dumas GA, Beaudoin L, Drouin G. In situ mechanical behavior of posterior spinal ligaments in the lumbar region. J Biomech. 1987;20:301–10.
19. Chazal J, Tanguy A, Bourges M, et al. Biomechanical properties of spinal ligaments and a histological study of the supraspinal ligament in traction. J Biomech. 1985;18:167–76.
20. Iida T, Abumi K, Kotani Y, et al. Effects of aging and spinal degeneration on mechanical properties of lumbar supraspinous and interspinous ligaments. Spine J. 2002;2:95–100.
21. Mulholland RC, Sengupta DK. Rationale, principles and experimental evaluation of the concept of soft stabilization. Eur Spine J. 2002;11(Suppl. 2):S198–205.

7 Surgical Technique for Ligament Reconstruction Using Sagittal and Horizontal (SH) Ligament

Sang-Ha Shin, Shin-Jae Kim, and Chi-Su Park

Abstract

Spinal stenosis is a degenerative condition often requiring surgical decompression to alleviate neural compression. However, traditional decompression techniques can exacerbate spinal instability, leading to long-term complications such as recurrent stenosis or postoperative back pain. Fusion surgery is often employed to address these issues but may be overly invasive, particularly for elderly patients with mild instability or osteoporosis. The SHLee Ligament™, composed of polyethylene terephthalate and approved by Korea's Ministry of Food and Drug Safety, offers an innovative alternative. Designed for soft stabilization, this artificial ligament provides spinal support while preserving segmental motion, reducing the need for invasive fusion procedures. Its application is particularly suited for patients with mild instability or grade I degenerative spondylolisthesis, where maintaining spinal flexibility is critical. This chapter details the composition, surgical technique, and clinical outcomes associated with the SHLee Ligament™, emphasizing its effectiveness in stabilizing decompressed spinal segments. By integrating minimally invasive decompression with artificial ligament stabilization, this approach addresses the limitations of conventional methods, offering improved outcomes for patients with lumbar spinal stenosis. The SHLee Ligament™ represents a significant advancement in spine surgery, balancing stability and mobility while minimizing surgical invasiveness.

Keywords

Ligament reconstruction · SHLee ligament
Artificial ligament · Soft stabilization · Spinal stenosis

7.1 Introduction

Spinal stenosis is a prevalent degenerative spinal disorder that significantly diminishes the quality of life in elderly patients [1, 2]. It is characterized by the progressive narrowing of the spinal canal, leading to symptoms such as neurogenic claudication, lower back pain, and functional impairment [3]. With the aging population worldwide, the incidence of spinal stenosis is increasing, posing a substantial socioeconomic burden [4]. Current surgical treatments primarily focus on neural decompression, aiming to relieve nerve compression and restore functionality [5]. However, the anatomical

S.-H. Shin (✉) · S.-J. Kim
Department of Neurosurgery, Cheongdam Wooridul Spine Hospital, Seoul, Korea (Republic of)
e-mail: burrhoer@wooridul.co.kr

C.-S. Park
Department of Nurse Practitioner, Cheongdam Wooridul Spine Hospital, Seoul, South Korea

S.-H. Lee et al. (eds.), *Ligament Reconstruction for Spine*,
https://doi.org/10.1007/978-981-95-3971-0_7

and biomechanical complexity of spinal stenosis often extends beyond simple nerve impingement, involving compensatory changes in spinal structures to address underlying instability [6].

These compensatory mechanisms include facet joint hypertrophy, ligamentum flavum thickening, and disc degeneration, which together contribute to spinal stenosis [7–9]. While decompression effectively alleviates symptoms of neural compression, it often exacerbates preexisting spinal instability [10]. Over time, this can lead to complications such as postoperative back pain, recurrent stenosis, or progressive spondylolisthesis, particularly in cases where structural support is compromised [11, 12].

To mitigate these issues, fusion surgery is frequently employed to stabilize the spine [13]. However, this approach has limitations, especially for elderly patients with mild instability or grade I degenerative spondylolisthesis [14]. Fusion surgery is often invasive, increases the risk of adjacent segment disease, and may not be ideal for elderly patients with osteoporosis or other comorbidities [15]. These drawbacks have spurred interest in alternative strategies that balance decompression with stabilization while preserving spinal mobility.

Soft stabilization, performed concurrently with neural decompression, has emerged as a promising solution [16]. This approach addresses micro-instability without compromising the structural integrity of the disc or adjacent segments. Unlike fusion, soft stabilization allows for segmental motion, making it a less invasive and more biomechanically favorable option for a broad range of patients [17].

In this context, artificial ligaments have gained traction as effective tools for spinal stabilization. The SHLee Ligament™ (Prestigemedicare, GEMSKOREA, Korea), consisting of the Sagittal ligament and Horizontal ligament, represents a significant advancement in this domain. Made primarily from durable materials such as polyethylene terephthalate, the SHLee Ligament™ offers a robust yet flexible solution tailored for spinal applications. While literature specifically addressing the SHLee Ligament™ remains limited, it aligns with the growing body of work exploring dynamic stabilization devices designed to maintain motion while providing necessary support [18–20]. In this chapter, we aim to introduce the SHLee Ligament™, detail its unique design, and provide a comprehensive description of its surgical procedure, illustrating how it addresses the limitations of existing treatments and offers a novel paradigm for managing spinal stenosis.

7.2 Surgical Steps

7.2.1 Open Midline Decompression (OMD)

Please refer to
Part II, Chap. 11.

7.2.2 Ligament Reconstruction (LP)

The SHLee Ligament™ (Prestigemedicare, GEMSKOREA, Korea) is composed of the Sagittal ligament and the Horizontal ligament (Fig. 7.1). After sufficient hemostasis, Sagittal ligament is tied between the spinous processes of the index level in the longitudinal direction (Fig. 7.2a). Before tightening the ligament with a contractor device, the regional lordotic angle of the lumbar spine was set by changing the angle of the operating table. Then, 2-0 nylon sutures were placed near the center of the knot to prevent excessive extension of the spine. Horizontal ligament is wound once more in each interspinous space in the transverse direction to wrap the longitudinally tied artificial ligament (Fig. 7.2b, c). The surgical wound was closed after the surgery was completed.

The development of minimally invasive surgical (MIS) techniques, such as tubular or endoscopic decompression, has been a game-changer, providing less invasive options for addressing lumbar spinal stenosis (LSS) [21–23]. These techniques have successfully minimized tissue damage, reduced recovery times, and improved short-term outcomes [21, 22]. However, their limitations, particularly in elderly patients with multilevel LSS accompanied by instability,

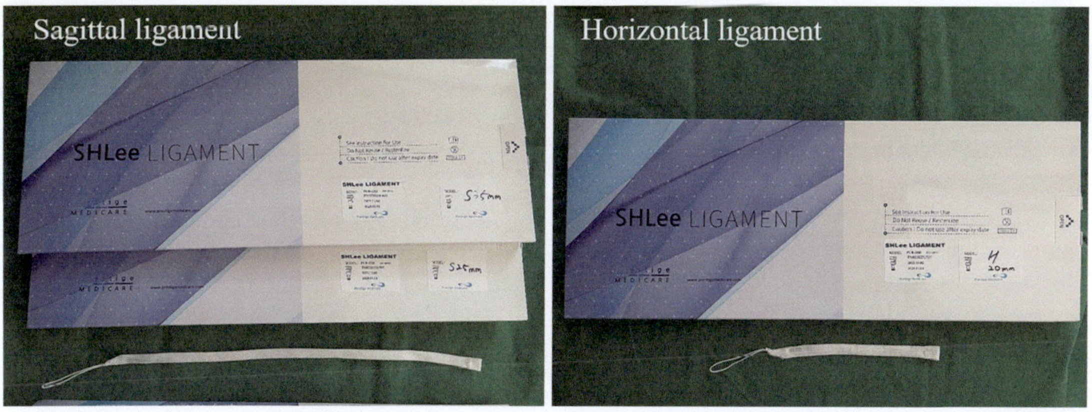

Fig. 7.1 Process of ligament reconstruction

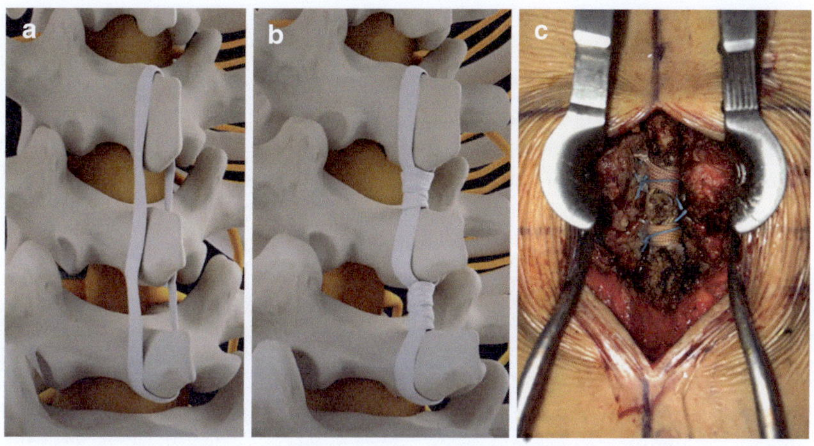

Fig. 7.2 Process of ligament reconstruction. (**a**) Sagittal ligament is tied at the index level of the spinous processes. (**b**) Horizontal ligament is tied around the longitudinal component at the interspinous spaces. (**c**) Surgical field of two-level ligament reconstruction after open midline decompression

remain significant. The structural compromises inherent in decompression procedures can lead to long-term complications, including progressive instability, recurrent stenosis, and persistent back pain, which undermine the benefits of initial intervention [10–12]. Alternative decompression techniques, such as spinous splitting laminectomy and contralateral decompression methods, have been proposed to mitigate these issues [24–26]. While these approaches have shown efficacy in achieving adequate decompression [24–26], they still fail to address the core problem of spinal instability. Decompression alone, regardless of technique, may result in a biomechanically weakened spine, predisposing patients to further degeneration or the need for revision surgery [4, 10, 11].

To address these challenges, soft stabilization techniques utilizing artificial ligaments have emerged as a promising solution [16, 17, 19, 27]. Unlike fusion, which sacrifices segmental motion, soft stabilization provides structural support while maintaining spinal flexibility. This approach is particularly advantageous for elderly patients or those with mild instability, such as grade I degenerative spondylolisthesis, where preserving motion is critical for maintaining overall spinal function and quality of life [15, 16, 19].

Artificial ligaments have a well-established history in orthopedic applications, particularly in knee and shoulder surgeries, where they have demonstrated durability and effectiveness [28, 29]. However, their application in spine surgery has gained attention only recently [16, 17, 27]. The SHLee Ligament™ (Prestigemedicare, GEMSKOREA, Korea), primarily composed of polyethylene terephthalate, represents a significant advancement in this field. Its approval by the MFDS (The Ministry of Food and Drug Safety in Korea) underscores its clinical viability. This ligament's unique design allows it to provide robust support while accommodating the dynamic movements of the spine, thus reducing the mechanical stresses that often lead to long-term complications in decompressed segments [16, 17, 27].

Several studies have documented the clinical and radiological outcomes of ligamentoplasty in spine surgery, reporting reduced rates of recurrent stenosis, improved pain scores, and enhanced functional outcomes compared to decompression alone [16, 17, 19, 27]. Moreover, soft stabilization with artificial ligaments has been shown to reduce the likelihood of adjacent segment disease, a common complication associated with fusion procedures [17, 27]. These findings highlight the potential of ligament reconstruction as a transformative approach in the management of LSS.

Despite these promising developments, several challenges remain. The long-term durability of artificial ligaments in spinal applications needs further investigation, particularly in diverse patient populations with varying degrees of instability [4, 16, 17, 19, 27]. Additionally, the cost-effectiveness of ligamentoplasty compared to traditional fusion or decompression techniques warrants further analysis to ensure its accessibility and widespread adoption [10, 15].

In conclusion, while MIS techniques and alternative decompression methods have revolutionized the management of LSS, their limitations necessitate complementary strategies to address spinal instability. Soft stabilization using artificial ligaments, such as the SHLee Ligament™, offers a balanced solution by combining structural support with the preservation of motion. Continued research and clinical validation will be essential to optimizing this approach and establishing it as a standard of care in spine surgery.

7.3 Summary

The SHLee Ligament™ offers a novel approach to managing lumbar spinal stenosis by combining open midline decompression (OMD) with soft stabilization. Unlike fusion surgery, it preserves spinal motion while addressing instability. This chapter highlights its design, surgical application, and promising outcomes, providing an effective alternative for patients with mild instability or osteoporosis.

References

1. Deyo RA, Mirza SK, Martin BI. Back pain prevalence and visit rates: estimates from U.S. national surveys, 2002. Spine (Phila Pa 1976). 2006;31(23):2724–7.
2. Kalichman L, Cole R, Kim DH, et al. Spinal stenosis prevalence and association with symptoms: the Framingham study. Spine J. 2009;9(7):545–50.
3. Genevay S, Atlas SJ. Lumbar spinal stenosis. Best Pract Res Clin Rheumatol. 2010;24(2):253–65.
4. Deyo RA, Cherkin DC, Loeser JD, et al. Morbidity and mortality in association with operations on the lumbar spine: the influence of age, diagnosis, and procedure. J Bone Joint Surg Am. 1992;74(4):536–43.
5. Försth P, Ólafsson G, Carlsson T, et al. A randomized, controlled trial of fusion surgery for lumbar spinal stenosis. N Engl J Med. 2016;374(15):1413–23.
6. Adams MA, Roughley PJ. What is intervertebral disc degeneration, and what causes it? Spine (Phila Pa 1976). 2006;31(18):2151–61.
7. Issack PS, Cunningham ME, Pumberger M, Hughes AP, Cammisa FP Jr. Degenerative lumbar spinal stenosis: evaluation and management. J Am Acad Orthop Surg. 2012;20(8):527–35.
8. Zhang L, Chen R, Chen Q, et al. Hypertrophy of ligamentum flavum in lumbar spine stenosis associated with the increased expression of connective tissue growth factor. J Spinal Disord Tech. 2011;24(7):401–6.
9. Urban JP, Roberts S. Degeneration of the intervertebral disc. Arthritis Res Ther. 2003;5(3):120–30.
10. Yang JC, Kim SG, Kim TW, Park KH. Analysis of factors contributing to postoperative spinal instability after lumbar decompression for spinal stenosis. Korean J Spine. 2013;10(3):149–54.
11. Kleinstück FS, Fekete TF, Jeszenszky D, et al. The influence of preoperative back pain on the outcome of lumbar decompression surgery. Spine (Phila Pa 1976). 2011;36(2):E134–41.
12. Kim HJ, Chun HJ, Kang KT, et al. The biomechanical influence of the facet joint orientation and the facet tropism in the lumbar spine. Spine J. 2013;13(10):1301–8.

13. Harris IA, Traeger A, Stanford R, Maher CG, Buchbinder R. Lumbar spine fusion: what is the evidence? Intern Med J. 2018;48(12):1430–4.
14. Koenig S, Jauregui JJ, Shasti M, Jazini E, Koh EY, Banagan KE, et al. Decompression versus fusion for grade I degenerative spondylolisthesis: a meta-analysis. Glob Spine J. 2019;9(2):155–61.
15. Park P, Garton HJ, Gala VC, et al. Adjacent segment disease after lumbar or lumbosacral fusion: review of the literature. Spine (Phila Pa 1976). 2004;29(17):1938–44.
16. Cakir B, Richter M. Dynamic stabilization of the lumbar spine. Curr Orthop. 2007;21(4):270–7.
17. Stoll TM, Dubois G, Schwarzenbach O. The dynamic neutralization system for the spine: a multi-center study of a novel non-fusion system. Eur Spine J. 2002;11(Suppl 2):S170–8.
18. Khoueir P, Kim KA, Wang MY. Classification of posterior dynamic stabilization devices. Neurosurg Focus. 2007;22(1):E3.
19. Fay LY, Wu JC, Tsai TY, et al. Dynamic stabilization for degenerative spondylolisthesis: evaluation of radiographic and clinical outcomes. Clin Neurol Neurosurg. 2016;144:60–7.
20. Shim CS, Lee SH, Park SH, Whang JH. Soft stabilization with an artificial intervertebral ligament in grade I degenerative spondylolisthesis: comparison with instrumented posterior lumbar interbody fusion. Int J Spine Surg. 2007;1(3):118–24.
21. Foley KT, Smith MM. Microendoscopic discectomy. Tech Neurosurg. 1997;3:301–7.
22. Kim HS, Park JY. Endoscopic spine procedures. Korean J Spine. 2017;14(1):1–4.
23. Ng KKM, Cheung JPY. Is minimally invasive surgery superior to open surgery for treatment of lumbar spinal stenosis? A systematic review. J Orthop Surg (Hong Kong). 2017;25(2):1–11.
24. Watanabe K, Hosoya T, Shiraishi T, et al. Lumbar spinous process-splitting laminectomy for lumbar canal stenosis. Tech Orthop. 2005;20(2):153–9.
25. Yeung YK, Park CW, Jun SG, Park JH, Tse AC. Comparative cohort study for expansion of lateral recess and facet joint injury after biportal endoscopic ipsilateral decompression and contralateral decompression. Asian Spine J. 2022;16(4):560–6.
26. Lee DH, Lee DG, Park CK, Jang JW, Hwang JS, Kim JY, et al. Saving stabilizing structure treatment with bilateral-contralateral decompression for spinal stenosis in degenerative spondylolisthesis using unilateral biportal endoscopy. Neurospine. 2023;20(3):931–9.
27. Schnake KJ, Schaeren S, Jeanneret B. Dynamic stabilization in addition to decompression for lumbar spinal stenosis with degenerative spondylolisthesis. Spine. 2006;31(7):442–9.
28. Gao K, Chen S, Wang L, et al. Anterior cruciate ligament reconstruction with LARS artificial ligament: a multicenter study with 3- to 5-year follow-up. Arthroscopy. 2010;26(4):515–23.
29. Legnani C, Ventura A, Terzaghi C, Borgo E, Albisetti W. Anterior cruciate ligament reconstruction with synthetic grafts: a review of literature. Int Orthop. 2010;34(4):465–71.

Application of Ligament Reconstruction in Combination with Interlaminar or Interspinous Device

8

Junseok Bae

Abstract

The combination of ligament reconstruction with interlaminar or interspinous devices represents an innovative approach to treating degenerative spinal conditions, particularly in elderly patients with chronic low back pain and spinal stenosis. Recent studies, particularly those published after 2020, have offered deeper insights into the efficacy and safety of this approach. These include advancements in patient outcomes and surgical methodologies validated through longitudinal research and meta-analyses. This chapter examines the technical aspects, clinical outcomes, and biomechanical rationale of this combined approach. The integration of ligament reconstruction with dynamic stabilization devices provides a less invasive alternative to traditional fusion surgery while maintaining spinal stability and potentially reducing adjacent segment degeneration.

Keywords

Ligament reconstruction · Interlaminar device
Interspinous device · Spinal stenosis
Minimally invasive surgery

J. Bae (✉)
Department of Neurosurgery, Cheongdam Wooridul Spine Hospital, Seoul, Korea (Republic of)
e-mail: jsbaemd@gmail.com

8.1 Introduction

As the population ages, the incidence of degenerative spinal conditions continues to rise. Traditional fusion surgery, while effective, may lead to complications such as adjacent segment disease and hardware failure, particularly in elderly patients with compromised bone quality. Newer comparative studies highlight that dynamic stabilization techniques can achieve similar or improved outcomes with reduced risk of adjacent segment degeneration and hardware-related issues, thereby offering a compelling alternative in carefully selected cases. The combination of ligament reconstruction with interlaminar or interspinous devices offers a novel solution that aims to preserve motion while providing adequate stabilization [1–3].

8.2 Presentation of the Patient

8.2.1 Patient Selection

The selection of appropriate patients for combined ligament reconstruction and dynamic stabilization requires careful consideration of multiple factors. The ideal candidates are typically patients who present with chronic low back pain that has been unresponsive to conservative treatment for at least 6 months. These patients should demonstrate radiological evidence of spinal stenosis

S.-H. Lee et al. (eds.), *Ligament Reconstruction for Spine*,
https://doi.org/10.1007/978-981-95-3971-0_8

and/or disc degeneration on imaging studies. It is crucial that they do not exhibit significant instability or spondylolisthesis, as these conditions may require more aggressive stabilization techniques. Additionally, patients should not have undergone prior lumbar fusion surgery at the target level, as this would complicate the procedure and potentially compromise outcomes [1].

8.2.2 Contraindications

Several conditions serve as absolute contraindications to this combined approach. Active infection anywhere in the body, but particularly in the surgical site, presents an unacceptable risk and must be fully resolved before considering surgery. Severe osteoporosis significantly increases the risk of hardware failure and poor outcomes, making it a major contraindication. Patients with significant spinal deformity or high-grade spondylolisthesis are not suitable candidates, as these conditions typically require more extensive corrective procedures. Prior fusion at the target level also precludes this approach, as it fundamentally alters the biomechanics and surgical approach.

8.3 Preoperative Planning

8.3.1 Imaging Studies

Comprehensive preoperative imaging is essential for surgical planning and patient selection. Standing radiographs in anteroposterior and lateral views, along with dynamic flexion–extension films, provide crucial information about segmental motion, overall spinal alignment, and potential instability. These studies help determine the extent of mechanical dysfunction and guide the selection of appropriate implant sizes (Fig. 8.1).

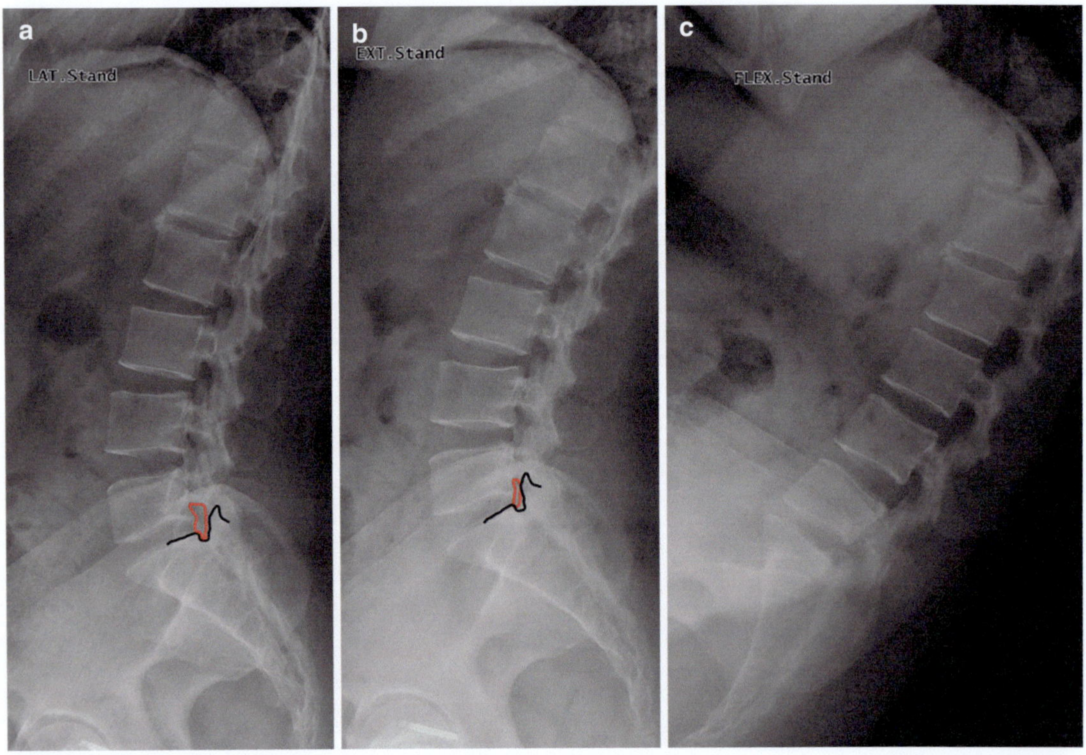

Fig. 8.1 Preoperative dynamic X-ray shows instability of index segment. (**a**; neutral, **b**; Extension, **c**; Flexion) Note the disc height narrowing on extension view causing superior articular process (black line) impinging neural foramen (red line)

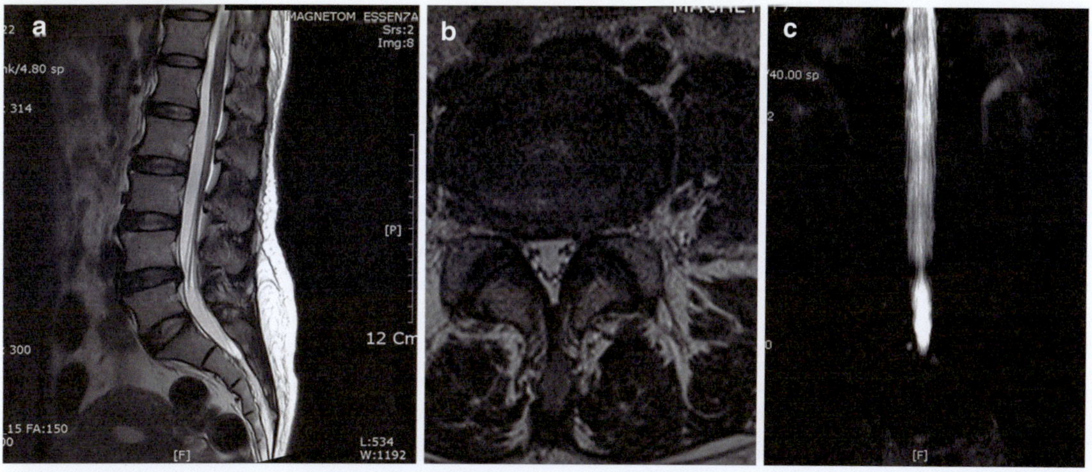

Fig. 8.2 Preoperative sagittal (**a**) and axial (**b**) MRI shows disc degeneration and stenosis at the L4–5 level. MR myelography (**c**) shows partial signal block representing central canal stenosis

Magnetic resonance imaging (MRI) serves as the primary tool for evaluating neural compression and soft tissue pathology. It allows detailed assessment of the degree of stenosis, extent of disc degeneration, and condition of the facet joints. The presence and severity of facet arthropathy, in particular, can influence the choice of decompression technique and implant type (Fig. 8.2).

Computed tomography (CT) may be necessary to evaluate bone quality and detail the bony anatomy. This is particularly important when assessing the integrity of the spinous processes and laminae that will serve as anchor points for the reconstruction. CT imaging can also help rule out occult fractures or other bony abnormalities that might compromise the surgical outcome.

8.3.2 Device Selection

The choice between interlaminar and interspinous devices depends largely on the specific pathology and anatomical considerations of each case. Interlaminar devices are particularly well-suited for cases requiring direct decompression, as they provide stability while allowing access to the spinal canal. These devices work in concert with the reconstructed ligament to maintain physiological motion patterns. In contrast, interspinous devices may be more appropriate for cases where indirect decompression is sufficient, particularly in elderly patients with less severe stenosis. The final device selection must take into account the patient's anatomy, the specific level of pathology, and the intended degree of decompression.

8.4 Surgical Steps

8.4.1 Patient Positioning and Approach

The procedure begins with careful positioning of the patient prone on a Wilson frame, which helps maintain proper lumbar lordosis and provides adequate access to the surgical site. After confirming the target level under fluoroscopic guidance, a midline incision of approximately 3–4 centimeters is made. The paraspinal muscles are then carefully dissected in a subperiosteal fashion to expose the required anatomy while minimizing tissue trauma.

8.4.1.1 Decompression Phase

During the decompression phase, the supraspinous ligament is preserved whenever possible, as it plays a crucial role in maintaining the posterior tension band. The ligamentum flavum is meticulously removed to achieve adequate neural decompression. The extent of decompression is tailored to the specific pathology present, with careful attention paid to preserving the integrity of the facet joints, which are essential for maintaining segmental stability.

8.4.2 Device Placement

The selection of the appropriate implant size is crucial and is determined through careful trialing. The interspinous or interlaminar space is prepared according to the manufacturer's specifications, taking care to avoid damage to the spinous processes or laminae. The dynamic stabilization device is then inserted under direct visualization, with fluoroscopic guidance used to confirm optimal positioning and alignment (Figs. 8.3 and 8.4).

8.4.2.1 Ligament Reconstruction

The ligament reconstruction phase begins with careful preparation of the attachment sites, ensuring adequate bony surface for optimal integration. The artificial ligament is passed through previously prepared channels, with attention to maintaining proper orientation and avoiding twist in the construct. The tension of the ligament is carefully adjusted to provide stability while

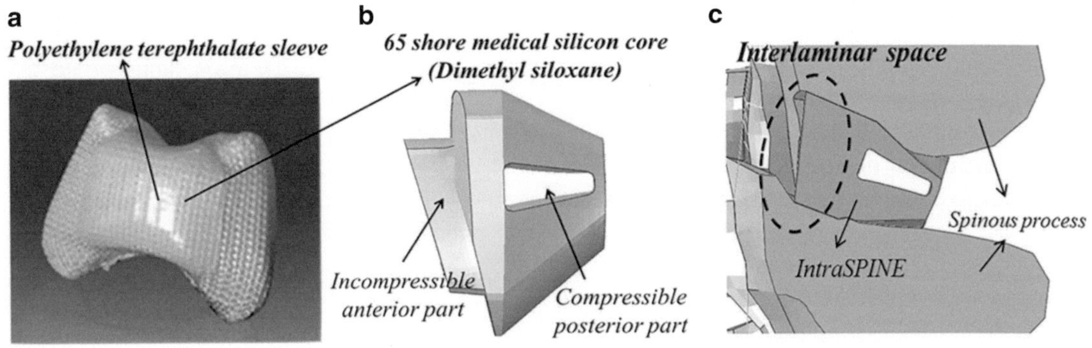

Fig. 8.3 The interlaminar dynamic spacer (IntraSPINE). (**a**) Perspective view. (**b**) Lateral view. (**c**) Sagittal view. The rigid incompressible anterior part positioned between the laminae (dotted circle), and the soft rear part (tunneled) is compressible. (Courtesy of Cousin Biotech, France)

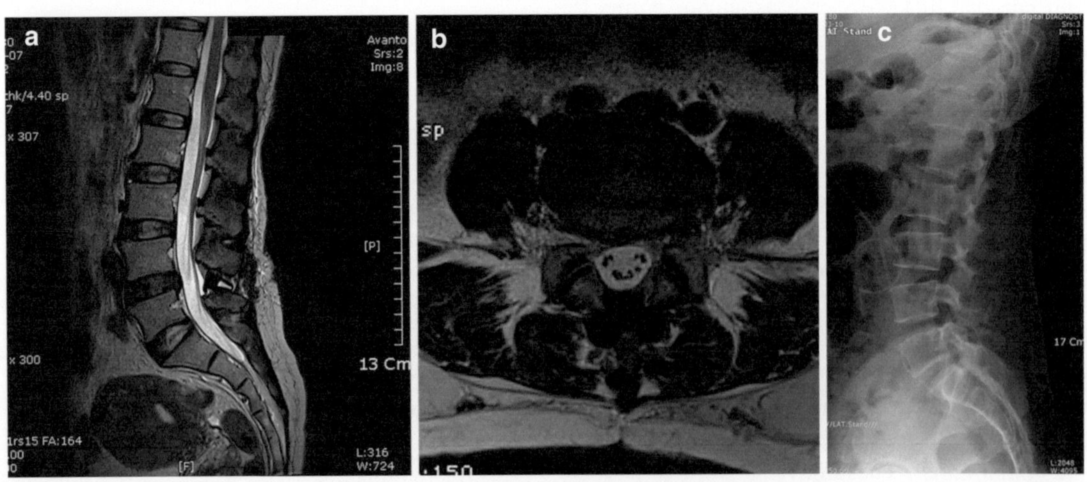

Fig. 8.4 Postoperative image after decompression and ligmentoplasty with interlarminar device. Sagittal (**a**) and axial (**b**) MRI shows decompression of central canal and lateral X-ray (**c**) shows stabilized state of L4–5 level

maintaining physiological motion. Final testing is performed to verify both stability and range of motion before proceeding to closure.

Additional Surgical Notes and Techniques (Incorporating IntraSPINE® Experience)

The use of interlaminar spacers such as IntraSPINE® has demonstrated promising outcomes for chronic low back pain associated with black disc and facet syndrome. This device is particularly effective when combined with preoperative dynamic X-rays and block tests to assess facet joint functionality.

Illustration

Case 1. A preoperative and postoperative image of the lumbar spine treated with IntraSPINE®, showcasing alignment and stability improvements (Fig. 8.5).

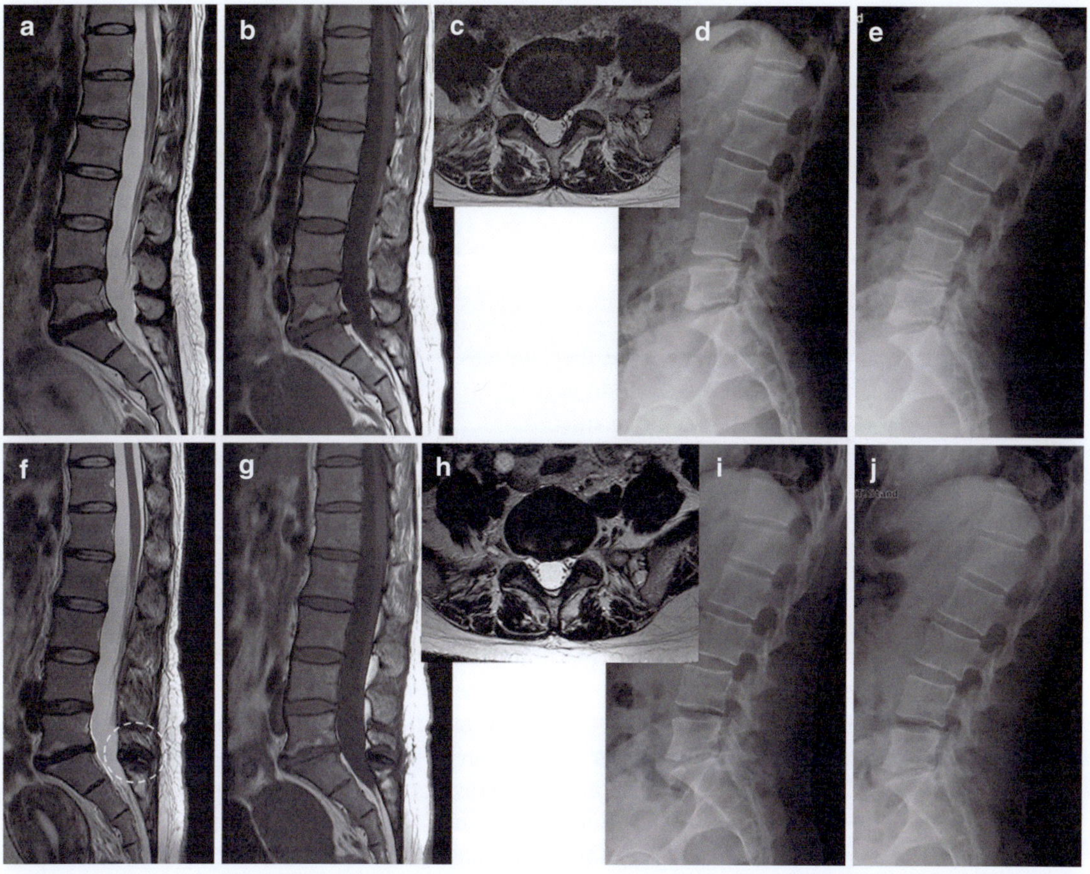

Fig. 8.5 A case presentation of a 37-year-old woman with chronic low back pain for 18 months before surgery. Preoperative magnetic resonance imaging (**a**–**c**) and flexion–extension radiography (**d**, **e**) showing disc degeneration and central protrusion at the L5-S1 level. Modic change (type 1) at the L5 and S1 vertebra can be seen. At the 24-month postoperative follow-up, magnetic resonance imaging (**f**–**h**) and dynamic radiography (**i**, **j**) were performed, showing remodeling of the protruded disc at the L5-S1 and decreased bone edema at the vertebral body. Note the dynamic spacer is located within the laminar space (round dot). At the final follow-up, the visual analog scale for back and leg pain decreased from 7 to 1 and 5 to 1, respectively, and the Oswestry Disability Index score decreased from 28% to 18%

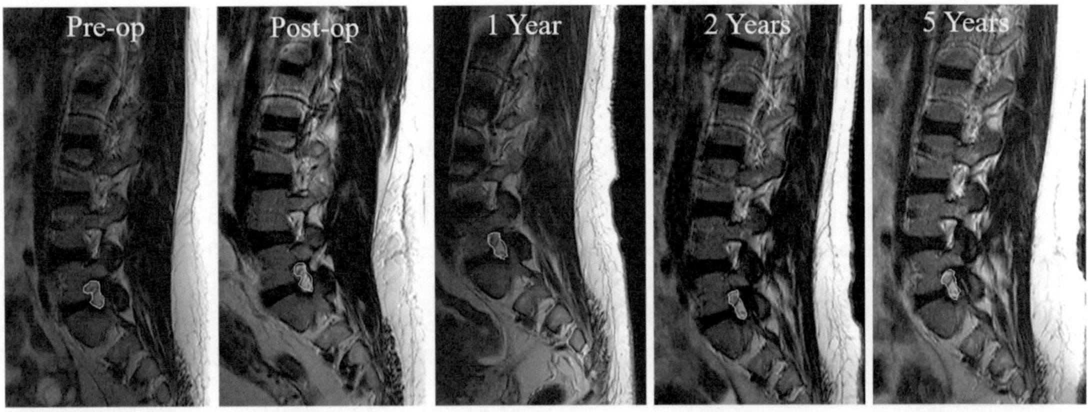

Fig. 8.6 5-year follow-up MRI shows foraminal dimension is maintained after interlaminar stabilization at the L4–5 level

Case 2. Illustration of long-term follow-up showing improvement of foraminal dimension after IntraSPINE placement (Fig. 8.6)

8.4.3 Wound Closure

Thorough irrigation of the surgical site is performed to remove any debris and minimize the risk of infection. The decision to place a drain is based on the extent of the dissection and the surgeon's preference. The wound is then closed in layers, with particular attention to achieving good approximation of the fascia. A sterile dressing is applied, and the patient is prepared for transfer to the recovery area.

8.5 Commentary

8.5.1 Biomechanical Considerations

The integration of ligament reconstruction with dynamic stabilization devices creates a unique biomechanical environment that offers several significant advantages over traditional fusion techniques. This combined approach successfully maintains physiological motion patterns while providing necessary stability to the spinal segment. The dynamic nature of the construct helps distribute loads more evenly across the spinal segment, particularly reducing the stress on facet joints that often occurs with rigid fixation [1, 4]. By preserving natural motion patterns, this technique also helps minimize the risk of adjacent segment degeneration, a common concern with traditional fusion procedures. The immediate stability provided by the construct allows for early mobilization while supporting the healing process.

8.5.2 Surgical Technique Considerations

Success with this combined approach heavily depends on several key technical aspects of the procedure. Patient selection remains the cornerstone of achieving optimal outcomes, with careful attention paid to both clinical and radiological criteria. The tensioning of the artificial ligament requires particular finesse—excessive tension can restrict normal motion and potentially lead to implant failure, while insufficient tension may not provide adequate stability [5, 6]. When performing the decompression, surgeons must strike a careful balance between achieving adequate neural decompression and maintaining sufficient bone stock for secure implant fixation. The quality of the patient's bone should always inform the choice of fixation method and implant size. Early mobilization should be encouraged postoperatively, but with appropriate guidance to prevent excessive early stress on the construct.

8.5.3 Potential Complications and Management

Complications associated with this technique can be categorized into three main groups, each requiring specific prevention strategies and management approaches. Recent studies indicate that device-related complications, including implant migration (2–5% incidence), loosening (3–7%), and spinous process fracture (up to 2%), can often be minimized through careful patient selection and precise surgical techniques, particularly concerning bone quality and implant sizing. Immediate surgical complications such as wound infection (1–3%), dural tears (less than 1%), and neurological injury (0.5–2%) require vigilant monitoring and prompt intervention when identified. Long-term complications, including adjacent segment degeneration (10–15% over 5 years), loss of correction, and hardware failure (5–10%), underscore the necessity of regular follow-up imaging and clinical assessment. Early recognition and tailored interventions remain pivotal in managing these potential complications effectively [1, 3–5].

8.5.4 Clinical Outcomes and Evidence Base

Current clinical evidence strongly supports the efficacy of this combined approach. Studies have consistently demonstrated significant improvements in Oswestry Disability Index (ODI) scores, with many patients achieving substantial clinical benefit thresholds. Visual Analog Scale (VAS) pain scores typically show marked reduction, both for back and leg pain components. Patient satisfaction rates remain consistently high, particularly when compared to traditional fusion procedures. Notably, the complication rates associated with this technique appear lower than those reported for conventional fusion surgery, especially regarding adjacent segment degeneration and hardware-related issues. Recent longitudinal studies and meta-analyses further validate these findings, highlighting sustained clinical improvements and reduced complication rates over 5- to 10-year follow-ups. These studies also emphasize the importance of precise patient selection and optimized surgical techniques to maximize long-term benefits.

References

1. Bae J, Lee SM, Lee SH, et al. The likelihood of reaching substantial clinical benefit following an Interlaminar dynamic spacer for chronic low Back pain: a clinical and radiological analysis of a prospective cohort. World Neurosurg. 2017; https://doi.org/10.1016/j.wneu.2017.02.083.
2. Lee S-H, Lee J-H, Hong S-W, Chung S-E, Yoo S-H, Lee H-Y. Spinopelvic alignment after interspinous soft stabilization with a tension band system in grade 1 degenerative lumbar spondylolisthesis. Spine. 2010;35:E691–701.
3. Guizzardi G, Petrini P, Morichi R, et al. Clinical results with IntraSPINE®. EC Orthopaedics. 2015;2:101–6.
4. Buric J, Pulidori M. Long-term reduction in pain and disability after surgery with the interspinous device for intervertebral assisted motion (DIAM) spinal stabilization system in patients with low back pain: 4-year follow-up from a longitudinal prospective case series. Eur Spine J. 2011;20:1304–11.
5. Lindsey DP, Swanson KE, Fuchs P, et al. The effects of an interspinous implant on the kinematics of the instrumented and adjacent levels in the lumbar spine. Spine. 2003;28:2192–7.
6. Lee SH, Seol A, Cho TY, Kim SY, Kim DJ, Lim HM. A systematic review of interspinous dynamic stabilization. Clin Orthop Surg. 2015;7:323–9.

Polyethylene Terephthalate as an Artificial Ligament and Its Various Medical Applications

9

Shin-Jae Kim

Abstract

Polyethylene terephthalate (PET), a thermoplastic polymer, has emerged as a cornerstone in artificial ligament development due to its unique chemical structure, exceptional tensile strength, and biocompatibility. Its applications span diverse medical fields, particularly in orthopedics and spinal surgeries, such as anterior cruciate ligament (ACL) reconstruction and acromioclavicular (AC) joint repair. Recent innovations, including the SHLee ligament, have demonstrated PET's ability to overcome challenges in spinal stabilization. Despite its advantages, PET has limitations, including susceptibility to infection, which has led to the exploration of polypropylene-based alternatives. This chapter delves into PET's chemical properties, medical applications, and future prospects in artificial ligament development.

Keywords

Polyethylene terephthalate · Artificial ligament · SHLee ligament · Polypropylene Soft stabilization

S.-J. Kim (✉)
Department of Neurosurgery, Cheongdam Wooridul Spine Hospital, Seoul, Korea (Republic of)

9.1 Introduction

Polyethylene terephthalate (PET) is a synthetic polymer widely recognized for its unique combination of mechanical, chemical, and biological properties [1, 2]. Initially developed for industrial applications such as textiles and packaging, PET has transitioned into the medical field, where its adaptability has allowed it to meet the demanding requirements of modern healthcare [3]. PET's success in medicine is largely due to its biocompatibility, high tensile strength, chemical resistance, and ability to be tailored for specific applications [3–5].

In orthopedics, PET plays a transformative role, especially in the development of artificial ligaments [1, 6]. Traditional grafts—such as autografts and allografts—have limitations, including donor site morbidity, limited availability, and risks of rejection or infection [6, 7]. PET overcomes these challenges by offering a synthetic alternative that closely mimics the biomechanical properties of natural tissues [1, 6]. This quality is particularly valuable in anterior cruciate ligament (ACL) reconstruction and acromioclavicular (AC) joint repair, where PET-based ligaments have shown promising clinical outcomes [1, 6].

Beyond orthopedics, PET has significantly impacted spinal surgery, particularly in the stabilization of the spine [8–10]. The introduction of Liganove ligaments marked PET's entry into spi-

S.-H. Lee et al. (eds.), *Ligament Reconstruction for Spine*,
https://doi.org/10.1007/978-981-95-3971-0_9

nal applications, and recent advancements, such as the SHLee ligament, have further refined its utility [8–11]. These ligaments provide structural support while promoting tissue integration, addressing both the mechanical and biological needs of spinal decompression procedures [8, 9, 11]. PET's versatility extends even further into other medical domains, including cardiovascular devices, surgical sutures, prosthetics, and regenerative medicine, where its lightweight, durable, and chemically stable nature makes it indispensable [3, 4].

However, PET is not without limitations. Challenges such as susceptibility to infection and reduced resilience under repetitive stress have led researchers and clinicians to explore alternative materials like polypropylene (PP), which addresses some of PET's shortcomings while offering its own advantages [12]. Efforts continue to improve the properties of PET-based implants, whether through surface modifications, coatings, or hybrid materials, to enhance their biocompatibility, durability, and functionality [4, 12].

This chapter explores PET's chemical structure, its role in artificial ligament development, and its applications across various medical fields. Additionally, it discusses the limitations of PET and the potential of emerging technologies to overcome these challenges, ensuring that PET remains a cornerstone of medical innovation [3, 4].

9.2 Chemical Structure of PET

Polyethylene terephthalate (PET) is a thermoplastic polymer made from two main components: ethylene glycol (EG) and terephthalic acid (TPA) [3]. These components form ester linkages (-COO-) in a condensation reaction, producing water as a by-product [3]. PET's linear polymer structure allows tight molecular packing, enabling the polymer to be processed into highly crystalline or amorphous forms. Highly crystalline PET is rigid and durable, whereas less crystalline PET is more flexible and transparent, allowing it to be tailored for various medical applications [3].

The molecular structure of PET includes ester bonds and aromatic rings, which confer resistance to hydrolysis, durability in wet environments, stiffness, and thermal stability [1]. PET's melting point of approximately 250 °C ensures stability during high-temperature sterilization processes like autoclaving, while its glass transition temperature (Tg) of about 70–80 °C provides flexibility at higher temperatures [9]. PET's hydrophobic nature and low moisture absorption help it maintain mechanical strength in moist environments, making it reliable for long-term implantation [1, 3]. Additionally, PET's lightweight nature reduces the overall burden on patients, and its transparency allows visual monitoring of implanted devices [11].

The molecular weight of PET significantly affects its tensile strength and durability. High molecular weight PET is ideal for load-bearing applications like artificial ligaments, whereas lower molecular weight PET facilitates easier processing for devices like sutures or surgical threads [6]. PET's recyclability also supports sustainable medical device production, aligning with environmental considerations [3, 11].

In summary, PET's chemical structure underpins its high strength, durability, chemical resistance, hydrophobicity, and flexibility, making it a versatile and reliable material for medical applications, including artificial ligaments and other orthopedic devices [1, 3, 6].

9.3 Unique Properties of PET in Medical Applications

PET's combination of physical, chemical, and biological properties makes it particularly suitable for artificial ligaments and numerous other medical devices [1, 3, 9, 11]:

1. *Biocompatibility*: PET interacts minimally with the immune system, reducing allergic reactions and blood incompatibility. Its smooth surface lowers thrombogenic risk, making it suitable for vascular grafts and artificial ligaments [3, 6].
2. *Chemical Resistance*: PET resists a wide range of chemicals and biological enzymes, maintaining stability in the body's biochemi-

cal environment and enduring various sterilization processes.

3. *High Tensile Strength and Durability*: PET's robust tensile strength supports load-bearing applications, essential for artificial ligaments and tendons subjected to repetitive stress [1].
4. *Ease of Processing*: PET can be woven, braided, or extruded to replicate the biomechanical behavior of natural tissues, enabling customized solutions [3, 11].
5. *Lightweight*: PET's low density reduces implant weight, minimizing physical burden and enhancing tissue integration [9].
6. *Transparency*: PET's transparency allows visual monitoring during and after surgical procedures, aiding in diagnostics and device assessment [11].
7. *High Melting Point (250 °C)*: PET remains stable during autoclaving and other high-temperature sterilization methods, preserving its structural integrity [1, 3].
8. *Low Moisture Absorption*: PET's hydrophobic nature prevents swelling, ensuring consistent mechanical strength and long-term stability [3].

Collectively, these properties ensure PET's versatility and reliability in medical applications, from artificial ligaments to vascular grafts and beyond [1, 3, 9, 11].

9.4 Medical Applications of PET

PET's adaptability across a range of medical fields reflects its biocompatibility, mechanical strength, and chemical stability [1, 6]:

9.4.1 Medical Implants and Artificial Structures (Fig. 9.1)

1. *Cardiovascular Stents*: PET-based stents maintain vascular patency and resist deformation, suitable for long-term implantation.
2. *Surgical Meshes*: PET meshes used in hernia repair offer lightweight support and promote tissue integration.
3. *Artificial Ligaments and Tendons*: PET ligaments in orthopedic reconstruction, such as ACL repair, mimic the biomechanical properties of natural ligaments.

9.4.2 Medical Packaging (Fig. 9.2)

PET's inertness and durability make it ideal for packaging pharmaceuticals, surgical instruments, and medical devices. Its transparency and low moisture absorption ensure product sterility and prevent contamination.

9.4.3 Surgical and Therapeutic Tools (Fig. 9.3)

1. *Sutures and Surgical Threads*: PET sutures combine tensile strength and biocompatibility, supporting wound healing and maintaining structural integrity.
2. *Orthopedic Artificial Joints*: PET components in artificial joints enhance function and durability due to their strength and low friction properties.

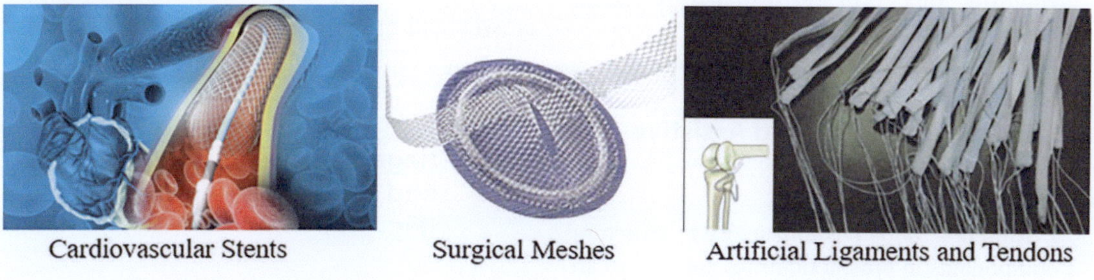

Fig. 9.1 Medical implants and artificial structures using PET

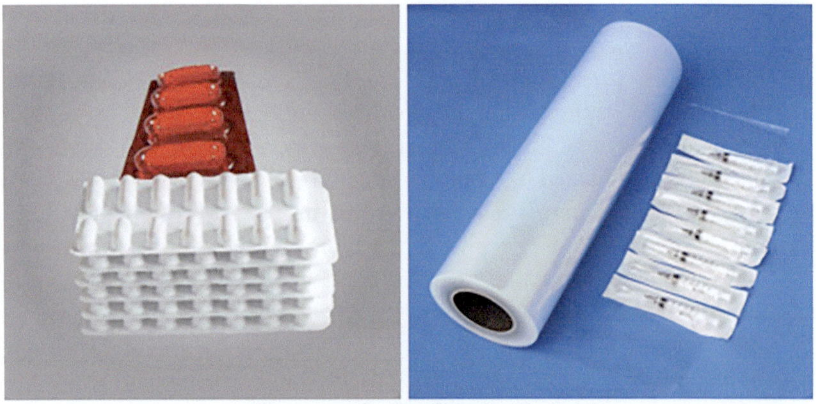

Pharmaceutical and Device Packaging

Fig. 9.2 Medical packaging using PET

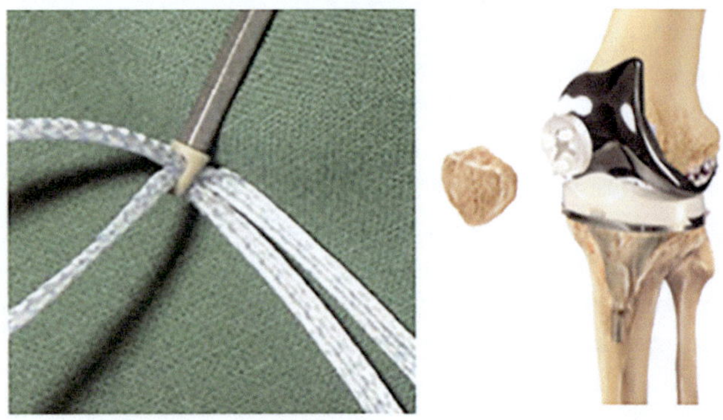

Sutures and Surgical Threads   Orthopedic artificial joint

Fig. 9.3 Surgical and therapeutic tools using PET

9.4.4 Medical Textiles and Fabrics (Fig. 9.4)

1. *Filters and Textile Products*: PET filters in blood purification and respiratory devices maintain performance under chemical and mechanical stresses.
2. *Artificial Blood Vessels*: PET vascular grafts resist biological degradation, enabling long-term performance in vascular surgeries.

9.4.5 Rehabilitation and Assistive Devices (Fig. 9.5)

1. *Prosthetics and Orthotics*: PET structural components in prosthetic limbs and braces are both strong and lightweight, improving patient comfort.
2. *Rehabilitation Aids*: PET-based materials in dynamic splints and mobility aids provide strength and flexibility for patient comfort and mobility.

9.4.6 Dental Applications (Fig. 9.6)

Temporary Dental Prosthetics PET's transparency and strength make it suitable for temporary crowns and bridges, offering structural integrity and ease of fabrication.

9.4.7 Regenerative Medicine and Tissue Engineering (Fig. 9.7)

Cell Culture Scaffolds PET scaffolds support cell attachment, proliferation, and differentiation,

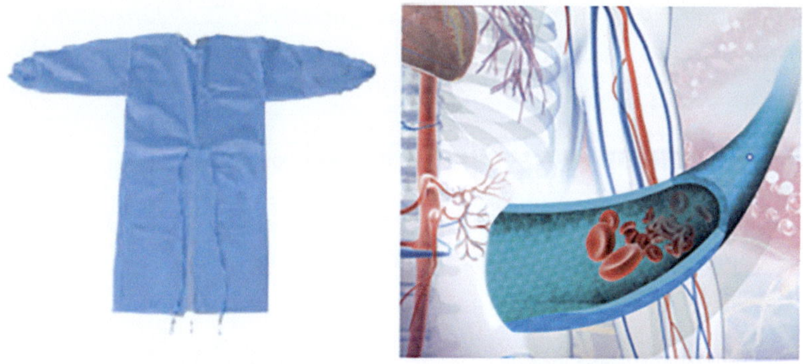

Filters and Textile Products Artificial Blood Vessels

Fig. 9.4 Medical textiles and fabrics using PET

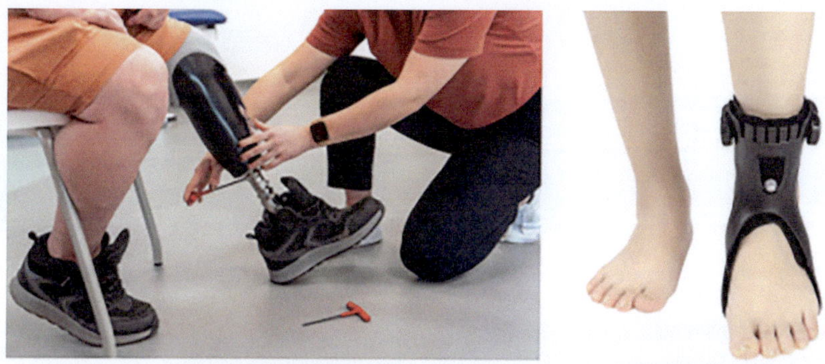

Prosthetics and Orthotics Rehabilitation Aids

Fig. 9.5 Rehabilitation and assistive devices using PET

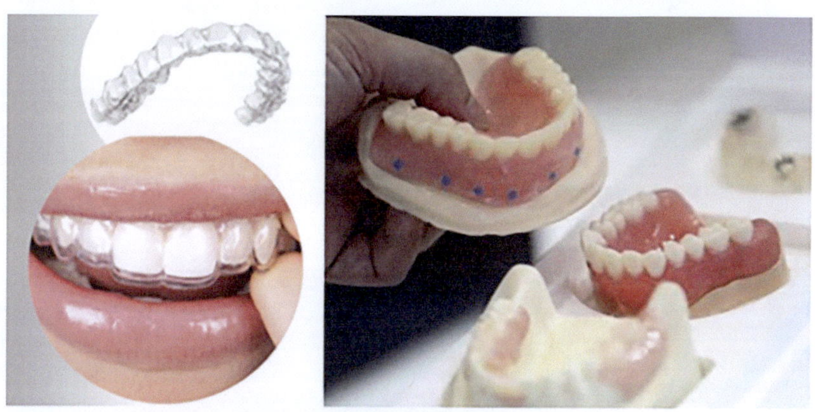

Temporary Dental Prosthetics

Fig. 9.6 Dental applications using PET

aiding in tissue engineering and regenerative medicine.

9.4.8 Implantable Devices (Fig. 9.8)

1. *Pacemakers*: PET housings protect pacemaker components from bodily fluids, ensuring long-term reliability.
2. *Neurostimulators*: PET encapsulates neurostimulator electronics, maintaining device performance and integration.

9.4.9 Orthopedic Applications (Fig. 9.9)

1. *Anterior Cruciate Ligament (ACL) Reconstruction*: PET ligaments restore joint

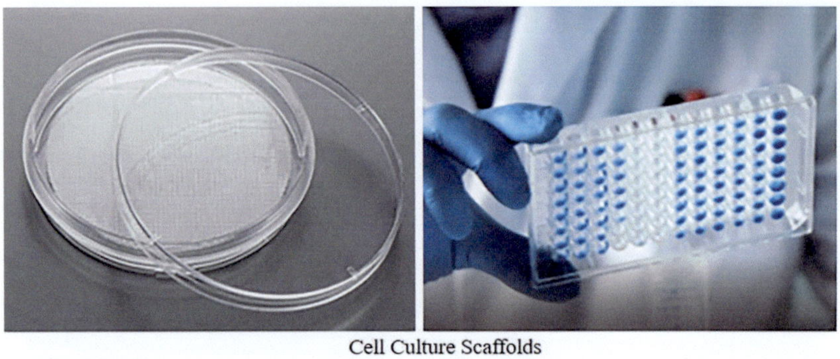

Fig. 9.7 Regenerative medicine and tissue engineering using PET

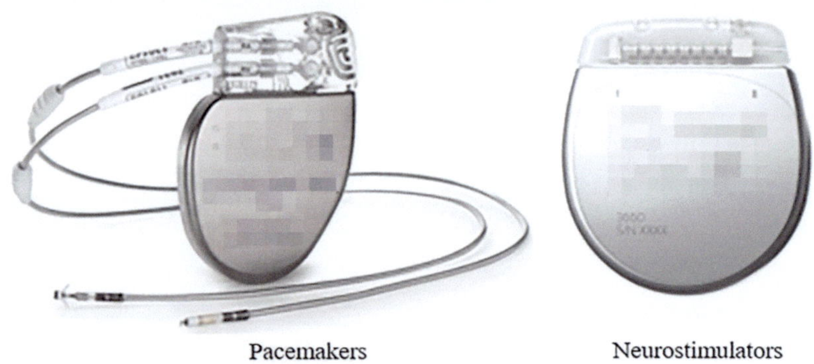

Fig. 9.8 Implantable devices using PET

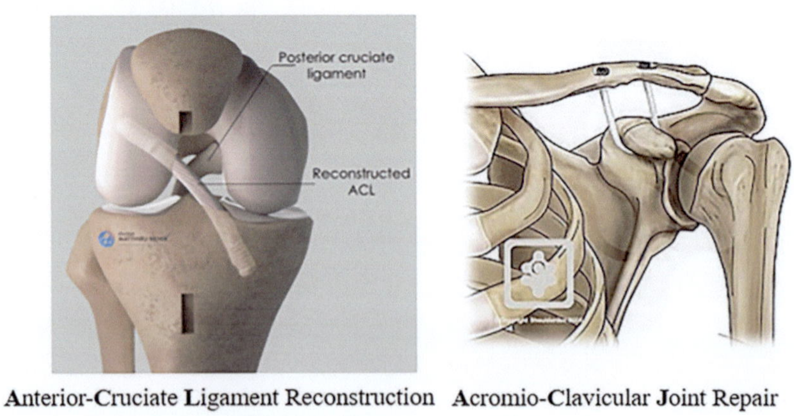

Fig. 9.9 Orthopedic artificial ligament using PET

stability and reduce complications compared to traditional grafts.
2. *Acromioclavicular (AC) Joint Repair*: PET-based systems effectively stabilize the AC joint, improving patient outcomes.

9.4.10 Spinal Applications (Fig. 9.10)

PET's role in spinal surgery evolved with systems like Liganove, introducing PET ligaments for spinal stabilization. The SHLee ligament further refines this approach by improving biomechanical properties and tissue integration. Designed for Open Midline Decompression (OMD) procedures, the SHLee ligament restores structural support after lamina resection while preserving facet joint integrity and ensuring effective neural decompression.

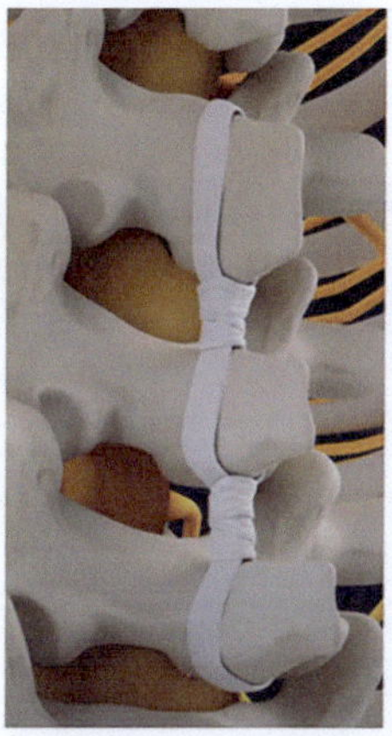

SHLee ligament (Sagittal ligament + Horizontal Ligament)

Fig. 9.10 Spinal artificial ligament (SHLee ligament) using PET

9.5 Limitations of PET and Emerging Alternatives

Despite PET's advantages, certain limitations persist [11]:

1. *Susceptibility to Infection*: PET's hydrophobic surface can promote bacterial colonization, increasing postoperative infection risk. Surface modifications or antimicrobial coatings are explored to mitigate this issue.
2. *Wear and Fatigue*: Prolonged use in high-mobility areas may lead to material fatigue or microdamage, affecting long-term reliability.
3. *Resilience*: PET's resilience is somewhat limited compared to natural tissues and some synthetic alternatives, impacting performance in dynamic stress environments [1].

Polypropylene (PP) has emerged as a promising alternative, offering enhanced infection resistance, improved resilience, and faster tissue integration. Quicker cellular adhesion and closure of surgical sites reduce complications such as seroma formation. Although PP addresses some PET shortcomings, more research is required to confirm its long-term biocompatibility and durability in diverse clinical scenarios [13].

9.6 Future Directions

Integrating PET with emerging technologies could further enhance its role in artificial ligament development and other medical applications [1, 3, 10]:

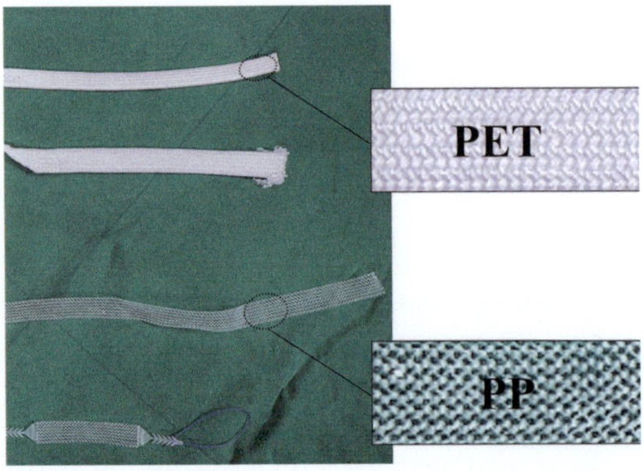

Fig. 9.11 Polypropylene (PP) has slightly lower tensile strength compared to PET; it demonstrates significantly lower infection rates, higher resilience, and faster tissue integration

1. *3D Printing*: Allows for patient-specific designs, optimizing anatomical fit and mechanical performance.
2. *Regenerative Medicine*: Combining PET scaffolds with growth factors and stem cells could promote tissue regeneration and biological integration.
3. *Smart Materials*: Incorporating bioactive coatings or antimicrobial properties could address infection risks and improve overall functionality.
4. *Alternative material*: Although polypropylene (PP) has slightly lower tensile strength compared to PET, it demonstrates significantly lower infection rates, higher resilience, and faster tissue integration. These properties make PP-based artificial ligaments a promising alternative material that can address several limitations of PET (Fig. 9.11).

These advancements aim to overcome PET's current limitations, expand its applications, and ensure it remains integral to the evolution of medical technologies [9–11, 13].

9.7 Summary

Polyethylene terephthalate (PET) has become a pivotal material in the medical field, offering exceptional versatility and reliability across multiple specialties. In orthopedics, PET provides a synthetic alternative to traditional grafts, delivering high tensile strength, biocompatibility, and durability—qualities that have made it particularly effective in anterior cruciate ligament (ACL) reconstruction and acromioclavicular (AC) joint repair. In these applications, PET-based implants restore joint stability and often facilitate faster patient recovery. PET's influence is equally notable in spinal surgery, where it has revolutionized decompression procedures. Beginning with Liganove ligaments, PET-based solutions have evolved into advanced devices like the SHLee ligament, offering improved tissue integration and mechanical support. These innovations address critical challenges in spinal decompression surgeries, ensuring better functional restoration and long-term patient outcomes. Beyond orthopedics and spinal applications, PET is integral to various medical devices, including cardiovascular stents, surgical sutures, regenerative medicine scaffolds, and prosthetics. Its lightweight nature, transparency, and resistance to chemical degradation enable PET to meet a diverse range of clinical needs. Despite its many advantages, PET is not without limitations. Susceptibility to infection and reduced resilience under repetitive stress highlight areas requiring further improvement. Alternative materials, such as polypropylene (PP), are emerging to complement PET by providing enhanced infection resistance, faster tissue integration, and greater resilience. Nonetheless, PET remains indispensable in healthcare. Ongoing advancements in material science and manufacturing techniques, such as 3D printing and regenerative medicine, promise to further enhance PET's integration with biological tissues and broaden its applications. PET not only bridges the gap between traditional and modern surgical materials but also paves the way for new possibilities in medical device design and patient care.

References

1. Gao K, Chen S, Wang L, et al. Anterior cruciate ligament reconstruction with LARS artificial ligament: a multicenter study with 3- to 5-year follow-up. Arthroscopy. 2010;26(4):515–23.

2. Parchi PD, Ciapini G, Paglialunga C, Giuntoli M, Picece C, Chiellini F, et al. Anterior cruciate ligament reconstruction with LARS artificial ligament: clinical results after a long-term follow-up. Joints. 2018;6(2):75–9.
3. Hench LL, Polak JM. Third-generation biomedical materials. Science. 2002;295(5557):1014–7.
4. Gillespie RJ, Knapik DM, Akkus O. Biologic and synthetic grafts in the reconstruction of large to massive rotator cuff tears. J Am Acad Orthop Surg. 2016;24(12):823–8.
5. Wang CH, Hou W, Yan M, Guo ZS, Wu Q, Bi L, et al. Effects of artificial ligaments with different porous structures on the migration of BMSCs. Stem Cells Int. 2015;2015:702381.
6. Machotka Z, Scarborough I, Duncan W, Kumar S, Perraton L. Anterior cruciate ligament repair with LARS (ligament advanced reinforcement system): a systematic review. Sports Med Arthrosc Rehabil Ther Technol. 2010;2:29.
7. Lubowitz JH, Verdonk PC, Reid JB III, Verdonk R. Graft choice for anterior cruciate ligament reconstruction: a level I systematic review comparing failure rates and functional outcomes. Arthroscopy. 2013;29(9):1693–701.
8. Stoll TM, Dubois G, Schwarzenbach O. The dynamic neutralization system for the spine: a multi-center study of a novel non-fusion system. Eur Spine J. 2002;11(Suppl 2):S170–8.
9. Cakir B, Richter M. Dynamic stabilization of the lumbar spine. Curr Orthop. 2007;21(4):270–7.
10. Fay LY, Wu JC, Tsai TY, et al. Dynamic stabilization for degenerative spondylolisthesis: evaluation of radiographic and clinical outcomes. Clin Neurol Neurosurg. 2016;144:60–7.
11. Schnake KJ, Schaeren S, Jeanneret B. Dynamic stabilization in addition to decompression for lumbar spinal stenosis with degenerative spondylolisthesis. Spine. 2006;31(7):442–9.
12. Ibrahim AMS, Vargas CR, Colakoglu S, Nguyen JT, Lin SJ, Lee BT. Properties of meshes used in hernia repair: a comprehensive review of synthetic and biologic meshes. J Reconstr Microsurg. 2015;31(2):83–94.
13. Park P, Garton HJ, Gala VC, et al. Adjacent segment disease after lumbar or lumbosacral fusion: review of the literature. Spine (Phila Pa 1976). 2004;29(17):1938–44.

Clinical Outcomes of Ligament Reconstruction

10

Yoon Kwang Kwon

Abstract

Degenerative spondylolisthesis is a well-known cause of spinal stenosis, presenting challenges in treatment selection. While simple decompression or fusion are traditional surgical options, both carry risks of complications. At Wooridul Spine Hospital, an alternative surgical approach called ligament reconstruction has been developed. This procedure is particularly considered for patients with low-grade degenerative spondylolisthesis, where there is instability but not severe enough to necessitate fusion. However, it's important to note that ligament reconstruction is not suitable for all cases of degenerative spondylolisthesis. The decision to proceed with this or other treatment options depends on various factors, including the degree of vertebral slippage, the patient's symptoms, and overall spinal stability. This personalized approach ensures that each patient receives the most appropriate treatment for their specific condition. Consequently, ligament reconstruction can be a suitable minimally invasive surgical option for patients with stenosis and instability that is not severe enough to require fusion surgery.

Keywords

Degenerative spondylolisthesis · Spinal stenosis · Ligament reconstruction · Clinical outcomes · Complications

10.1 Introduction

Degenerative spondylolisthesis, a known cause of spinal stenosis, presents challenges in treatment selection. Traditional surgical options include simple decompression or fusion, both carrying risks of complications. Wooridul Spine Hospital offers an alternative: ligament reconstruction.

This procedure is considered for patients with low-grade degenerative spondylolisthesis, where instability exists but isn't severe enough to require fusion. However, it's not suitable for all cases of degenerative spondylolisthesis.

Lumbar spondylolisthesis is a condition where one vertebra in the lower back slips forward over the vertebra below it, potentially leading to back instability and pain, as well as leg pain due to nerve compression. Treatment options vary based on severity and symptoms, ranging from conservative management to surgical interventions.

Y. K. Kwon (✉)
Department of Neurosurgery, Gimpo Airport Wooridul Spine Hospital,
Gimpo Airport, Korea (Republic of)
e-mail: ykkwonmd@snu.ac.kr

S.-H. Lee et al. (eds.), *Ligament Reconstruction for Spine*,
https://doi.org/10.1007/978-981-95-3971-0_10

The decision to proceed with ligament reconstruction or other treatments depends on factors such as the degree of vertebral slippage, patient symptoms, and overall spinal stability. This personalized approach ensures each patient receives the most appropriate treatment for their specific condition.

By offering ligament reconstruction, Wooridul Spine Hospital provides an additional option in the spectrum of treatments for degenerative spondylolisthesis, potentially benefiting patients who fall between the need for conservative management and more invasive surgical procedures.

The advantages of ligament reconstruction include being less invasive compared to conventional decompression or fusion surgeries, with reduced operation time and decreased blood loss. Therefore, it can be considered suitable for elderly patients or those with underlying medical conditions.

Ligament reconstruction has shown overall pain improvement in patients with mild stenosis accompanied by degenerative spondylolisthesis who complain of lower back pain and leg pain [1–5].

At Seoul Gimpo Airport Wooridul Spine Hospital, a clinical study was conducted on 298 patients who underwent ligament reconstruction between 2014 and 2023. The average follow-up period was 28 months. When examining the clinical outcomes for back pain and leg pain, back pain decreased from NRS 7.34 to 2.40, and leg pain from NRS 7.28 to 2.51, both showing statistically significant improvements (Table 10.1). A comparative study was also conducted on the improvement of clinical symptoms among 102 patients with level 1 central stenosis with degenerative spondylolisthesis. The study included 58 patients who underwent LP (Ligament Reconstruction) and 44 patients who underwent simple decompression. The group that received LP showed significant improvement compared to the group that underwent UBL (Unilateral Laminotomy Bilateral Decompression). In the LP group, back pain improved from an NRS (Numeric Rating Scale) of 6.83 to 2.17, while leg pain improved from an NRS of 6.52 to 2.01 (Table 10.2).

Table 10.1 Change in improvements in back pain and leg pain after ligament reconstruction

Variable		DS
Back Pain VAS	Preop	7.34 ± 1.15
	Postop	2.40 ± 0.86
	Difference	4.94 ± 0.95
	p value	**<0.001**
Leg Pain VAS	Preop	7.91 ± 0.65
	Postop	2.66 ± 0.79
	Difference	5.25 ± 0.88
	p value	**<0.001**

Disc height and change in disc height is measured in millimeters
Intragroup significance compared with preoperative value, $P < 0.01$
VAS Visual Analogue Scale

Lee et al. conducted a study on 556 patients from three institutions in three countries, with an average follow-up of 48.9 months. Using the MacNab criteria to evaluate clinical outcomes, they reported an 80.4% success rate [1].

Furthermore, in a study comparing ligament reconstruction with PLIF (Posterior Lumbar Interbody Fusion) surgery, Lee et al. reported statistically significant improvements in both back and leg pain [2]. In another comparison with a laminotomy group, they also found statistically significant results for both back and leg pain [3].

In the study conducted at Seoul Gimpo Airport Wooridul Spine Hospital, the average operation time was 159 minutes per level, and the average intraoperative blood loss was 312 ml per level (Table 10.3). This is less than the average operation time of 210 minutes for single-level fusion reported by Kim et al. [6], and less than the average blood loss of 350 ml per level for fusion surgery reported by Chanbour et al. [7].

Radiological studies have also shown good results. A comparison of anterior translation progression between a group that underwent simple decompression and a group that underwent ligament reconstruction at Seoul Gimpo Airport Wooridul Spine Hospital showed an average progression of 1.23 mm in the ligament reconstruction group compared to 3.27 mm in the simple decompression group, which was statistically significant.

Table 10.2 The degree of improvement in back pain and leg pain for each type of surgery

Variable		LP	UBE	*p* value
Back pain NRS	Preop	6.83 ± 1.23	7.34 ± 1.19	0.014
	Postop	2.17 ± 1.15	4.14 ± 1.47	<0.001
	Difference	4.66 ± 1.50	3.30 ± 1.73	<0.001
	p value	**<0.001**	**<0.001**	
Leg pain NRS	Preop	6.52 ± 1.27	7.57 ± 1.37	<0.001
	Postop	2.05 ± 1.64	3.93 ± 1.92	<0.001
	Difference	4.47 ± 1.75	3.64 ± 1.95	0.026
	p value	**<0.001**	**<0.001**	

Disc height and change in disc height is measured in millimeters
Intragroup significance compared with preoperative value, $P < 0.01$
LP Ligament Reconstruction
UBE Unilateral Biportal Endoscopic decompression
NRS Numeric Rating Scale

Table 10.3 The operation time and intraoperative blood loss according to the level of ligament reconstruction surgery

Operation time					
	Level I	Level II	Level III	Level V	Total average
Average time (min)	132	189	264	248	159.17

Intraoperative blood loss					
	Level I	Level II	Level III	Level V	Total average
Average bleeding (ml)	261	353	552	400	312

Operative time includes anesthesia time
Operative time is measured in minutes

Hong et al. also compared radiological results with a simple decompression group, reporting significant increases in lumbar lordosis and segmental lordosis in the ligament reconstruction group. Symptomatic instability occurred in only 4.3% of the ligament reconstruction group compared to 27.8% in the simple decompression group, showing significant results [3].

Lee et al. compared with a PLIF group and reported statistically significant increases in sacral slope and decreases in pelvic tilt in the ligament reconstruction group compared to the PLIF group [2].

In addition, Lee et al. divided the ligament reconstruction group into two subgroups based on the degree of symptom improvement and compared the differences. They reported significant improvements in lumbar lordosis and segmental lordosis in the group with improved symptoms compared to the group without improvement, attributing this to an important role in pain relief and functional improvement. Therefore, they suggested that careful patient selection is necessary for patients with low preoperative segmental lordosis values [3].

In another study, Lee et al. reported that the tension band effect through ligament reconstruction could limit flexion in patients, which could be effective in preventing late recurrent stenosis and resultant radicular pain due to worsening instability. Based on these results, they argue that the preoperative extension potential of the corresponding segment could be a prognostic factor for predicting postoperative clinical outcomes [5].

All complications possible in general spine surgery can occur in ligament reconstruction. Among the 298 patients surveyed at Seoul Gimpo Airport Wooridul Spine Hospital, complications occurred in 26 patients (8.7%). The most common complication was re-stenosis, occurring in 16 patients (5.37%). Other complications included infection in 4 patients (1.34%), dural tear in 3 patients (1.01%), recurrent disc herniation in 2 patients (0.67%), and spinous fracture in 1 patient (0.34%). Among these, 20 patients (6.71%) with re-stenosis and infection underwent fusion surgery.

In a multicenter study, Lee et al. reported major complications such as hematoma and infection, with an incidence rate of 1.5%. Reoperation was performed in 2.3% of cases [1].

10.2 Summary

Ligament reconstruction can be a suitable minimally invasive surgical option for patients with instability that is not severe enough to require fusion surgery. The decision to proceed with ligament reconstruction or other treatments depends on factors such as the degree of vertebral slippage, patient symptoms, and overall spinal stability.

References

1. Lee S-H, Enes M, Hoogland T. Soft stabilization with interspinous artificial ligament for mildly unstable lumbar spinal stenosis: a multicenter comparison. Arch Orthop Trauma Surg. 2010;130(11):1335–41.
2. Lee S-H, Lee J-H, Hong S-W, Chung S-E, Yoo S-H, Lee H-Y. Spinopelvic alignment after interspinous soft stabilization with a tension band system in grade 1 degenerative lumbar spondylolisthesis. Spine (Phila Pa 1976). 2010;35(15):E691–701.
3. Hong S-W, Lee H-Y, Kim KH, Lee S-H. Interspinous ligamentoplasty in the treatment of degenerative spondylolisthesis: midterm clinical results. J Neurosurg Spine. 2010;13(1):27–35.
4. Lee S-H, Lee J-H, Hong S-W, Shim CS, Chung S-E, Yoo S-H, Lee H-Y. Factors affecting clinical outcomes in treating patients with grade 1 degenerative spondylolisthesis using interspinous soft stabilization with a tension band system: a minimum 5-year follow-up. Spine (Phila Pa 1976). 2012;37(7):563–72.
5. Lee S-H, Lee H-Y, Baek OK, Bae JS, Yoo S-H, Lee J-H. Clinical significance of achieving a flexion limitation with a tension band system in grade 1 degenerative spondylolisthesis: a minimum 5-year follow-up. Spine (Phila Pa 1976). 2015;40(6):E349–58.
6. Kim BD, Hsu WK, De Oliveira GS Jr, Saha S, Kim JYS. Operative duration as an independent risk factor for postoperative complications in single-level lumbar fusion: an analysis of 4588 surgical cases. Spine (Phila Pa 1976). 2014;39(6):510–20.
7. Chanbour H, Chen JW, Roth SG, Stephens BF, Abtahi AM, Zuckerman SL. How much blood loss is too much for a 1-level open lumbar fusion? Int J Spine Surg. 2023;17(1):146–55.

Part II

Various Decompression Technique Combined with Ligament Reconstruction

Microscopic Open Midline Decompression

11

Shin-Jae Kim

Abstract

Open midline decompression (OMD) is a revolutionary surgical technique designed to optimize neural decompression while preserving critical spinal structures. Traditional methods such as partial laminectomy and unilateral approach bilateral laminectomy (UBL) often require partial resection of the facet joints, leading to complications like postoperative instability and chronic back pain. OMD addresses these issues by utilizing a tunneling approach to remove the ligamentum flavum en bloc, achieving thorough decompression without compromising facet joint integrity. This preservation significantly reduces the risk of postoperative complications and helps maintain spinal stability, offering a clear advantage over conventional techniques. Additionally, OMD creates a wide interlaminar space, providing an ideal surgical field for ligamentoplasty (LP). This synergy between OMD and LP enables simultaneous decompression and stabilization, resulting in improved patient outcomes and reduced recovery times. This chapter explores the principles and surgical methodology of OMD, detailing how its innovative approach minimizes complications and maximizes effectiveness. By emphasizing facet joint preservation and its compatibility with LP, OMD is establishing itself as a preferred method for achieving optimal outcomes in spinal decompression surgeries.

Keywords

Open midline decompression · Ligament reconstruction · Spinal stenosis · Microscopic lumbar decompression · Facet joint preservation

11.1 Introduction

As global life expectancy continues to rise, the aging population faces a growing prevalence of lumbar spinal stenosis (LSS), a degenerative condition that typically emerges after the age of 50 [1, 2]. Studies estimate that LSS affects up to 11% of the general population and is the leading cause of spinal surgery in individuals over 65 years of age [3, 4]. Patients with LSS often present with chronic back pain, leg numbness, and neurogenic claudication, substantially impairing their quality of life [3, 5]. Although conservative management options—including physical therapy, pharmacological interventions, and epidural injections—have long been the mainstay of treatment, these approaches frequently fail to provide sustained relief for many elderly patients [6].

S.-J. Kim (✉)
Department of Neurosurgery, Cheongdam Wooridul Spine Hospital, Seoul, Korea (Republic of)

S.-H. Lee et al. (eds.), *Ligament Reconstruction for Spine*,
https://doi.org/10.1007/978-981-95-3971-0_11

With an increasing emphasis on enhancing quality of life in older adults, surgical intervention has emerged as a proactive alternative [7]. However, elderly patients often have multiple comorbidities, making extended surgical procedures under general anesthesia particularly risky [8]. In cases of multilevel LSS, the presence of spinal instability further complicates treatment. Traditional approaches have been limited primarily to decompression, which effectively alleviates neural compression but often overlooks underlying instability. Over time, this can lead to recurrent stenosis, persistent back pain, or progression of spinal deformities [9, 10].

Minimally invasive surgical (MIS) techniques, such as tubular or endoscopic decompression, have revolutionized LSS management by reducing tissue damage and shortening recovery times [11]. Despite these advances, MIS techniques frequently fail to adequately address the structural instability commonly encountered in multilevel LSS, particularly in elderly patients. Alternative decompression methods, including spinous splitting laminectomy and contralateral decompression, have been proposed but may still leave the spine vulnerable to long-term instability [12, 13]. To overcome these challenges, soft stabilization techniques using artificial ligaments have gained traction. Initially developed for orthopedic surgeries—such as knee and shoulder stabilization—artificial ligamentoplasty is now being explored for spinal applications [14, 15]. By providing spinal support while preserving motion, artificial ligamentoplasty offers a less invasive alternative to fusion surgery [16].

In this study, we introduce the microscopic open midline decompression (OMD) technique as a novel approach that addresses both neural decompression and spinal instability. By removing hypertrophied ligamentum flavum and decompressing the lateral recess through an interspinous window, OMD minimizes invasiveness while preserving critical structures such as the facet joint complex and spinous-laminar arch [17]. This preservation reduces intraoperative bone bleeding and lowers the risk of iatrogenic instability [18]. When combined with ligamentoplasty, OMD provides robust stabilization and has shown particular promise for elderly patients with multilevel LSS [16, 17]. This chapter examines the rationale, technique, and clinical outcomes of combining OMD with ligament reconstruction, offering a compelling solution for managing complex cases of lumbar spinal stenosis.

11.2 Presentation of the Patient

An 85-year-old male patient suffered from low back pain and neurogenic claudication, which became aggravated after a 10-meter walk. The patient had been experiencing diminished perianal sensation for the past 2 years, accompanied by bowel and bladder dysfunction. The patient has a medical history of hypertension, diabetes mellitus, and Parkinson's disease, which was diagnosed 3 years ago and is currently under treatment. Additionally, the patient was undergoing treatment for severe osteoporosis, with a BMD of −3.8. The physical examination revealed toe gait and hop test difficulties. The patient exhibited generalized weakness in both lower extremities, with motor strength particularly reduced to grade 4 in hip flexion and ankle dorsiflexion. Preoperative MRI shows severe spinal stenosis from L2-2-3-4 level with signal blocking at the same level (Fig. 11.1). Preoperative dynamic X-ray revealed Grade 1 L4-5 degenerative spondylolisthesis, along with instability (Fig. 11.2).

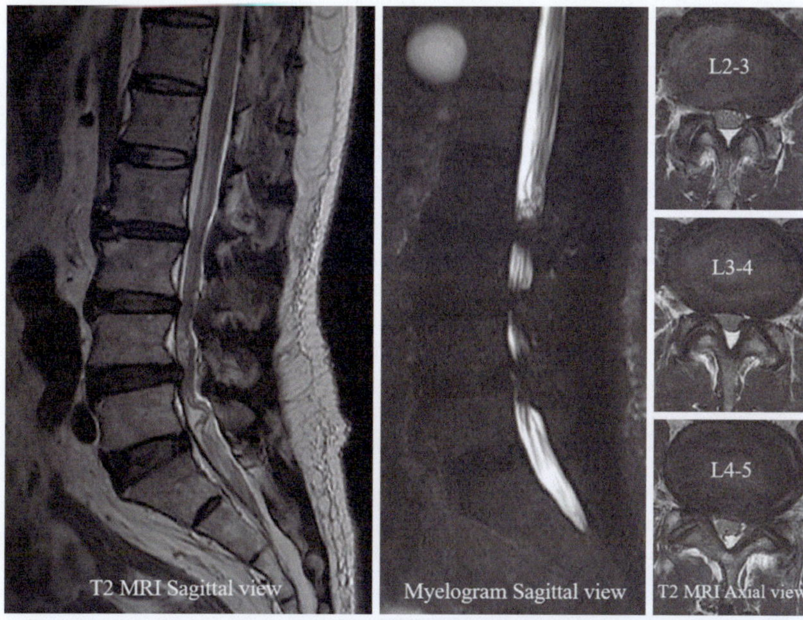

Fig. 11.1 Preoperative MRI and myelogram show spinal stenosis from L2 to L5

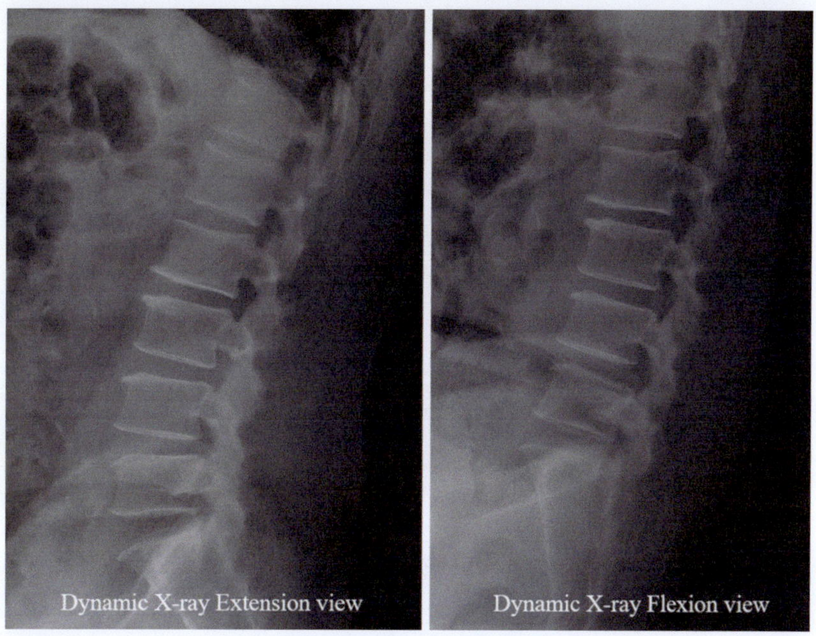

Fig. 11.2 Preoperative dynamic X-ray shows instability and grade 1 degenerative spondylolisthesis at L4–5 level

11.3 Preoperative Planning

The patient had L4-5 degenerative spondylolisthesis with instability, but the spondylolisthesis was mild at Grade 1, and the foraminal stenosis was not severe. Considering the patient's advanced age, underlying disease (especially Parkinson's disease), and osteoporotic bone condition, it was determined that decompression of the central canal, rather than multilevel fusion surgery, could be expected to provide sufficient symptom relief with shorter and faster recovery. The myelogram revealed significant signal blocking (Fig. 11.1), indicating reduced CSF flow at the L2-3-4-5, which were determined as the surgical target levels.

11.4 Surgical Steps

11.4.1 Open Midline Decompression (OMD)

(A) *Initial Dissection*

Under general anesthesia, the patient was positioned prone on a Wilson frame to optimize surgical exposure. Following sterile preparation and draping, a midline skin incision was made, extending from the center of the upper spinous process to the lower margin of the lower spinous process at the targeted level (Fig. 11.3a). The fascia on the left side was incised approximately 0.5 cm lateral to the midline, and the para-spinal muscles were meticulously dissected. Using monopolar cautery, the supraspinous and interspinous ligaments were detached from the spinous processes. These detached ligament complexes were then utilized to facilitate the dissection of the contralateral para-spinal muscles. A self-retaining retractor was placed to maintain clear access to the interspinous space.

(B) *Creation of the Interspinous Window*

Soft tissue was thoroughly removed using monopolar cautery and a high-speed drill to establish the "interspinous window" (Fig. 11.3a). Under microscopic guidance, decompression began at the caudal spinous base and extended laterally toward the medial pedicle (Fig. 11.3b, c).

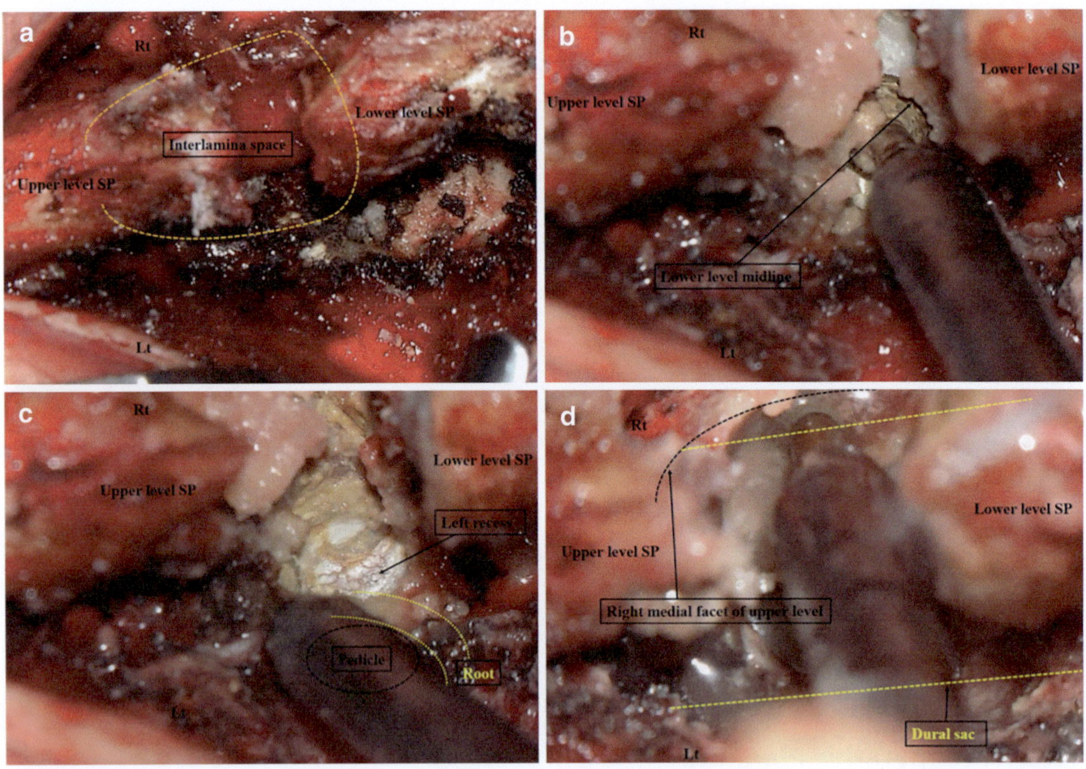

Fig. 11.3a Process of open midline decompression. (**a**) Bilateral muscle dissection is performed to expose the spinous processes (SP) from the upper to the lower levels of the target segment. (**b**) Midline drilling is initiated at the lower level to expose the underlying dural sac, providing clear access for further decompression. (**c**) The lateral recess at the lower level is drilled, extending to the medial wall of the pedicle until it is fully exposed and detached. (**d**) Using the contralateral "interspinous window," the medial facet of the upper level is carefully drilled with an undercutting technique. This approach minimizes facet destruction while effectively decompressing the lateral recess

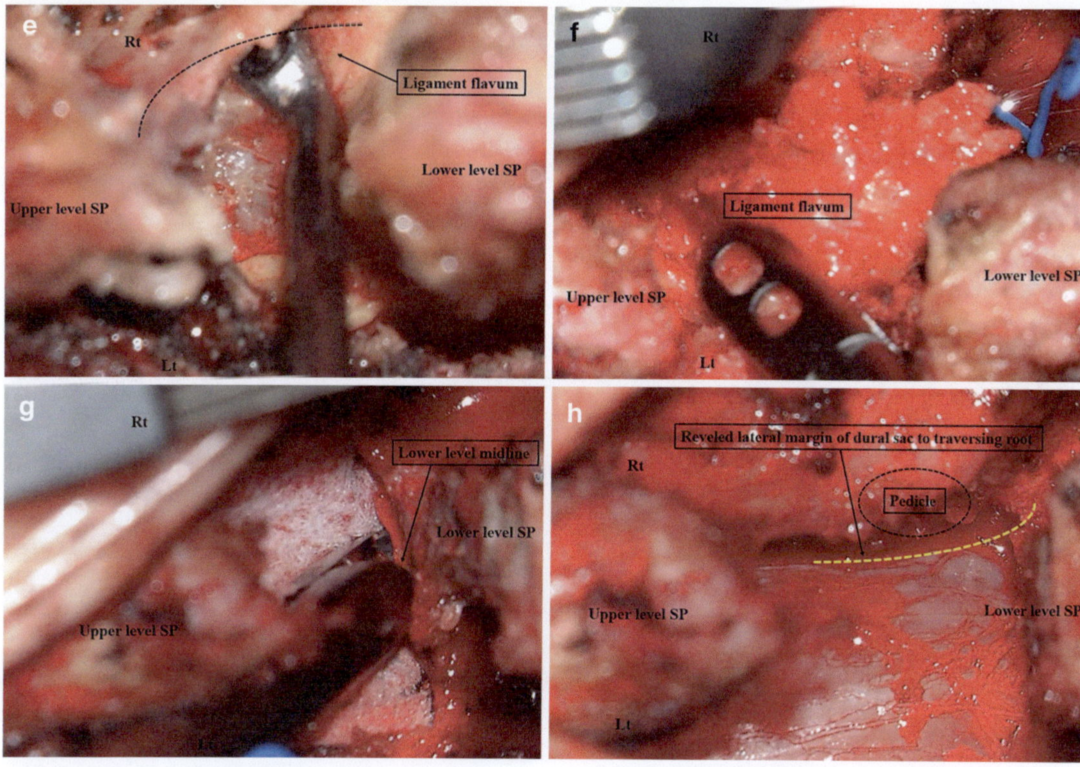

Fig. 11.3b Process of open midline decompression continued. (**e**) Once adequate drilling is completed, the ligamentum flavum is carefully detached from the lamina using a curette with gentle technique. (**f**) The ligamentum flavum is removed en bloc to ensure thorough decompression. (**g**) Additional bony decompression is performed on the upper and lower laminae to enhance exposure above the dural sac. (**h**) The decompression is verified by confirming that the dural sac and both traversing nerve roots are fully relieved of pressure

Cranial decompression was performed by undercutting the cranial lamina with a high-speed drill. Medial facetectomy was performed to decompress the lateral recess using a contralateral decompression approach (Fig. 11.3d). In cases of foraminal stenosis, additional decompression of the neural foramen was performed as needed.

(C) *Preservation of Structural Integrity*

To maintain structural stability, particular attention was given to preserving the spino-laminar junction, minimizing the risk of spinous process fractures post-decompression. The contralateral approach enabled effective decompression of the lateral recess and foramen while preserving the facet joint.

(D) *En Bloc Flavectomy.*

The hypertrophied ligamentum flavum (LF) was carefully detached en bloc from its cranial and caudal attachments on the lamina (Fig. 11.3e, f). This step was performed meticulously to ensure complete removal of the LF while maintaining the integrity of surrounding structures.

(E) *Additional Bony Decompression*

Following flavectomy, further bony decompression was performed on the upper and lower laminae to ensure adequate decompression of the dural sac and traversing nerve roots (Fig. 11.3g, h). This comprehensive decompression strategy aimed to achieve optimal neural decompression while preserving overall spinal stability.

11.4.2 Ligament Reconstruction (LP)

Please refer to

Part I, Chap. 7.

After surgery, the patient's neurologic claudication and cauda equina symptoms showed significant improvement. Postoperative MRI confirmed that sufficient nerve decompression was achieved with minimal damage to the facet joints (Fig. 11.4). The myelogram also confirmed a significant improvement in CSF flow postoperatively. Postoperative dynamic X-ray showed instability improvement at L4–5 level (Fig. 11.5). Sagittal translation decreased from 7.4 mm to 4.1 mm at L4–5. Sagittal angulation increased from −2.4° to 10.1° (Fig. 11.6). The patient was discharged after suture removal 1 week postoperatively.

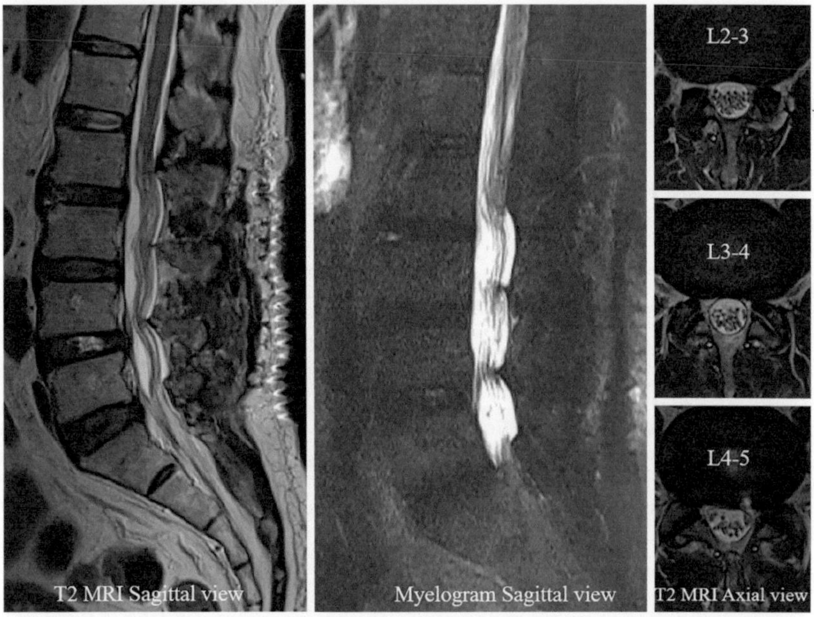

Fig. 11.4 Postoperative MRI shows well-decompressed dural sac with CSF flow improvement

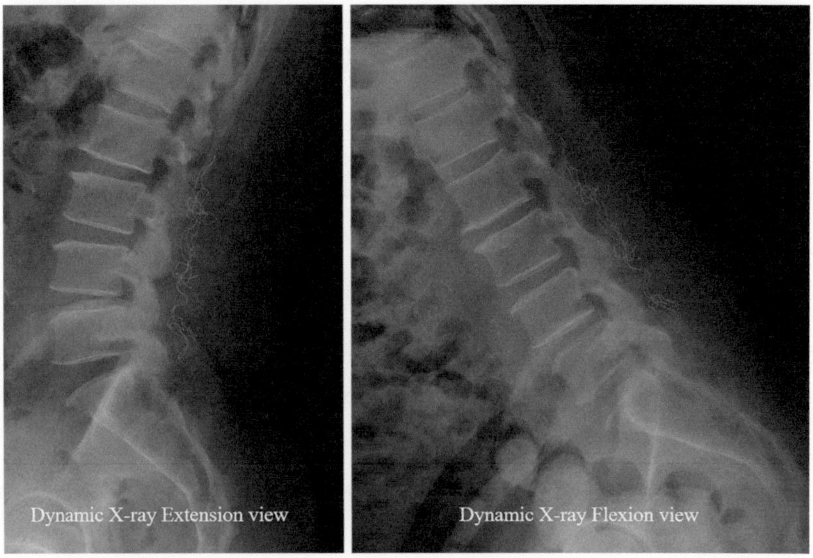

Fig. 11.5 Postoperative dynamic X-ray shows instability improvement at L4–5 level

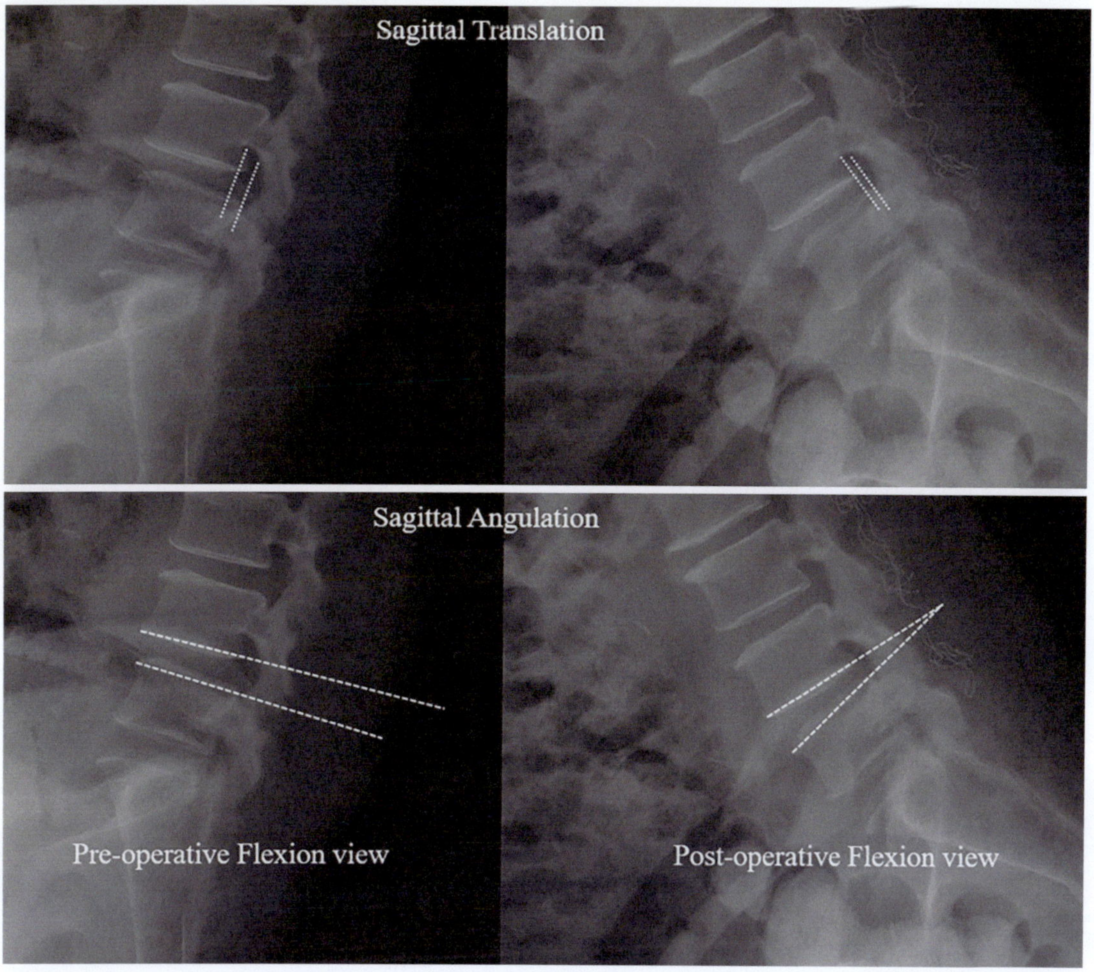

Fig. 11.6 Sagittal translation decreased from 7.4 mm to 4.1 mm at L4–5. Sagittal angulation increased from −2.4° to 10.1°

11.5 Commentary

Facet joint preservation is fundamental to achieving optimal outcomes in spinal surgery, as these joints play a critical role in maintaining spinal stability and regulating motion [19]. The long-term consequences of facet joint removal, including postoperative pain, progressive spinal instability, and the development of degenerative changes in adjacent segments, underscore the importance of preserving these structures [19, 20]. These complications can severely impact a patient's quality of life, particularly in younger individuals who require sustained spinal functionality over an extended period [21]. Traditional decompression techniques, such as partial laminectomy and unilateral approach bilateral laminectomy (UBL), often necessitate partial resection of the facet joints to relieve neural compression [12, 13]. While effective in the short term, such approaches increase the likelihood of chronic complications, including persistent back pain and spinal deformities [9, 20]. Long-term studies have highlighted the correlation between facet joint removal and accelerated spine degeneration, emphasizing the need for surgical methods that minimize disruption to these critical structures [4, 22]. Open midline decompression (OMD) represents a transformative advancement in addressing this challenge [17]. Unlike traditional techniques, OMD prioritizes facet joint preservation without compromising the effectiveness of neural decompression [14]. The procedure begins with the removal of the interspinous ligament and creates a surgical pathway through the interlaminar space. Using a microscopic tunneling approach, the cranial lamina is carefully undercut, and the hypertrophied ligamentum flavum removed en bloc. This technique fully opens the interlaminar space and enables access to the lateral recesses at shallow angles, minimizing facet joint resection. By maintaining the structural integrity of the facet joints, OMD significantly reduces the risks of postoperative instability and chronic back pain [17]. An additional advantage of OMD lies in its compatibility with ligamentoplasty (LP) [16]. The widened interlaminar space created during OMD provides an ideal surgical field for LP, allowing simultaneous neural decompression and stabilization. This synergy addresses both neural compression and segmental instability, offering a comprehensive solution for patients with lumbar spinal stenosis (LSS) [16, 23]. By enhancing spinal stability without sacrificing motion, LP in conjunction with OMD is particularly suitable for patients with mild to moderate instability who may not benefit from more invasive fusion procedures [15, 23]. Recent studies have increasingly recognized the clinical benefits of OMD combined with LP. Patients undergoing this combined approach report superior outcomes, including reduced rates of recurrent stenosis, improved postoperative functionality, and lower incidences of adjacent segment disease [15, 17, 23]. Moreover, the emphasis on facet preservation aligns with the growing trend in spinal surgery to adopt techniques that balance structural stability with maintaining natural spinal motion [19, 20]. This is especially important for elderly patients, who often present with multilevel LSS and comorbidities, as less invasive procedures reduce surgical risks and promote faster recovery.

In summary, OMD represents a paradigm shift in spinal decompression surgery, offering a refined approach that combines effective neural decompression with the preservation of critical spinal structures [14, 17]. Its compatibility with LP further enhances its utility, providing a holistic solution to the dual challenges of instability and neural compression [15, 16, 23]. By reducing the risks of long-term complications while improving patient outcomes, OMD sets a new benchmark for surgical innovation in the treatment of LSS.

References

1. Deyo RA, Mirza SK, Martin BI. Back pain prevalence and visit rates: estimates from U.S. national surveys, 2002. Spine (Phila Pa 1976). 2006;31(23):2724–7.
2. Kalichman L, Cole R, Kim DH, et al. Spinal stenosis prevalence and association with symptoms: the Framingham Study. Spine J. 2009;9(7):545–50.
3. Genevay S, Atlas SJ. Lumbar spinal stenosis. Best Pract Res Clin Rheumatol. 2010;24(2):253–65.
4. Deyo RA, Cherkin DC, Loeser JD, et al. Morbidity and mortality in association with operations on the lumbar spine: the influence of age, diagnosis, and procedure. J Bone Joint Surg Am. 1992;74(4):536–43.
5. Ishimoto Y, Yoshimura N, Muraki S, Yamada H, Nagata K, Hashizume H, et al. Prevalence of symptomatic lumbar spinal stenosis and its association with physical performance in a population-based cohort in Japan: the Wakayama Spine Study. Osteoarthr Cartil. 2012;20(10):1103–8.
6. Chou R, Loeser JD, Owens DK, et al. Interventional therapies, surgery, and interdisciplinary rehabilitation for low back pain: an evidence-based clinical practice guideline. Spine (Phila Pa 1976). 2009;34(10):1066–77.
7. Försth P, Ólafsson G, Carlsson T, et al. A randomized, controlled trial of fusion surgery for lumbar spinal stenosis. N Engl J Med. 2016;374(15):1413–23.
8. White HJ, Bradley J, Hadgis N, Wittke E, Piland B, Tuttle B, et al. Predicting patient-centered outcomes from spine surgery using risk assessment tools: a systematic review. Curr Rev Musculoskelet Med. 2020;13(3):247–63.
9. Kleinstück FS, Fekete TF, Jeszenszky D, et al. The influence of preoperative back pain on the outcome of lumbar decompression surgery. Spine (Phila Pa 1976). 2011;36(2):E134–41.
10. Bellini CM, Galbusera F, Raimondi MT, Mineo GV, Brayda-Bruno M. Biomechanics of the lumbar spine after dynamic stabilization. J Spinal Disord Tech. 2007;20(6):423–9.
11. Kim HS, Park JY. Endoscopic spine procedures. Korean J Spine. 2017;14(1):1–4.
12. Watanabe K, Hosoya T, Shiraishi T, et al. Lumbar spinous process-splitting laminectomy for lumbar canal stenosis. Tech Orthop. 2005;20(2):153–9.
13. Toyoda H, Nakamura H, Konishi S, Dohzono S, Kato M, Matsuda H. Clinical outcome of microsurgical

bilateral decompression via unilateral approach for lumbar canal stenosis: minimum five-year follow-up. Spine (Phila Pa 1976). 2011;36(5):410–5.
14. Cakir B, Richter M. Dynamic stabilization of the lumbar spine. Curr Orthop. 2007;21(4):270–7.
15. Gao K, Chen S, Wang L, et al. Anterior cruciate ligament reconstruction with LARS artificial ligament: a multicenter study with 3- to 5-year follow-up. Arthroscopy. 2010;26(4):515–23.
16. Stoll TM, Dubois G, Schwarzenbach O. The dynamic neutralization system for the spine: a multi-center study of a novel non-fusion system. Eur Spine J. 2002;11(Suppl 2):S170–8.
17. Fay LY, Wu JC, Tsai TY, et al. Dynamic stabilization for degenerative spondylolisthesis: evaluation of radiographic and clinical outcomes. Clin Neurol Neurosurg. 2016;144:60–7.
18. Cakir B, Carazzo C, Schmidt R, et al. Adjacent segment mobility after rigid and dynamic instrumentation of the lumbar spine. Spine (Phila Pa 1976). 2009;34(12):1287–91.
19. Kim HJ, Chun HJ, Kang KT, et al. The biomechanical influence of the facet joint orientation and the facet tropism in the lumbar spine. Spine J. 2013;13(10):1301–8.
20. Yang JC, Kim SG, Kim TW, Park KH. Analysis of factors contributing to postoperative spinal instability after lumbar decompression for spinal stenosis. Korean J Spine. 2013;10(3):149–54.
21. Panjabi MM. The stabilizing system of the spine. Part II. Neutral zone and instability hypothesis. J Spinal Disord. 1992;5(4):390–6.
22. Park P, Garton HJ, Gala VC, et al. Adjacent segment disease after lumbar or lumbosacral fusion: review of the literature. Spine (Phila Pa 1976). 2004;29(17):1938–44.
23. Schnake KJ, Schaeren S, Jeanneret B. Dynamic stabilization in addition to decompression for lumbar spinal stenosis with degenerative spondylolisthesis. Spine. 2006;31(7):442–9.

Bilateral Partial Hemi-Laminectomy

12

Shin Young Lee and Sang-Ho Lee

Abstract

Spinal canal stenosis is a common pathologic condition in old age. Generally, spinal disorders which contain both stenosis and spondylolisthesis bring many kinds of social problems and require a large amount of financial costs (Atlas SJ et al., Spine 21(15):1787–1794, 1996; Biswas KC et al., Proc Inst MechEng Part H J Eng Med 233:1292–1298, 2019; Cornefjord M, Eur Spine J 9(6):563–570, 2000). Most patients who have spinal disorder receive a conservative treatment initially. However, patients who have not improved after long-term conservative treatment have to consider surgical treatment eventually. Spinal canal stenosis may occur alone or be accompanied by degenerative spondylolisthesis. In case of patients with degenerative spondylolisthesis above grade 2, proper treatment is not easy because of severe vertebral body slippage (Pan A et al., Eur Spine J 25:1522–1532, 2016; Schaeren S et al., Spine 33:E636–42, 2008; Shim CS et al., Spine Arthroplasty Soc J 1(3):118–124, 2007). For many patients who suffer from neurologic intermittent claudication and leg pain, various treatment methods are introduced from percutaneous procedures to deformity surgeries which require reconstruction of vertebral bodies and decompression of spinal canal using a microscope (Biswas JK, Proc Inst MechEng Part H J Eng Med. 2019;233:1292–1298; Christie SD, Spine, 30(16 Suppl): S73–S78, 2005; Rhee J et al. J Neurosurg Spine 17(5):453–458, 2012). The author introduces the method of obtaining successful clinical results using bilateral partial hemi-laminectomy using a microscope and endoscope among several methods.

Keyword

Spinal canal stenosis · Microscopic canal decompression · Degenerative spondylolisthesis · Bilateral hemilaminectomy · Artificial interspinous ligament

Supplementary Information The online version contains supplementary material available at https://doi.org/10.1007/978-981-95-3971-0_12.

S. Y. Lee (✉)
Department of Neurosurgery, Daegu Wooridul Spine Hospital, Daegu, Korea (Republic of)
e-mail: creutz@naver.com

S.-H. Lee
Department of Neurosurgery, Cheongdam Wooridul Spine Hospital, Seoul, Korea (Republic of)
e-mail: sh500909@wooridul.co.kr

S.-H. Lee et al. (eds.), *Ligament Reconstruction for Spine*,
https://doi.org/10.1007/978-981-95-3971-0_12

12.1 Introduction

Lumbar spinal stenosis is a relatively well-known aging process that generally occurs in the elderly over 60 years of age and causes the spinal canal compression by physical and anatomical problems. Lumbar spinal stenosis is also typically derived from degenerative facet-joint arthrosis, ligamentum flavum hypertrophy, and disc bulging, leading to compression of the spinal canal [1, 4, 9].

The main pathologic etiology is the degenerative process of the spine and intervertebral discs. As a result, the diameter of the spinal canal get narrower, and neurologic deficits, which are compressive clinical symptoms of the thecal sac and neuromuscular muscles, arise in the motor and sensory nervous bundles [12]. Spinal stenosis is more common in women. The Incidence of degenerative spondylolisthesis shows four times more in women than that of men. The treatment of lumbar stenosis is divided into a nonsurgical method and a surgical method, and a minimally invasive spinal surgery technique is added to the basic concept of conventional spinal surgery. It is less harmful to the patient but has the similar surgical result compared with classical technique [2, 17].

The surgical treatment of lumbar stenosis was announced in 1893 by Lane, who performed laminectomy for the first time. Since then, clinical surgical results have rapidly increased due to the improvement of surgical instruments such as microscopes and spinal endoscopes [6, 19].

The incidence of facet joint violation was relatively higher in performing spinal surgery using a microscope than performing it under an endoscope. In this chapter, the author introduces a good method that can effectively decompress the spinal canal and lateral recess while minimizing a damage to the posterior facet joints. The main strategy of this method is to expand the spinal canal by removing the upper laminar, lower laminar, facet joint, and yellow ligament of the opposite side of the field of view from both sides [24]. These surgical procedures can benefit by sufficiently decompressing the spinal canal and securing the stability of the spine [12, 28].

The names of the opposite side decompression have been called in various ways. For example, crossed unilateral bi-hemilaminectomy (X-UBL) named by BJ Jung and JK Kim, midline canal decompression with contralateral laminectomy named by SH Lee, and bilateral hemi-laminectomy named by the author. In addition, various surgical names are recently emerging [17, 18, 30].

12.2 Presentation of the Patient

A 67-year-old woman presented with chronic back pain with neurologic intermittent claudication and 8/10 on visual analog scale. Patient complained severe sciatica with sole paresthesia showing intractable neuropathic pain. Sciatica was dominant at left side than right side that presented especially at the night time and decreased at the day time. Preoperative plain x-ray and CT scan showed mild degenerative spondylolisthesis with calcified central disc herniation at the level of L4-5 (Figs. 12.1, 12.2 and 12.3). Preoperative magnetic resonance imaging and myelogram showed spinal canal stenosis with thecal sac compression (Figs. 12.4, 12.5 and 12.6). Preoperative electromyography (EMG) revealed no definitive abnormal finding. Patient received a microscopic contralateral partial hemilaminectomy at the level of L4-5. Hypertrophic ligament flavum was resected under direct visualization using curette and Kerrison punch. Epidural drain was left to evacuate epidural hematoma after bilateral hemilaminectomy. Postoperative MRI and CT showed full decompression of spinal canal (Figs. 12.7 and 12.8). Postoperatively, the patient's sciatica and neurologic claudication were much improved. There are no definitive postoperative complications at the surgery level.

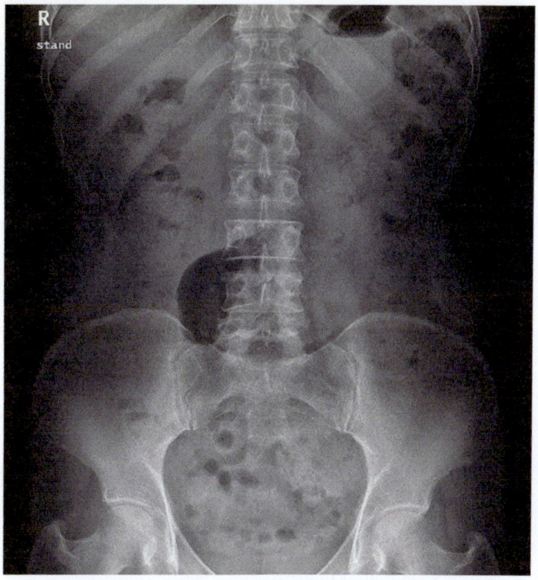

Fig. 12.1 Preoperative plain anterior-posterior radiograph showing bony spur of L4, L5 vertebral bodies

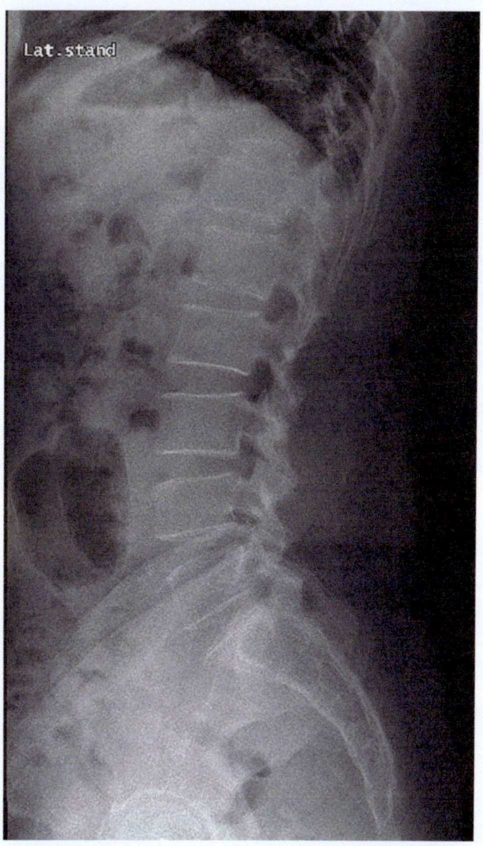

Fig. 12.2 Preoperative plain lateral radiograph showing mild degenerative spondylolisthesis at the level of L4 on L5

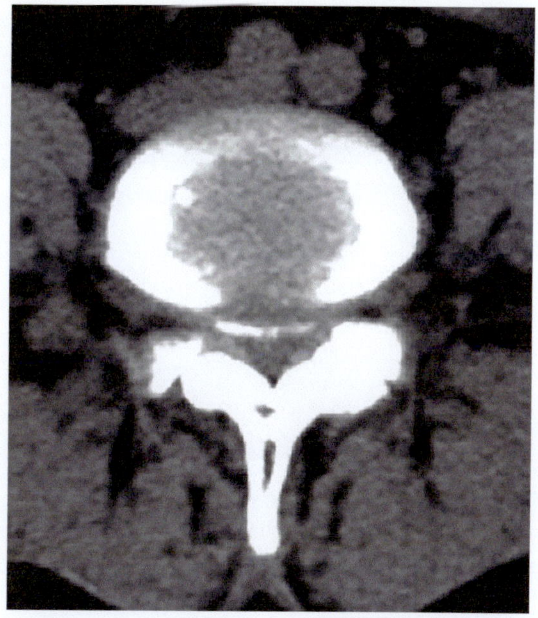

Fig. 12.3 Preoperative CT scan axial view showing calcified central disc herniation at L4-5 level

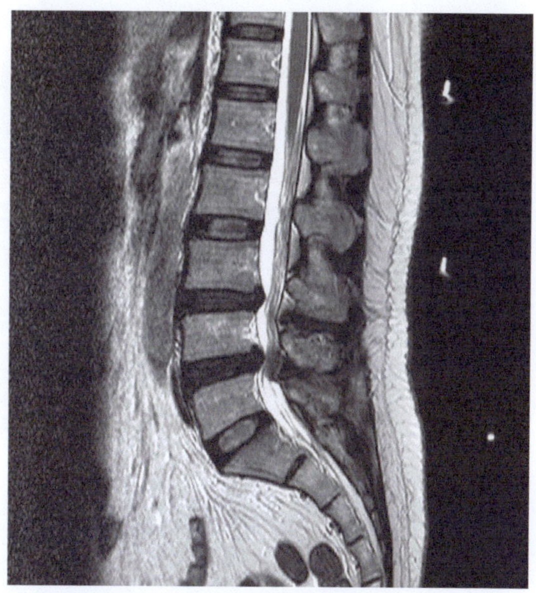

Fig. 12.4 Preoperative sagittal MRI showing mild degenerative spondylolisthesis with canal stenosis at the level of L4 on L5

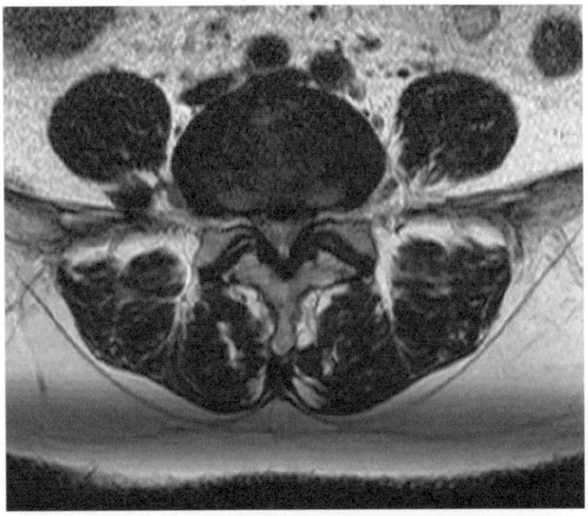

Fig. 12.5 Preoperative axial MRI showing spinal canal stenosis with facet hypertrophy at L4-5 level

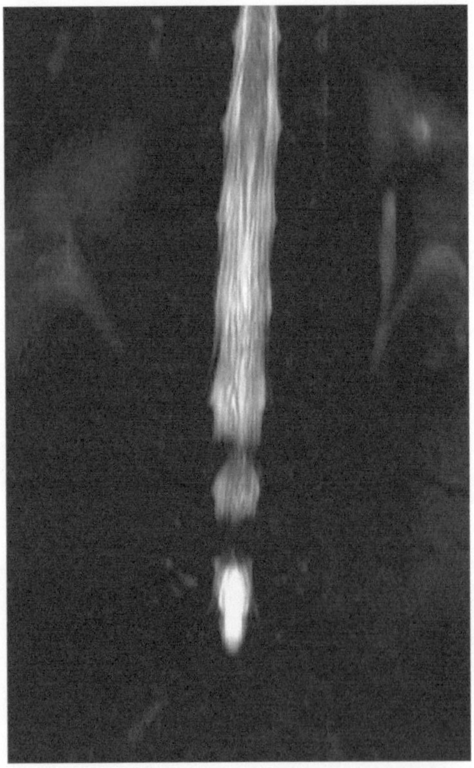

Fig. 12.6 Preoperative MR myelogram showing total signal block at L4-5 level

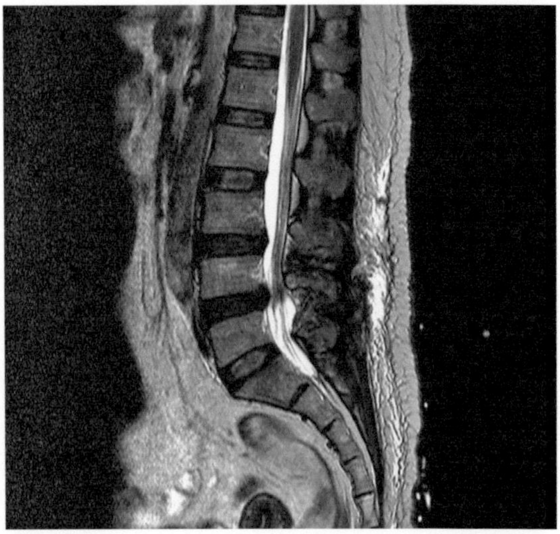

Fig. 12.7 Postoperative sagittal MRI showing well-decompressed spinal canal at L4-5 level

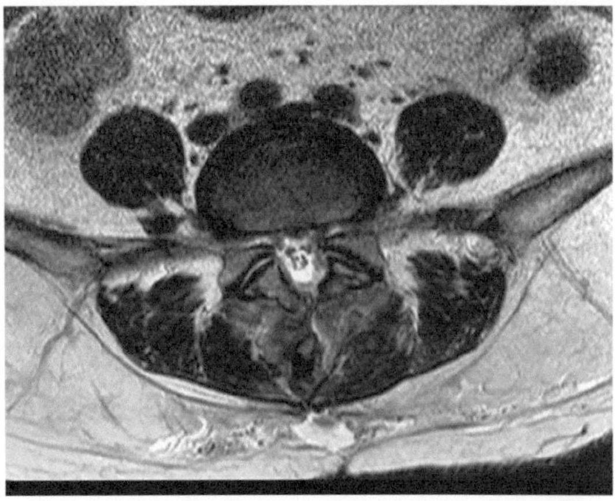

Fig. 12.8 Postoperative axial MRI showing well-expanded thecal sac with minimally violated facet joints at L4-5 level

12.3 Preoperative Planning

Preoperative planning for treating spinal canal stenosis or lateral recess stenosis by bilateral hemi-laminectomy is similar to that of endoscopic spinal procedures.

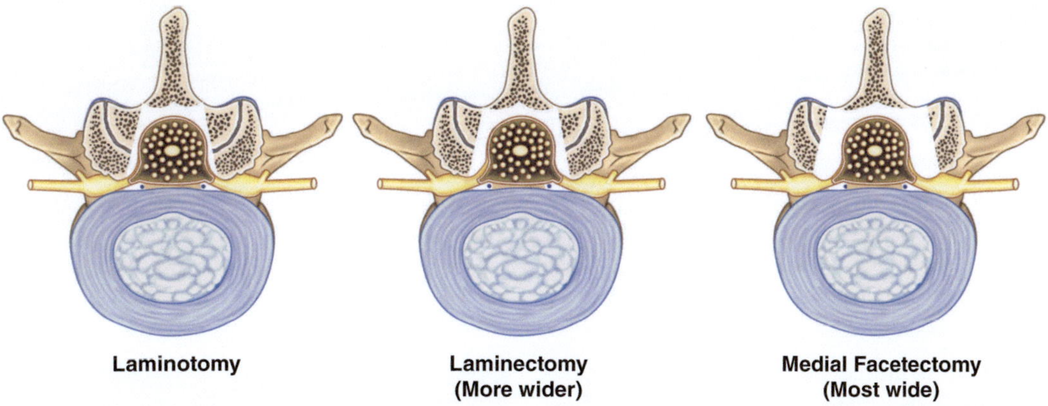

Fig. 12.9 Illustration of the range of laminectomy from hemi-laminotomy to medial facetectomy

Previously, patients with medical problems or elderly patients were subject to surgery avoidance, but the introduction of minimally invasive spinal surgery tends to reduce many obstacles. Recently, the concept of micro-invasive spinal surgery has become widely known, and many announcements have been made on various surgical instruments and surgical methods [10, 11]. However, detailed research and analysis of these are still insufficient. If the patient weighs more complaints on low back pain rather than radiating pain in the lower extremities and spinal instability is likely to progress, the author recommends fusion surgery rather than decompression surgery [13]. If the elderly female patient has low bone density (BMD), preoperative anti-osteoporosis drugs which can reduce postoperative spinal instability and complications must be considered.

Preoperative radiography contains a flexion and extension views should be performed to carefully evaluate the spinal instability that may occur after surgery. In general, medial facetectomy of less than one-third of the facet joints does not significantly affect spinal instability, but removal of more than half of the facet joints may result in iatrogenic instability [14, 15, 26]. And facet orientation is an important point, and you should be more careful when operating on patients with sagittal orientation than patients with coronal orientation. The range from hemi-laminotomy to medial facetectomy is as follows (Fig. 12.9).

It is important to determine whether the canal stenosis is due to ligamentum flavum buckling or the lateral process stenosis due to facet hypertrophy. If the patient has both ligamentum flavum buckling and lateral recess stenosis, fusion surgery may be considered in this severe case. [3, 23, 30].

12.4 Surgical Steps (Illustration, Photos, Videos)

This procedure was done under general anesthesia. The patients were positioned in the prone position on a Wilson frame with flexed hips and knees for the contralateral bilateral hemi-laminectomy procedure [21, 25, 26].

Bilateral hemi-laminectomy is more effective for lateral process stenosis with thickened facet than central canal stenosis. This surgical method aims to preserve the posterior joint more efficiently with partial decompression and maintain the posterior ligament complex (PLC) structure while relieving canal compression compared to extensive laminectomy [13, 16].

Although a part of the lower part of the interspinous ligament is removed, The point to keep in mind in this surgical technique is the preservation of spinous bone [29]. The ligamen-

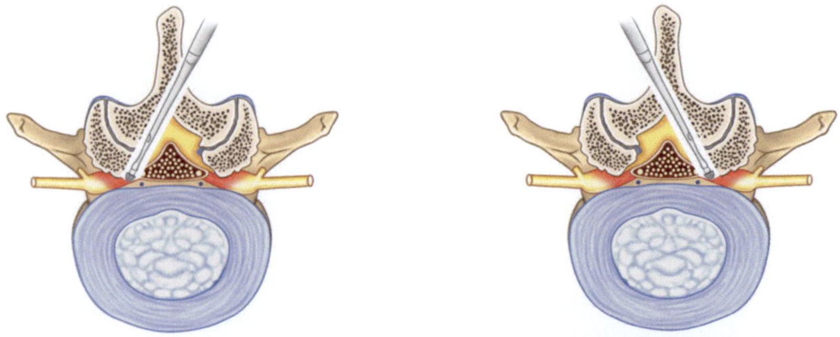

Fig. 12.10 Illustration showing contralateral hemilaminectomy in each side using a high-speed drill

tum flavum is ultimately removed while removing a part of the inner side of the posterior facet joint by undercutting using a small-head high-speed diamond burr (Primado 2, NSK-Nakanishi Surgical) and Kerisson punch (Fig. 12.10).

This method requires removal of the ligamentum flavum flap on the opposite side for prevention of sacrificing the base of the spinous process [31–33].

1. *Assessment of Proper Surgical Level*
   - After fluoroscopic localization of correct surgical level, the initial skin incision was placed 2–3 cm midline, as verified on the intraoperative fluoroscopic posterior-anterior view.
   - A surgical access corridor was made on opening level, identifying the intermuscular plane between the longissimus and iliocostalis, also easily identified by manual palpation. A self-retaining retractor was placed on top of the facet joint complex to initiate decompression of spinal canal.
2. *Dissection of Paraspinal Muscles*
   - To perform muscle dissection, periosteal dissector was applied in the subosteal plane in order to reduce paravertebral muscle injury. A muscle-splitting dissection technique was used to facilitate tubular retractor placement in the posterior lumbar spine [35].
   - At this point, the surgeon can select various types of retractors such as Caspar, Magana, Duval, Cerebellar, and Tubular retractors (METRx system, Medtronic Sofamor Danek). The purpose of the dissection is to confirm the surgical anatomy; lower half of the upper lamina, upper half of the lower lamina, and medial side of the facet joint.

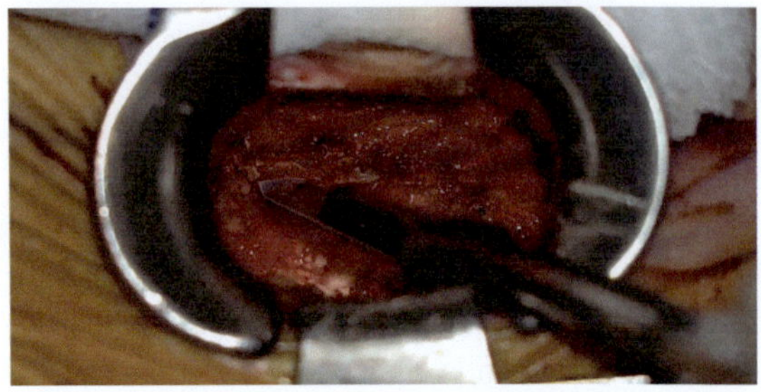

Fig. 12.11 Intraoperative microscopic view showing incision the lower part of the interspinous ligament with a surgical knife

3. *Detection of Ligamentum Flavum*
   - If lamina, facet, and yellow ligament are sufficiently checked, then an incision on the lower part of the interpersonal ligament with a surgical knife should be performed (Fig. 12.11).
   - After incising the lower part of the interspinous ligament, it is sometimes possible to observe the adhesion of the yellow ligament that occurred after epidural steroid injection.
   - In this case, the epidural fat disappears and the dura surface of thecal sac and ligamentum flavum may adhere severely, so the surgeon must be careful of dural tear when performing epidural dissection (Fig. 12.12).

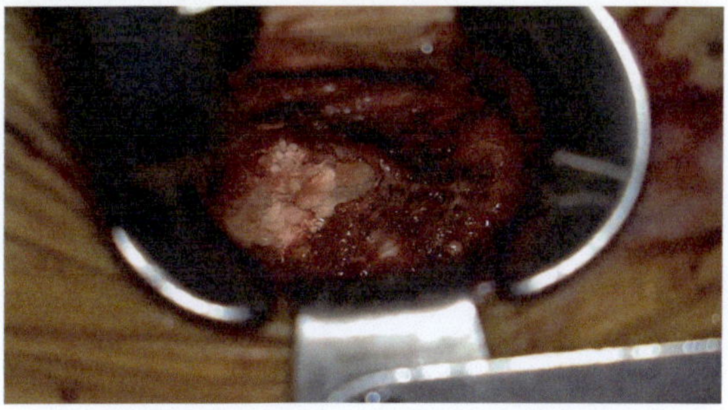

Fig. 12.12 Intraoperative microscopic view showing the adhesion of the yellow ligament that occurred after epidural steroid injection

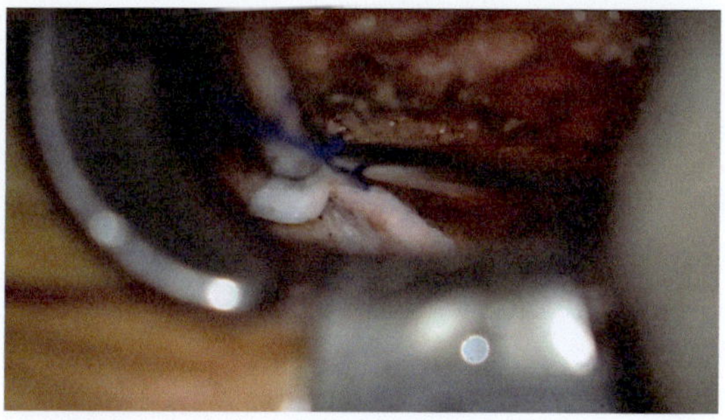

Fig. 12.13 Intraoperative microscopic view showing insertion of the cottonoid paddy in the epidural space to prevent possible dural tear during drilling

4. *Contralateral Drilling of Opposite Laminae*
   - The next surgical step is to perform a contralateral hemi-laminectomy by removing the superior edge of the inferior laminar.
   - For drilling, using a small burr is advantageous for facet preservation and is generally used when a 2 mm or 3 mm burr is mounted on a high-speed drill (Primado 2, NSK-Nakanishi Surgical) [34].
   - The most important point to be aware of when you are drilling is not to violate the ipsilateral facet joint, which you can achieve through maximal preservation of remnant facet joint after contralateral partial hemi-laminectomy [24, 27].
   - Before drilling, it is recommended to place the cottonoid paddy in the epiural space to prevent possible dural tear during drilling. After drilling is finished, detect the lower part of the yellow ligament with a large curette and make sure the epidural fat covers the dura well (Figs. 12.13 and 12.14).
   - The decompression of lateral recess was additionally performed to allow for simple resection in the same segment, performing an undercutting of the adjacent facet joint junction.
5. *Total Removal of Ligamentum Flavum*
   - After detecting the lower part of the ligamentum flavum(LF), carefully remove the ligamentum flavum in an en bloc manner using Kerisson punch and curette.
   - Removal of the ligamentum flavum exposes the epidural space with an epidural vein and epidural fat covering the dura of the thecal sac medially and the nerve root laterally (Fig. 12.15).
   - Finally, the contra-lateral hemi-laminectomy is completed by removing the remnant ligamentum flavum of the upper lamina located close to the midline.

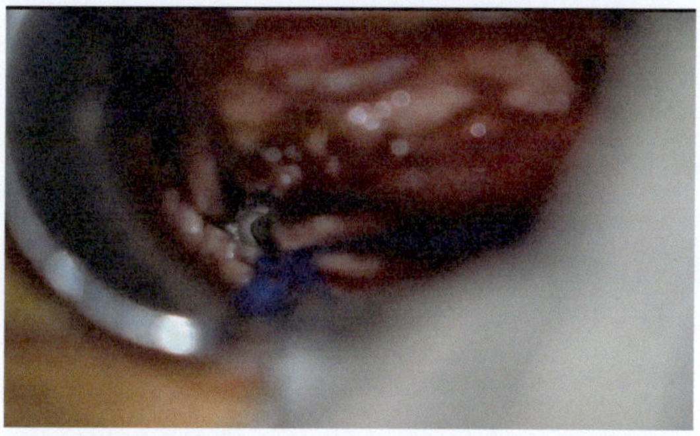

Fig. 12.14 Intraoperative microscopic view showing drilling of contralateral facet joint using 2 mm burr with high-speed drill

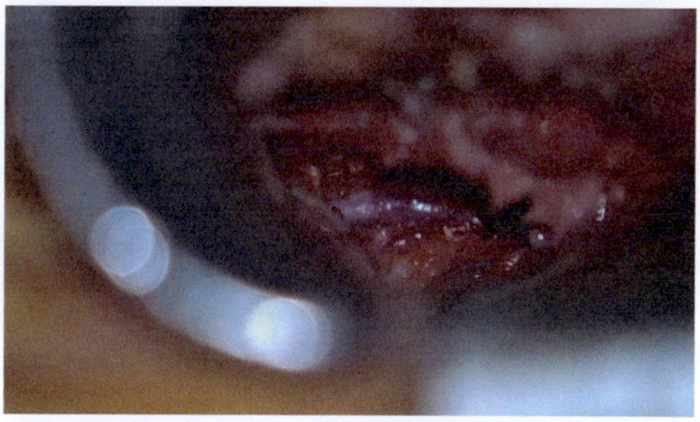

Fig. 12.15 Intraoperative microscopic view showing contralateral epidural vein and dorsal epidural fat

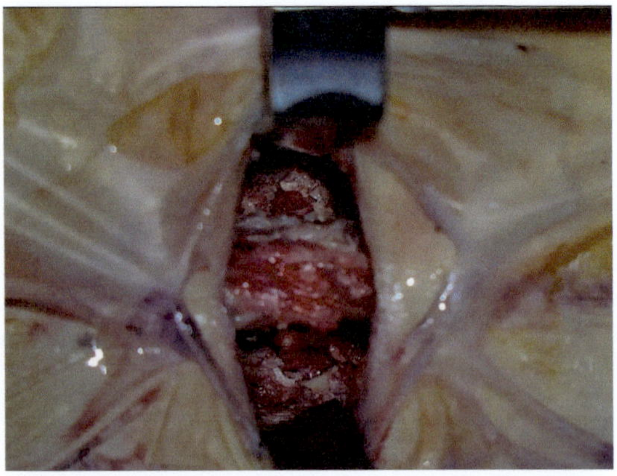

Fig. 12.16 Photograph showing well-decompressed thecal sac and exiting roots with minimally violated facet joints

6. *Artificial Ligament*
   - The contralateral hemi-laminectomy is also performed in the same way, and finally, check whether the exiting root is decompressed.
   - Bleeding control was made on epidural vein and epidural fat, which can reduce the shrinkage of the thecal sac by slowly performing hemostasis with hemostatic agents such as Floseal(Baxter), Hemofence Hemostatic(BMI Korea), and Tachosil(Baxter) rather than cauterizing with bipolar cautery (Fig. 12.16).
   - In an elderly patient with mild spondylolisthesis, soft stabilization with artificial interspinous ligament(SH Lee ligament, Gems Korea) would be concluded to represent an effective prevention of increased post-decompression instability with reliable reproducibility (Fig. 12.17) [5, 22, 30, 34, 36].

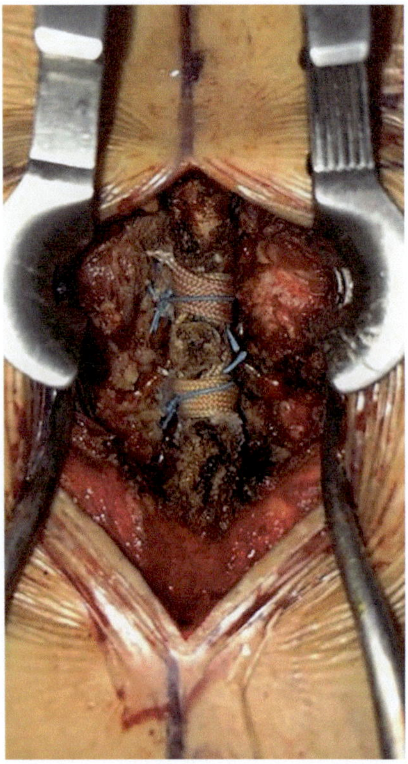

Fig. 12.17 Photograph showing soft stabilization with artificial ligament, utilizing the knot of the ligament to separate the spinous processes

12.5 Commentary

1. Bilateral hemi-laminectomy is an easy-to-learn procedure with a relatively short learning curve.
2. Surgical indications should be applied well, and if this surgical method is performed in patients with severe spinal stenosis, the surgeon has to consider that postoperative cauda

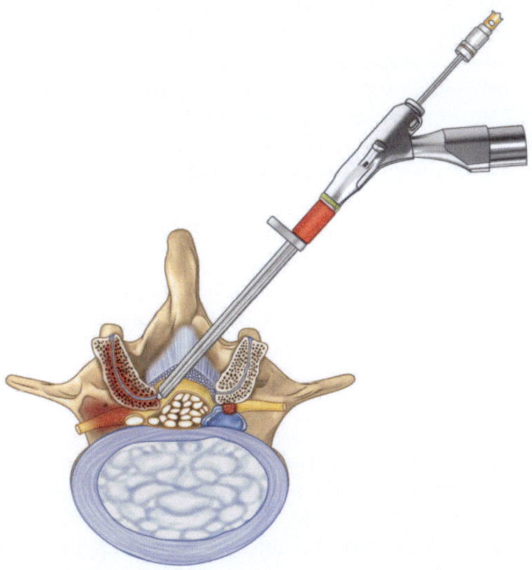

Fig. 12.18 Illustration showing contralateral hemilaminectomy using a full-endoscopic instrument

equina syndrome may occur due to swelling of cauda equinae.

3. After drilling with a 2 mm burr, the spinal canal is decompressed by detecting the ligament flavum. If there is a severe adhesion between the thecal sac and ligamentum flavum, the surgeon must be careful of dural tear.
4. In case of a patient with high obesity, paraspinal muscle injury may be occurred after surgery. so the author recommend endoscopic bilateral hemi-laminectomy using an full-endoscopic instrument which muscle damage can be minimized (Fig. 12.18).
5. Artificial interspinous ligament (SH ligament, Gems Korea) is sometimes used in combination when there is a spinal stenosis accompanied by mild spondylolisthesis [7, 8, 17, 18, 20].
6. Contralateral hemi-laminectomy can be done in various ways with microscopes, tubular retractor and endoscopes, each with its advantages and disadvantages [19].

References

1. Atlas SJ, Deyo RA, Keller RB, Chapin AM, Patrick DL, Long JM, DE Singer. The Maine Lumbar Spine Study, Part III. 1-year outcomes of surgical and nonsurgical management of lumbar spinal stenosis. Spine. 1996;21(15):1787–94.
2. Biswas JK, Roy S, Rana M, Halder S. A comparison of rigid, semirigid and fexible spinal stabilization devices: a finite element study. Proc Inst MechEng Part H J Eng Med. 2019;233:1292–8.
3. Booth KC, Bridwell KH, Eisenberg BA, Baldus CR, Lenke LG. Minimum 5-year results of degenerative spondylolisthesis treated with decompression and instrumented posterior fusion. Spine. 1999;24:1721–7.
4. Bouknaitir JB, Carreon LY, Brorson S, Pedersen CF, Andersen MO. WideLaminectomy, SegmentalBilateralLaminotomies, or unilateral hemilaminectomy for lumbar spinal stenosis: five-year patient-reported outcomes in propensity-matched cohorts. Spine (Phila Pa 1976). 2021;46(21):1509–15.
5. Christie SD, Song JK, Fessler RG. Dynamic interspinous process technology. Spine. 2005;30(16 Suppl):S73–8.
6. Cornefjord M, Byrod G, Brisby H, Rydevik B. A long-term (4- to 12-year) follow-up study of surgical treatment of lumbar spinal stenosis. Eur Spine J. 2000;9(6):563–70.
7. Fassio B, Cohen R, Beguin C, Jucopilla N. Treatment of degenerative lumbar spinal instability L4–L5 by interspinous ligamentoplasty. Rachis. 1991;3:465–74.
8. Fehlings MG, Chua SY. Interspinous ligamentoplasty. J Neurosurg Spine. 2010;13(1):24–5.
9. Garner MD, Wolfe SJ, Kuslich SD. Development and preclinical testing of a new tension-band device for the spine: the Loop system. Eur Spine J. 2002;11(Suppl 2):S186–91.
10. Hadlow SV, Fagan AB, Hillier TM, Fraser RD. The Graf ligamentoplasty procedure. Comparison with posterolateral fusion in the management of low back pain. Spine. 1998;23:1172–9.
11. Horan J, Husien MB, Bolger C. Bilateral laminotomy through a unilateral approach (minimally invasive) versus open laminectomyforlumbarspinal stenosis. Br J Neurosurg. 2021;35(2):161–5.
12. Iguchi T, Kurihara A, Nakayama J, Sato K, Kurosaka M, Yamasaki K. minimum 10-year outcome of decompressive laminectomy for degenerative lumbar spinal stenosis. Spine. 2000;25(14):1754–9.
13. Kaech DL, Woodtli MD. Interspinous U fixation in spinal stenosis and lumbar disc surgery. European

Association of Neurosurgical Societies. Grand-Duche de Luxembourg; 2006.
14. Mueller K, Fayed I, Spitz S, Nair N, Voyadzis J-M, Sandhu FA. Contralateral minimally invasive laminectomy for resection of a synovial cyst: 2-dimensional operative video. Oper Neurosurg. 2002;19(1):E63-E64.
15. Lawrence S, Llewellyn S, Hunt H, Cowin G, Sturgess DJ, Reutens D. Anatomy of the lumbar interspinous ligament: findings relevant to epidural insertion using loss of resistance. Reg Anesth Pain Med. 2021;46(12):1085–90.
16. Lee J, Hida K, Seki T, Iwasaki Y, Minoru A. An inter spinous process distractor (X STOP) for lumbar spinal stenosis in elderly patients: preliminary experiences in 10 consecutive cases. J Spinal Disord Tech. 2004;17(1):72–7.
17. Lee SH, Lee IM, Sung KH, Sung YS, Kim JS. Comparison of posterior interbody fusion, posterolateral fusion, and inter spinous ligamentoplasty for degenerative lumbar instability. J Neurosurg. 1997;86:424A.
18. Lee SH, Kim JS. comparison of ligamentoplasty to rigid fixation for degenerative lumbar instability. J Minim Invasive Spinal Tech. 2002;2(1):10–4.
19. Mitha R, Mahan MA, Patel RP, Colan JA, Leyendecker J, Zaki MM, Harake ES, Kathawate V, Kashlan O, Konakondla S, Huang M, Elsayed GA, Hafez DM, Pennicooke B, Agarwal N, Hofstetter CP, Ogunlade J. Lumbar endoscopic unilateral laminectomy for bilateral decompression in degenerative spondylolisthesis. World Neurosurg. 2024;191:e644–51.
20. Onda A, Otani K, Konno S, Kikuchi S. Mid-term and long term follow-up data after placement of the Graf stabilization system for lumbar degenerative disorders. J Neurosurg Spine. 2006;5(1):26–32.
21. Overdevest G, Vleggeert-Lankamp C, Jacobs W, Thomé C, Gunzburg R, Peul W. Effectiveness of posterior decompression techniques compared with conventional laminectomy for lumbarstenosis. Eur Spine J. 2015;24(10):2244–63.
22. Pan A, Hai Y, Yang J, Zhou L, Chen X, Guo H. Adjacent segment degeneration after lumbar spinal fusion compared with motion preservation procedures: a metaanalysis. Eur Spine J. 2016;25:1522–32.
23. Papp T, Porter RW, Aspden RM, Shepperd JAN. An in vitro study of the biomechanical effects of flexible stabilization on the lumbar spine. Spine. 1997;22:151–5.
24. Parchi PD, Evangelisti G, Vertuccio A, Piolanti N, Andreani L, Cervi V, et al. Biomechanics of Interspinous devices. Biomed Res Int. 2014;2014:1–7.
25. Pietrantonio A, Trungu S, Famà I, Forcato S, Miscusi M, Raco A. Long-term clinical outcomes after bilateral laminotomy or total laminectomy for lumbar spinal stenosis: a single-institution experience. Neurosurg Focus. 2019;46(5):E2.
26. Rahman M, Summers LE, Richter B, Mimran RI, Jacob RP. Comparison of techniques for decompressive lumbar laminectomy: the minimally invasive versus the "classic" open approach. Minim Invasive Neurosurg. 2008;51(2):100–5.
27. Rhee J, Anaizi AN, Sandhu FA, Voyadzis JM. Minimally invasive resection of lumbar synovial cysts from a contralateral approach. J Neurosurg Spine. 2012;17(5):453–8.
28. Schaeren S, Broger I, Jeanneret B. Minimum four-year follow-up of spinal stenosis with degenerative spondylolisthesis treated with decompression and dynamic stabilization. Spine. 2008;33:E636–42.
29. Shepherd DE, Leahy JC, Mathias KJ, Wilkinson SJ, Hukins DW. Spinous process strength. Spine. 2000;25(3):319–23.
30. Shim CS, Lee SH, Park SH, Whang JH. Soft stabilization with an artificial intervertebral ligament in grade I degenerative spondylolisthesis: comparison with instrumented posterior lumbar interbody fusion. Spine Arthroplasty Soc J. 2007;1(3):118–24.
31. Swanson KE, Lindsey DP, Hsu KY, Zucherman JF, Yerby SA. The effects of an interspinous implant on intervertebral disc pressures. Spine. 2003;28:26–32.
32. Talwar V, Lindsey DP, Fredrick A, Hsu KY, Zucherman JF, Yerby SA. Insertion loads of the X STOP interspinous process distraction system designed to treat neurogenic intermittent claudication. Eur Spine J. 2006;15(6):908–12.
33. Voydeville G, Diop A, Lavaste F, Girard F, Hardy P. Experimental lumbar instability and artificial ligament. Eur J OrthopSurgTraumatol. 2000;10:167–76.
34. Wang H, Ma L, Yang D, Wang T, Liu S, Yang S, et al. Incidence and risk factors of adjacent segment disease following posterior decompression and instrumented fusion for degenerative lumbar disorders. Medicine (Baltimore). 2017;96:e6032.
35. Watanabe K, Matsumoto M, Ikegami T, Nishiwaki Y, Tsuji T, Ishii K, et al. Reduced postoperative wound pain after lumbar spinous process–split-ting laminectomy for lumbar canal stenosis: a randomized controlled study. J Neurosurg Spine. 2011;14:51–8.
36. Wilke HJ, Drumm J, Häussler K, Mack C, Steudel WI, Kettler A. Biomechanical effect of different lumbar interspinousim plants on flexibility and intradiscal pressure. Eur Spine J. 2008;17:1049–56.

Unilateral Laminotomy for Bilateral Decompression

13

Hyeong-Seok Oh

Abstract

This chapter presents a unilateral laminotomy technique for bilateral decompression (ULBD) of lumbar spinal stenosis. The procedure prioritizes preservation of paraspinal muscles and ligaments while achieving complete decompression of both sides of the spinal canal. Utilizing Caspar and tubular retractor to create surgical access minimizes tissue trauma and provides access. The authors detail surgical steps, including patient and surgeon positioning, incision, and methods for both central and lateral recess decompression, bilaterally. Advantages highlighted include promising neural decompression compared to endoscopic procedure, and reduced pain, shorter recovery time, and less blood loss compared to conventional laminectomy. It is also an available and effective technique for decompression of the contralateral foraminal stenosis and contralateral extruded disc.

Supplementary Information The online version contains supplementary material available at https://doi.org/10.1007/978-981-95-3971-0_13.

H.-S. Oh (✉)
Department of Neurosurgery, Busan Wooridul Spine Hospital, Busan, Korea (Republic of)
e-mail: bstonefive@naver.com

Keywords

Lumbar stenosis · Unilateral laminotomy · Contralateral decompression · Foraminal stenosis · Contralateral discectomy

13.1 Introduction

Lumbar spinal stenosis (LSS) is a common cause of chronic low back pain and neurogenic claudication, significantly impacting quality of life and imposing a considerable burden on healthcare systems [1, 2]. The condition arises from a narrowing of the spinal canal, often due to facet joint hypertrophy, disc degeneration, and ligamentum flavum thickening [3, 4]. Although open laminectomy has historically been the standard surgical approach, it involves extensive tissue dissection, causing significant muscle damage and potentially leading to postoperative instability, chronic back pain, and increased recovery time [4, 5]. Consequently, minimally invasive techniques, including endoscopic and microscopic approaches, have gained prominence as less-traumatic alternatives [6–8].

To address these shortcomings, minimally invasive surgical techniques have emerged as valuable alternatives Spinous process splitting laminectomy (SPSL) for lumbar canal stenosis, a minimally invasive technique aiming to preserve paraspinal muscles [9] (Fig. 13.1). While SPSL

S.-H. Lee et al. (eds.), *Ligament Reconstruction for Spine*,
https://doi.org/10.1007/978-981-95-3971-0_13

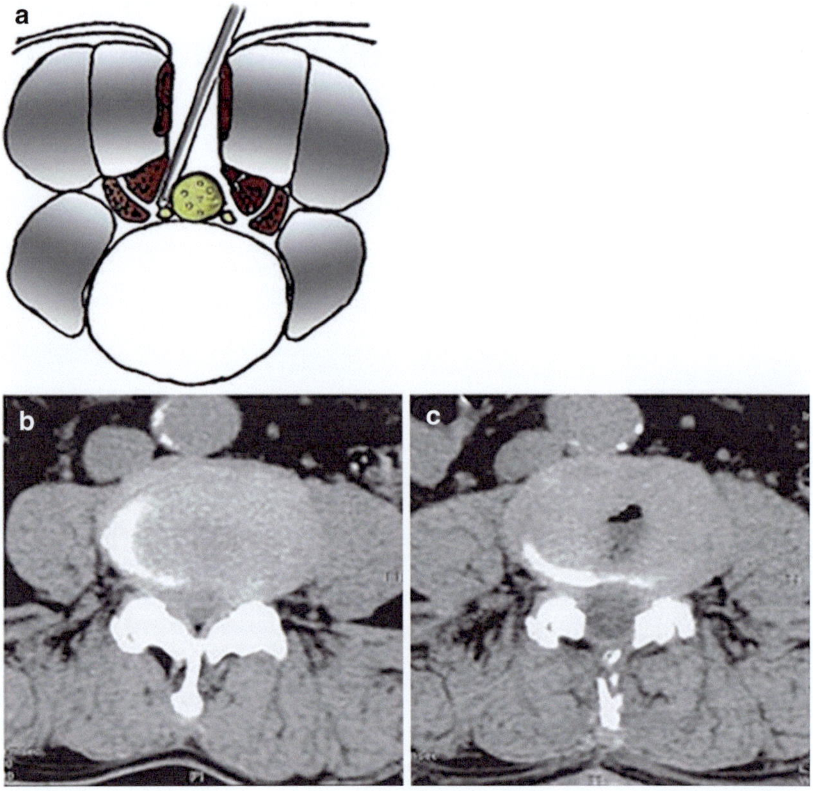

Fig. 13.1 Illustrations showing the technique of spinous process splitting laminectomy (**a**). After retracting the split spinous processes, decompression of the lumbar canal stenosis and/or discectomy was performed. Preoperative (**b**) and postoperative (**c**) computed tomography scans showing decompression of the lumbar canal stenosis using SPSL at the L4–5 level. Discectomy was performed on the right side simultaneously

offers benefits in minimizing muscle damage, incomplete decompression of the lateral recess and a relatively high re-herniation rate in patients with simultaneous discectomy may limit its effectiveness. In 2011, Central approach bilateral ligamentectomy (X-UBL) was introduced by the Wooridul hospital [10] (Fig. 13.2). The approach was from both sides in opposite directions. In this study, a total of 19 cases were enrolled. The advantage of it was maximal preservation of facet joint and no implantation, although the operation time was longer than ULBD.

This chapter focuses on a refined minimally invasive approach: unilateral laminotomy for bilateral decompression of lumbar spinal stenosis. This technique builds upon previous unilateral approaches, aiming to decompress both sides of the spinal canal through a single, smaller incision, minimizing tissue trauma [11]. The modern iteration utilizes the Caspar or tubular retractors to efficiently separate muscle fibers, facilitating optimal access to the surgical site with minimal tissue disruption.

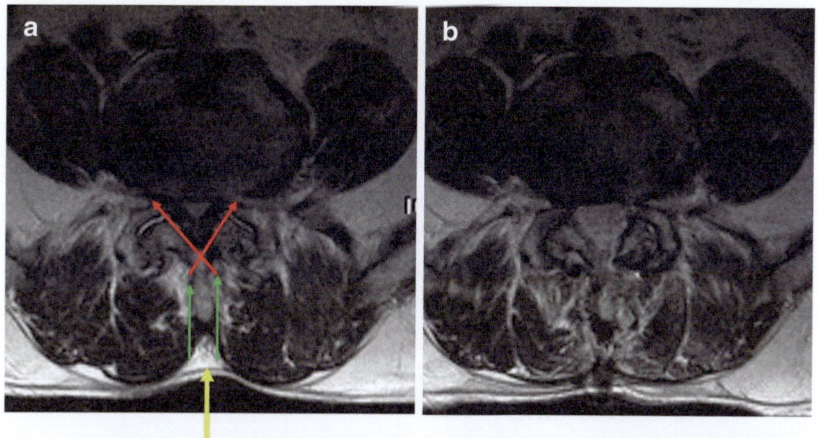

Fig. 13.2 Central approach bilateral ligamentectomy (X-UBL). A 73-year-old male patient presented with bilateral buttock and leg pain. Preop MR scan showed severe stenosis at L4/5 level (**a**). After bilateral ligamentectomy through contralateral approach, postop MR scan showed successful decompression (**b**)

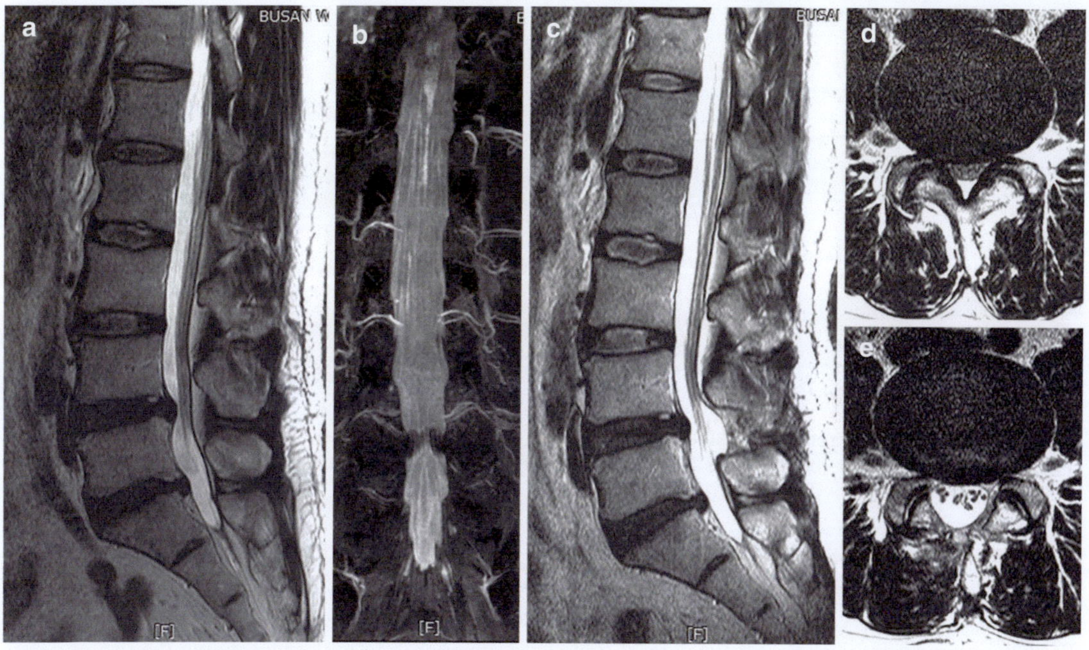

Fig. 13.3 Preoperative MR scan presented stenosis at L4/5 level and signal block at MR myelogrpahy (**a**, **b**, **d**). Postoperative MR scan, after Rt. approach ULBD, presented full decompression of thecal sac (**c**, **e**)

13.2 Presentation of the Patient

A 44 years old male suffered from bilateral leg pain (Rt. Main). Symptom onset 1 year and aggravation 3 months, preoperative and postoperative MR scans were presented (Fig. 13.3). He underwent Rt. side unilateral laminotomy bilateral decompression. Intraoperative video was presented (Video 13.1). His symptom was improved successfully.

13.3 Preoperative Planning

To maximize nerve decompression while minimizing removal of unnecessary bone and soft tissue, the exact area compressing nerve tissue must be thoroughly understood. Classifying the area compressing the nerve in lumbar spinal stenosis, McCulloch and Young's classification is usually cited [12] (Fig. 13.4). According to their classification method, when classifying from bottom to

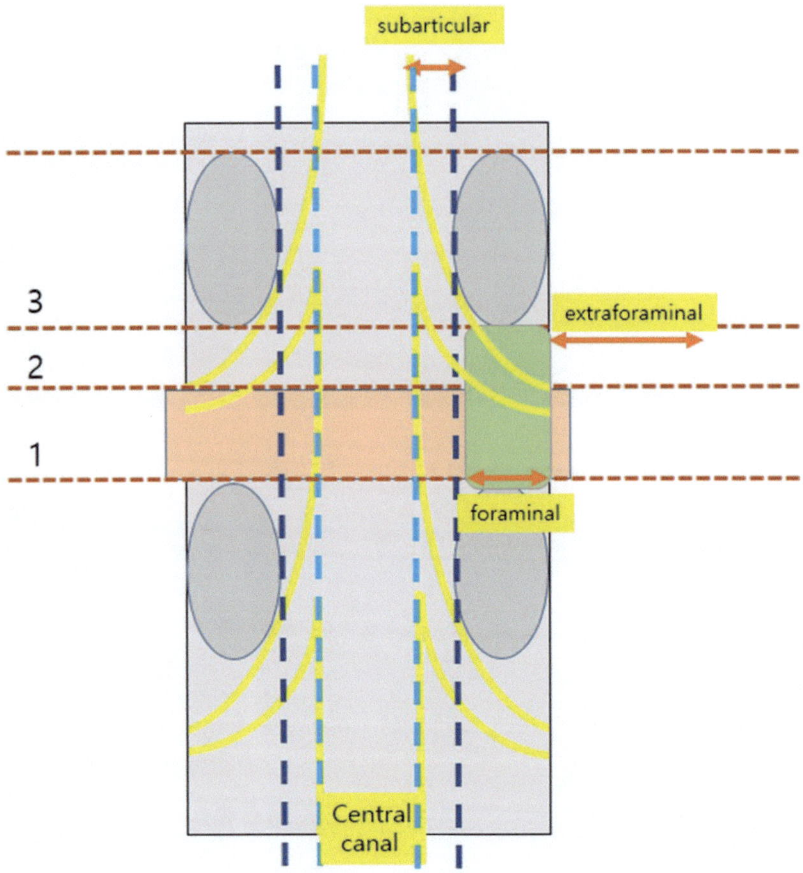

Fig. 13.4 McCulloch and Young's classification of nerve compression areas. 3 floor (floor 1—the disc, floor 2—foramen, floor 3—pedicle) and 3 zone (subarticular, foraminal zone, extraforaminal)

top, it can be divided into the disc floor, foramen floor, and pedicle, and when classifying from medial to lateral, first is the central zone. It is divided into a lateral zone, and the lateral zone can be further divided into a subarticular zone, a foraminal zone, and an extraforaminal zone.

To minimize postoperative pain and accelerate recovery, it is advantageous to use serial muscle-splitting retractors to spread the muscles apart, rather than performing subperiosteal dissection of the muscles from the bone. Finally, employing a tubular retractor completes the procedure.

Several methods exist for optimizing surgical visualization. One approach uses the METRx system (Fig. 13.5), where a tubular retractor is secured to the operating table, facilitating the use of a surgical microscope. Alternatively, a Caspar self-retaining retractor can be employed (Fig. 13.6). Numerous minimally invasive instruments from various manufacturers have been developed, many designed to facilitate visualization and manipulation within confined surgical fields.

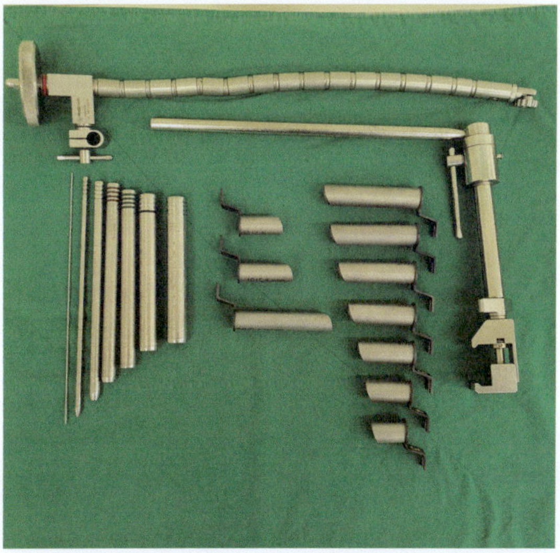

Fig. 13.5 Surgical equipment and instruments—METRx system

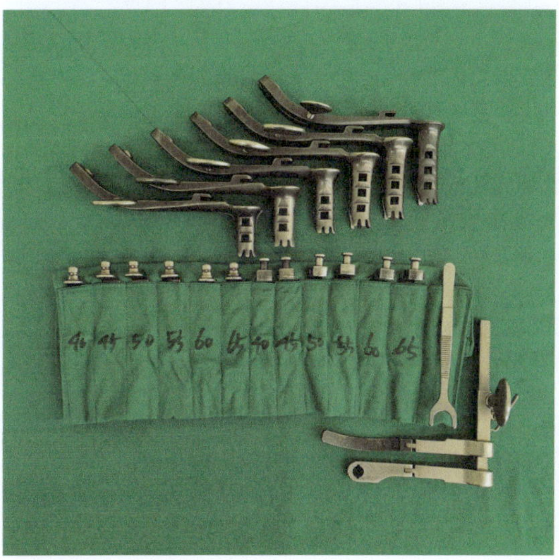

Fig. 13.6 Surgical equipment and instruments—Caspar self-retractor system

13.4 Surgical Steps

The surgical steps for minimally invasive unilateral laminotomy are as follows:

1. Patient and Surgeon Positioning: The patient is positioned prone with the lumbar spine flexed to widen the interlaminar spaces. A head down position is more advantageous for sublaminar undercutting and decompression. Surgeon positioning varies depending on experience, patient's symptom, foraminal stenosis, and lateral listhesis. The operating table may be angled to improve visualization of the contralateral side, allowing for decompression of the contralateral foraminal and lateral recess regions. For bilateral symptoms, a right-handed surgeon would typically position themselves on the patient's left side.
2. Skin Incision and Localization: A small skin incision (approximately 2.0–2.5 cm) is made slightly lateral to the midline at the target vertebral level, guided by C-arm fluoroscopy. A spinal needle is used to confirm the precise location before the incision.
3. Muscle dissection and Retractor Placement: Carefully muscle dissection are used; and make the space between the muscles. The Caspar retractor is then inserted and expand for secure to maintain optimal surgical exposure.
4. Ipsilateral partial laminotomy: A high-speed drill or Kerrison rongeurs are used to remove a portion of the ipsilateral lamina, creating an interlaminar window. Usually, the starting point of laminotomy is at midline cleft and then moved down. The ligamentum flavum is carefully separated from the dura using a curette and then excised using Kerrison rongeurs. The medial aspect of the inferior articular process of the vertebra below may also be partially removed for additional decompression in cases of ipsilateral subarticular stenosis.
5. Contralateral Decompression: The operating table is tilted to improve visualization of the contralateral side. Under microscopic view, the contralateral lamina is carefully thinned using a drill. Care is taken to avoid dural injury. The ligamentum flavum on the contralateral side is removed using Kerrison rongeurs. Decompression of the contralateral central canal and lateral recess proceeds similarly to the ipsilateral side, with careful attention to the exiting and traversing nerve roots.

6. Final Decompression and Wound Closure: The surgeon confirms adequate decompression on both sides using probes to assess the nerve roots' freedom of movement. Hemostasis is achieved, and the wound is meticulously closed in layers.

The precise techniques and steps may vary slightly based on individual surgeon preference, patient anatomy, and the specific challenges presented during the operation.

13.5 Commentary

The primary benefits of ULBD approach compared to bilateral decompression is reduced postoperative pain and morbidity and preservation of paraspinal muscles and ligaments. Moreover, compared to endoscopic surgery, microscopic nerve decompression can achieve safety and promise decompression, can be a method familiar to the operator, and can easily deal with complications such as dura tears.

13.5.1 Extended Indication

13.5.1.1 Lumbar Spinal Stenosis with Disc Herniation

The carbon dioxide pin point scalpel may facilitate the sophisticated discectomy in the narrow surgical field [13–15]. In case of lumbar stenosis with disc herniation, bilateral discectomy using a carbon dioxide laser could be an alternative and precise procedure for decompression of bilateral nerve root. It also tends to preserve the contralateral facet joint, the lamina, and the midline ligament structures, while widening spinal canal. Successful contralateral decompression hinges on achieving satisfactory ipsilateral decompression first, creating space for access. The extent of root sleeve retraction after contralateral decompression is also important, as contralateral compression may remain due to anterior lesions. CO2 laser facilitates precise discectomy in the limited surgical field, although it may cause iatrogenic annular tears on the contralateral side. However, laser-induced metaplasia is thought to potentially decrease reherniation rates. In summary, while offering a less invasive approach, the technique requires precise surgical skill and careful assessment of the relationship between ipsilateral and contralateral decompression (Fig. 13.7).

13.5.1.2 Contralateral Approach to Foraminotomy

This technique offers advantages over traditional ipsilateral approaches by providing excellent visualization of the contralateral foramen while preserving the facet joint, thus preventing iatrogenic instability. It is a minimally invasive, facet-sparing technique and is effective for treating radiculopathy from foraminal compression and allows for decompression of lumbar spinal stenosis and bilateral lateral recess decompression without the need for fusion (Fig. 13.8).

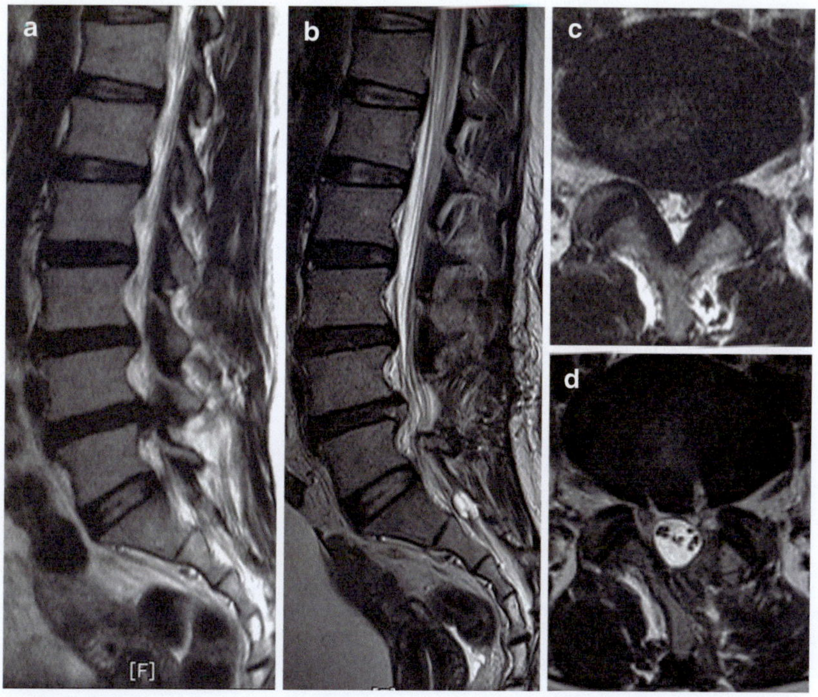

Fig. 13.7 CO2 Laser-assisted contralateral discectomy and decompression with UBLD Lt. A 56-year-old female presented with bilateral leg pain (Lt > Rt.). Symptom duration was 4 months. Neurogenic intermittent claudication presented after 10 minutes. Preop MR scan (**a**, **c**) presented L4/5 disc herniation bilaterally and stenosis. Postop MR scan (**b**, **d**) presented successful contralateral discectomy and decompression

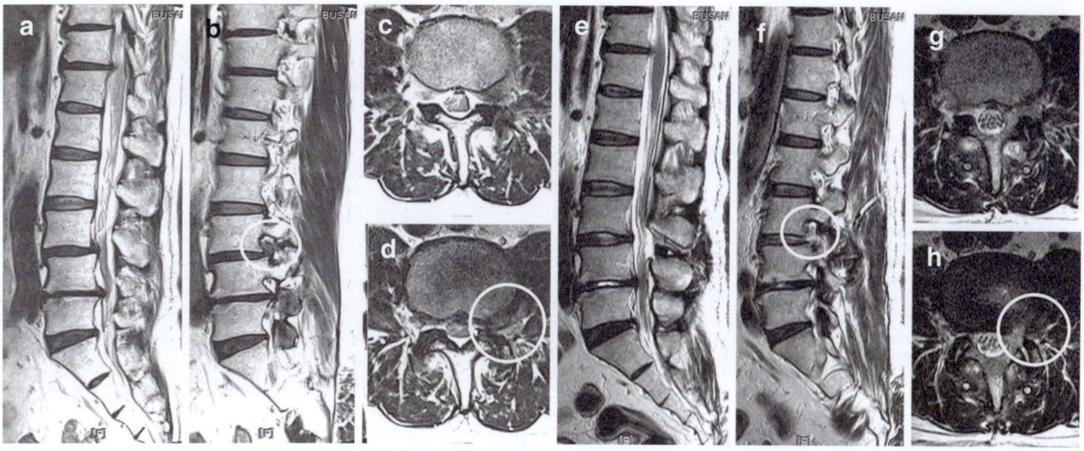

Fig. 13.8 Contralateral approach and decompression to foraminotomy. A 61-year-old male presented with Lt. buttock pain and Lt. leg atropic change. His symptom onset was 3 months earlier. Preoperative MR scan presented L3/4 listhesis with stenosis and Lt. foraminal disc (**a–d**). The operation was midline decompression L3/4 and foraminal decompression Rt. with disc removal. Postoperative MR scan presented successful removal of foraminal disc and central decompression (**e–h**)

13.6 Overall

Minimally invasive unilateral laminotomy for bilateral decompression offers a compelling alternative to traditional open laminectomy for appropriately selected patients with lumbar spinal stenosis. The reduced invasiveness translates to significant improvements in patient recovery and quality of life. However, the surgeon's experience, meticulous surgical technique, and careful patient selection are paramount to realize these benefits while mitigating potential limitations and complications.

References

1. Deyo RA, Mirza SK, Martin BI, Kreuter W, Goodman DC, Jarvik JG. Trends, major medical complications, and charges associated with surgery for lumbar spinal stenosis in older adults. JAMA. 2010;303:1259–65.
2. Udeh BL, Costandi S, Dalton JE, Ghosh R, Yousef H, Mekhail N. The 2-year cost-effectiveness of 3 options to treat lumbar spinal stenosis patients. Pain Pract. 2015;15:107–16.
3. Amundsen T, Weber H, Lilleas F, Nordal HJ, Abdelnoor M, Magnaes B. Lumbar spinal stenosis. Clin Radiol Features Spine (Phila Pa 1976). 1995;20:1178–86.
4. Weinstein J, Tosteson T, Lurie J, Tosteson A, Blood E, Hanscom B. Surgical versus nonsurgical therapy for lumbar spinal stenosis. N Engl J Med. 2008;358:794–810.
5. Datta G, Gnanalingham KK, Peterson D, Mendoza N, O'Neill K, Van Dellen J, McGregor A, Hughes SP. Back pain and dis ability after lumbar laminectomy: is there a relationship to muscle retraction? Neurosurgery. 2004;54:1413–20.
6. Lee CW, Yoon KJ, Ha SS. Comparative analysis between three different lumbar decompression techniques (microscopic, tubular, and endoscopic) in lumbar canal and lateral recess stenosis: preliminary report. Biomed Res Int. 2019;2019:6078469.
7. Overdevest G, Vleggeert-Lankamp C, Jacobs W, Thomé C, Gun Zburg R, Peul W. Effectiveness of posterior decompression techniques compared with conventional laminectomy for lumbar stenosis. Eur Spine J. 2015;24:2244–63.
8. Yagi M, Okada E, Ninomiya K, Kihara M. Postoperative outcome after modified unilateral-approach microendoscopic mid line decompression for degenerative spinal stenosis. J Neurosurg Spine. 2009;10:293–9.
9. Lee DY, Lee SH. Spinous process splitting laminectomy for lumbar canal stenosis : a critical appraisal. Minim Invas Neurosurg. 2008;51:204–7.
10. Kim JK, Lee SH Central approach and bilateral decompression for lumbar spinal canal stenosis. Friday teleconference in wooridul spine health hospital. 2012.
11. Hong SW, Choi KY, An Y, Baek OK, Wang JC, Lee SH, Lee HY. A comparion of unilateral and bilateral laminotomies for decompression of L4-5 spinal stenosis. Spine. 2011;36:E172–8.
12. McCollough JA, Young PH. Essentials of spinal microsurgery. Philadelphia: Lippincott-Raven Publishers; 1998.
13. Kim JS, Lee SH. Carbon dioxide (CO2) laser-assisted ablation of lumbar discal cyst. Photomed Laser Surg. 2009;27(6):837–42.
14. Lee DY, Lee SH. Carbon dioxide (CO2) laser-assisted microdiscectomy for extraforaminal lumbar disc herniation at the L5-S1 level. Photomed Laser Surg. 2011;29(8):531–5.
15. Kim JS, Oh HS, Lee SH. Usefulness of carbon dioxide laser for recurrent lumbar disc herniation. Photomed Laser Surg. 2012;30(10):568–72.

14 Lumbar Stenosis: Unilateral Biportal Endoscopic Surgery (UBE)

Ki Hyoung Moon

Abstract

Unilateral biportal endoscopic (UBE) decompression is a minimally invasive technique for treating degenerative lumbar stenosis. This method minimizes damage to normal lumbar structures while removing pathological lesions, enabling rapid patient recovery. This study aims to explore the UBE technique for treating spinal stenosis, focusing on preoperative preparation, surgical landmarks, procedural steps, and precautions. We will examine patient positioning, portal creation, and endoscopic visualization techniques. The decompression process, including laminectomy and flavectomy, will be detailed. Additionally, we will discuss the importance of maintaining proper saline irrigation pressure and strategies for complication avoidance. By understanding these aspects, surgeons can effectively utilize UBE for safe and efficient spinal stenosis treatment.

Keywords

Unilateral biportal endoscopic surgery · Spinal stenosis · Foraminal stenosis · Bilateral decompression · Contralateral foraminal decompression

K. H. Moon (✉)
Department of Neurosurgery, Gimpo Airport Wooridul Spine Hospital, Seoul, Korea (Republic of)
e-mail: enema1@hanmail.net

S.-H. Lee et al. (eds.), *Ligament Reconstruction for Spine*,
https://doi.org/10.1007/978-981-95-3971-0_14

14.1 Introduction

The history of the Unilateral Biportal Endoscopy (UBE) surgical technique has evolved as follows: In 1983, Kambin and Gellman attempted lumbar discectomy using arthroscopy, laying the foundation for minimally invasive spinal surgery [1]. In 1989, Schreiber et al. performed lumbar discectomy utilizing a bilateral dual-channel arthroscopic approach [2]. In 1996, De Antoni et al. pioneered the use of a dual-channel endoscopic surgery technique via a unilateral approach for the first time [1]. Compared to the conventional total laminectomy, this technique offered the advantage of reduced muscle injury and facet violation. In the 1990s, endoscopic treatment for disc herniation began in earnest.

In 2001, Dr. Abdul Gaffer presented the UBE technique at the American Academy of Orthopedic Surgeons meeting, which inspired Korean surgeons. Subsequently, Dr. Eum learned the UBE technique from Dr. Gaffar, introduced it to South Korea, and further developed it [3]. In the treatment of spinal stenosis, which has traditionally been performed using microscopic decompression, UBE technique can effectively decompress neural structures. Moreover, UBE offers the advantage of simultaneously decompressing contralateral foraminal stenosis within the same surgical field when it coexists.

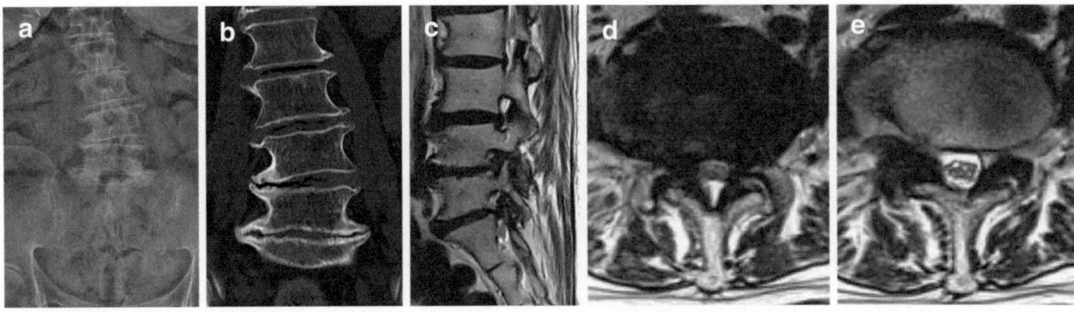

Fig. 14.1 The lumbar X-ray AP view shows decreased disc height at L4-5 on the right side (**a**) and the CT coronal reconstruction image demonstrates the same finding (**b**). On MRI, the T2 sagittal image reveals right foraminal stenosis at L4-5 (**c**) and the T2 axial image shows canal stenosis at L4-5 (**d**) and right foraminal stenosis (**e**)

14.2 Presentation of the Patient: Canal Stenosis

A 70-year-old female patient presents with low back pain and radiating leg pain that occurs during walking. Her neurogenic intermittent claudication (NIC) lasts approximately 5 minutes, and the pain subsides when sitting or lying down. MRI reveals L4-5 spinal stenosis with accompanying foraminal stenosis. X-rays show segmental coronal imbalance at L4-5, and CT images demonstrate unilateral disc height reduction (Fig. 14.1). Conservative treatment has been ineffective, so a decision has been made to perform a UBE approach at L4-5 for bilateral spinal canal decompression. Additionally, the contralateral foraminal stenosis will be decompressed using a contralateral sublaminar approach.

14.3 Preoperative Planning and Surgical Steps: Canal Stenosis

The surgery is performed with the patient in the prone position under general anesthesia or epidural anesthesia. This positioning allows for optimal access to the surgical site and helps to open the interlaminar window, facilitating the procedure.

Preoperative planning for skin incision and initial drilling in UBE decompression for lumbar spinal stenosis is a critical process that involves several key steps. The surgeon begins by using biplanar fluoroscopy to accurately determine and mark the index level on the patient's skin. It's essential to tilt the fluoroscope parallel to the disc space to obtain a true anterior-posterior image.

The target point is the spinolaminar junction at the index level (Fig. 14.2). Two small skin incisions are required, typically placed along the medial pedicle line and separated by about 2–3 cm. The first incision, intended for the viewing portal, should be approximately 5–6 mm in length. This portal will accommodate the arthroscope and allow for continuous normal saline irrigation. The second incision, serving as the working portal, should be slightly larger, about 8–10 mm, to facilitate instrument access and fluid outflow (Fig. 14.3).

After making of surgical working space around the spinolaminar junction, the initial target area for drilling is identified at the spinolaminar junction, where the spinous process meets the lower laminar margin of the superior vertebra. This serves as the starting point for the decompression procedure. The plan is to begin drilling by using a high-speed diamond burr, typically 3 or 4 mm in diameter at the spino-laminar junction, working from the lower margin of the lamina in a cranial direction. This approach aims to expose the origin of the ligamentum flavum and the underlying epidural fat.

During UBE decompression for lumbar spinal stenosis, the removal of the ligamentum flavum and decompression of lateral recess stenosis are crucial steps. During laminectomy, the important landmark that guides the surgeon is the "midline

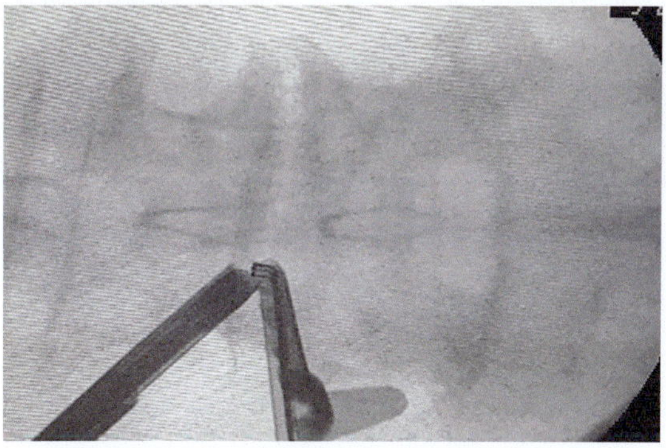

Fig. 14.2 When approaching L4-5 from the left side using UBE technique, the target point on the C-arm AP (anteroposterior) view is the spinolaminar junction of L4-5

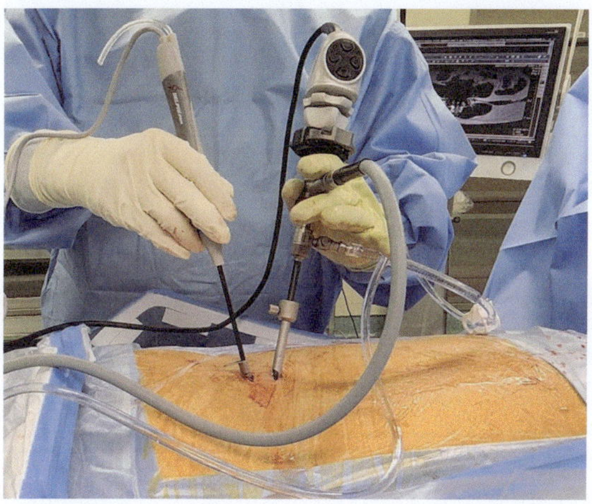

Fig. 14.3 Two small skin incisions (view portal and working portal) are required, typically placed along the medial pedicle line and separated by about 2–3 cm

cleft" of the ligamentum flavum. The ligamentum flavum has a butterfly-shaped appearance with a significant anatomical landmark called the "midline cleft" where it meets the ligament on the opposite side (Fig. 14.4). This cleft serves as a crucial landmark for identifying the midline location, even in patients with severe degenerative lumbar changes.

The superficial layer of the ligamentum flavum is then carefully separated from the lamina using a curette, moving from caudal to cranial. It's essential to preserve the deep layer initially to protect the underlying neural structures. The surgeon then uses a Kerrison punch or osteotome to

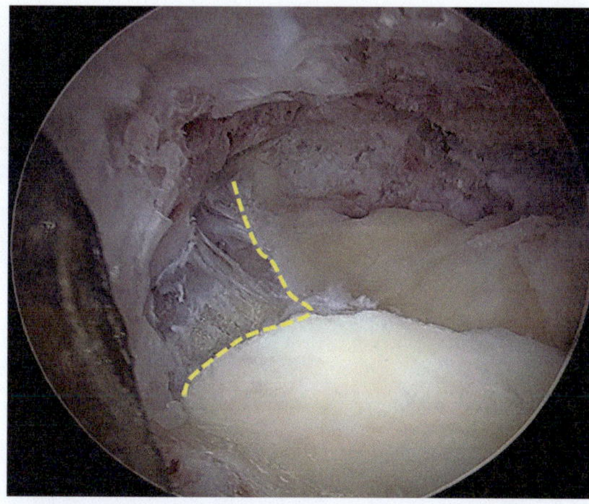

Fig. 14.4 The ligamentum flavum has a butterfly-shaped appearance (V-shaped) with a significant anatomical landmark called the "midline cleft" (dotted line) where it meets the ligament on the opposite side, and this cleft serves as a crucial landmark for identifying the midline location

detach the deep layer of the ligamentum flavum from its lower attachments.

For contralaterally spinal canal decompression, the surgeon employs an "over-the-top" technique. A blunt dissector is used to separate the ligamentum flavum from the contralateral lamina, keeping it intact with the dura for neural protection. The contralateral lateral recess is then decompressed using small, curved Kerrison punches or drill. To address the lateral recess stenosis, the surgeon performs a sublaminar medial facetectomy to preserve the integrity of the facet joint. A 3 mm or 4 mm diamond drill is used for bony decompression of the facet joint and lateral recess. The remaining ligamentum flavum is delicately resected using a curette or punch to completely relieve the neural structures on both sides.

To perform contralateral foraminal decompression, first, the position of the contralateral superior articular process (SAP) is identified. The upper margin of the pedicle (L5) where the SAP begins is then located using instruments such as a curette. Next, an angled osteotome is used to remove the SAP en bloc (Fig. 14.5). Following this, the ligamentum flavum surrounding the exiting nerve is removed, thereby decompressing the exiting nerve root.

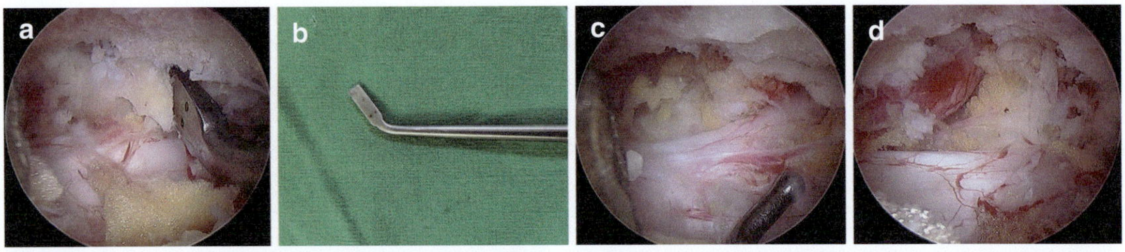

Fig. 14.5 The right L5 superior articular process (SAP) is being removed en bloc using a curved osteotome (**a**, **b**). After removal, the exiting L4 nerve root can be visualized (**c**). Within the same endoscopic view, both the exiting nerve root (L4) and the traversing nerve root (L5) can be simultaneously observed (**d**)

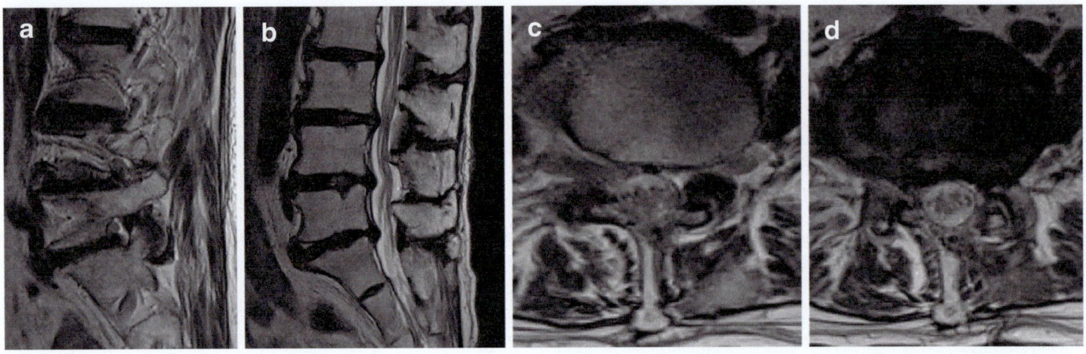

Fig. 14.6 Postoperative MRI findings: The T2 sagittal images demonstrate widening of the L4-5 foramen (**a**). On T2 axial images, the previously observed canal stenosis has been resolved (**b**). The axial images reveal that the right L4-5 foraminal stenosis has been alleviated (**c**). These axial images confirm the resolution of the bilateral canal stenosis that was present before the surgery (**d**)

Postoperative MRI confirmed that the canal stenosis and foraminal stenosis were resolved (Fig. 14.6).

14.4 Presentation of the Patient: Foraminal Stenosis

A 72-year-old female patient presents with low back pain and radiating leg pain that occurs during walking. Her neurogenic intermittent claudication (NIC) lasts approximately 2~3 minutes, and the pain subsides when sitting or lying down. MRI reveals L5-S1 foraminal and extraforaminal stenosis (Fig. 14.7). Conservative treatment has been ineffective, so a decision has been made to perform a UBE approach at L5-S1 through the Wiltse approach for foraminal decompression.

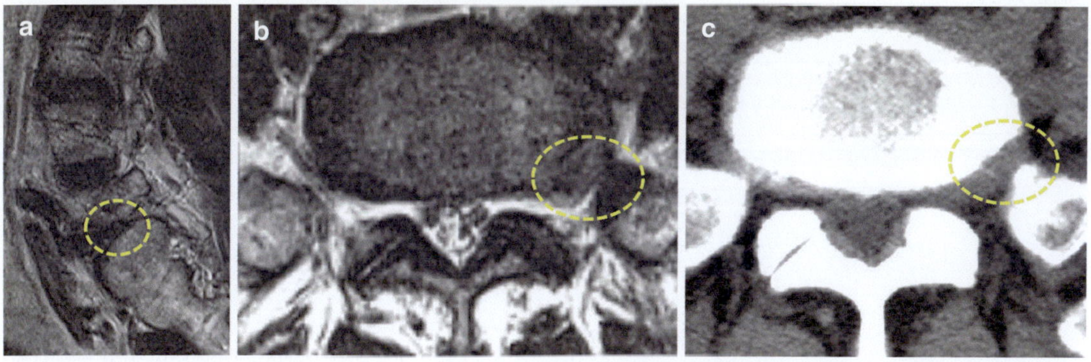

Fig. 14.7 Preoperative MRI: The T2 sagittal image reveals left extraforaminal stenosis at L5-S1 (**a**) and the T2 axial image shows the same finding (**b**), Preoperative CT: extra foraminal stenosis by alar (**c**)

14.5 Preoperative Planning and Surgical Steps: Foraminal or Extraforaminal Stenosis

UBE decompression using the Wiltse approach for foraminal or extraforaminal stenosis at L5-S1 in the lumbar spine is a minimally invasive technique that combines the benefits of endoscopic surgery with the muscle-sparing advantages of the Wiltse approach.

The procedure begins with the patient positioned prone on a radiolucent frame. The skin entry point is determined by targeting the isthmus, positioning it 1–2 cm lateral to the lateral margin of the pedicle, following the Wiltse approach (Fig. 14.8). This technique preserves the multifidus muscle and minimizes soft tissue damage. The surgeon then performs blunt dissection between the multifidus and longissimus muscles to access the lateral aspect of the facet joint.

An endoscope is introduced through one portal, while surgical instruments are inserted through the other. Using endoscopic burrs, the surgeon carefully removes part of the superior articular process and the superolateral portion of the pars interarticularis to widen the foramen. The hypertrophied ligamentum flavum and any protruding disc material are then removed using endoscopic instruments (Fig. 14.9). Throughout the procedure, the surgeon must exercise caution to preserve facet integrity, protect nerve roots, and maintain clear visualization. It's crucial to avoid excessive facet joint violation, which could lead to instability, and to carefully manipulate around the exiting and traversing nerve roots to prevent neurological complications.

Proper control of irrigation fluid pressure and outflow is essential to maintain a clear surgical field. The goal of the decompression is to achieve free mobilization of the exiting L5 nerve root. Meticulous hemostasis is performed throughout the procedure to prevent postoperative hematoma formation and ensure clear endoscopic visualization. When using radiofrequency or electrocautery devices, the surgeon must be mindful of the proximity to neural structures to avoid thermal damage. By combining the Wiltse approach with UBE techniques, surgeons can achieve effective decompression of foraminal and extraforaminal stenosis at L5-S1 while minimizing tissue damage (Fig. 14.10).

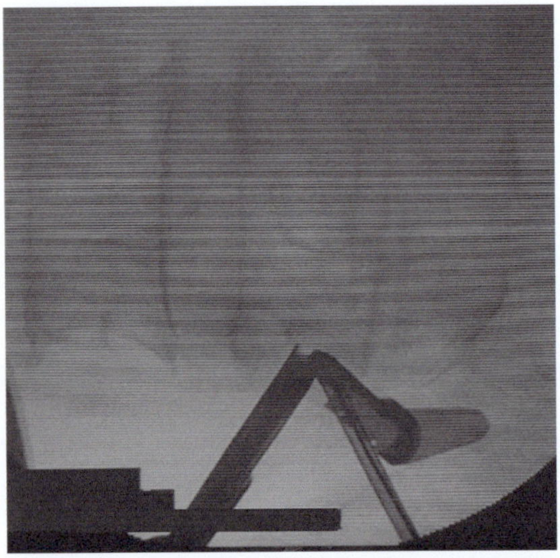

Fig. 14.8 Under C-arm guidance, the approach is made using the Wiltse technique, targeting the L5 isthmus

14.6 Commentary

When performing decompression surgery for spinal stenosis by UBE technique, several key points should be considered.

Neurological protection is paramount. During flavectomy of the target compartment, care must be taken to avoid injuring the nerve root that runs ventrally the lateral recess [4]. Dural tear prevention is crucial. Meticulous dissection is required when separating the ligamentum flavum from the dura or decompressing areas adjacent to the dura, as the risk of dural tear is high in these regions. This precaution helps prevent cerebrospinal fluid leakage [5, 6].

In the event of a dural tear, the appropriate management depends on the size of the tear. If the tear is large, open surgery is necessary to per-

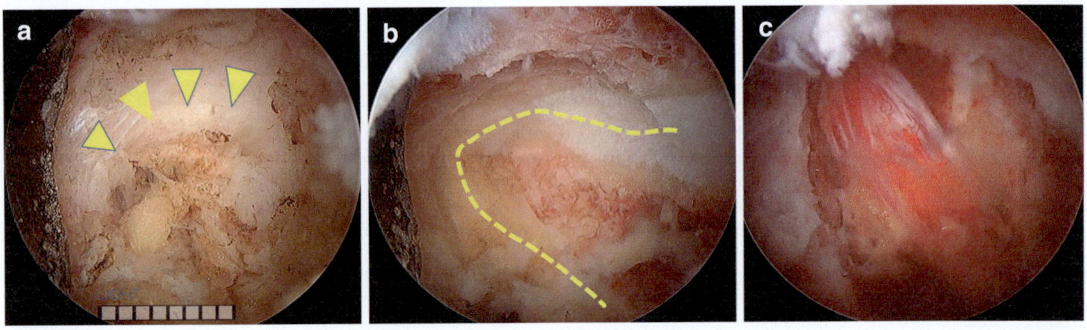

Fig. 14.9 In the endoscopic view, the isthmus of the left L5 (arrowheads) is observed (**a**) After endoscopic drilling, the area around the tip of the SAP (dotted line) is exposed (**b**). The ligamentum flavum is removed, and the L5 exiting nerve root is decompressed (**c**)

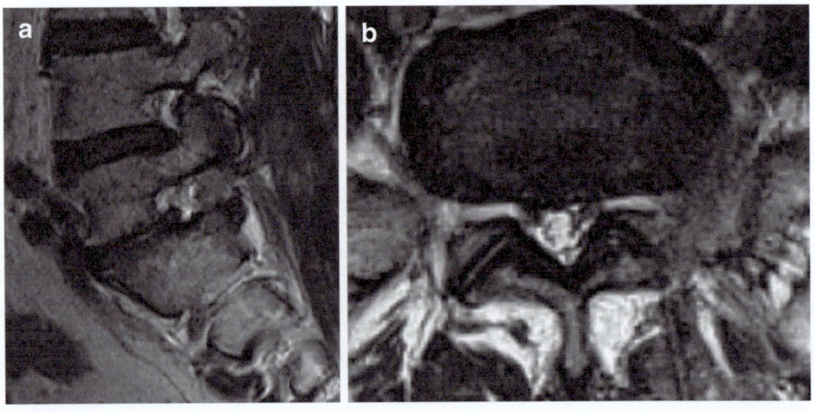

Fig. 14.10 Postoperative MRI findings: The T2 sagittal images demonstrate widening of the L5-S1 foramen (**a**) On T2 axial images, the previously observed extraforaminal stenosis has been resolved (**b**)

form a dural repair. However, for smaller tears, approximately 2-3 mm in size, the application of hemostatic agents such as TachoSil (tachocomb) may be sufficient to resolve the issue. This approach can often effectively seal small dural tears without the need for more invasive surgical intervention [7, 8].

Water pressure management is critical during UBE. It is recommended to maintain water pressure below 30 mmHg when possible to prevent complications such as increased intracranial pressure, which can lead to postoperative headaches, neck stiffness, seizures, and retroperitoneal fluid collection [9].

Hemostasis is crucial to prevent postoperative hematoma. Techniques such as en bloc removal of the ligamentum flavum and careful coagulation of bleeding sources should be employed [10]. Controlling bone bleeding that occurs during bone drilling with bone wax helps prevent postoperative hematoma formation.

Infection prevention should be prioritized, especially in high-risk patients such as those with diabetes, cancer, liver cirrhosis, chronic renal failure, advanced age, or long-term steroid use. These patients are more susceptible to postoperative inflammation and require special attention [4]. Generally, it is reported that the risk of infection in UBE surgery is very low due to the irrigation system [11]. Adequate decompression should be achieved while minimizing soft tissue and facet joint destruction to preserve segmental stability [5].

By adhering to these precautions and techniques, surgeons can safely and effectively perform UBE decompression for spinal stenosis while minimizing complications and preserving spinal stability.

References

1. Choi G, Pophale CS, Patel B, Uniyal P. Endoscopic spine surgery. J Korean Neurosurg Soc. 2017;60(5):485–97.
2. Antonacci CL, Zeng FR, Ford B, Wellington I, Kia C, Zhou H. A narrative review of endoscopic spine surgery: history, indications, uses, and future directions. J Spine Surg. 2024;10(2)
3. Eum JH, Heo DH, Son SK, Park CK. Percutaneous biportal endoscopic decompression for lumbar spinal stenosis: a technical note and preliminary clinical results. J Neurosurg Spine. 2016;24:602–7.
4. So J-Y, Park J-Y. Essential surgical techniques during unilateral biportal endoscopic spine surgery. J Minim Invasive Spine Surg Tech. 2023;8(2):186–97.
5. Pao J-L, Lin S-M, Chen W-C, Chang C-H. Unilateral biportal endoscopic decompression for degenerative lumbar canal stenosis. J Spine Surg. 2020;6(2):438–46.
6. Yu H, Zhao Q, Lv J, Liu J, Zhu B, Chen L, Jing J, Tian D. Unintended dural tears during unilateral biportal endoscopic lumbar surgery: incidence and risk factors. Acta Neurochir (Wien). 2024;166(1):95.
7. Park HJ, Kim SK, Lee SC, Kim W, Han S, Kang SS. Dural tears in percutaneous biportal endoscopic spine surgery: anatomical location and management. World Neurosurg. 2020;136:e578–85.
8. Lee HG, Kang MS, Kim SY, Cho KC, Na YC, Cho JM, et al. Dural injury in unilateral biportal endoscopic spinal surgery. Glob Spine J. 2021;11:845–51.
9. Kim JE, Choi DJ, Kim MC, Park EJ. Risk factors of postoperative spinal epidural hematoma after biportal endoscopic spinal surgery. World Neurosurg. 2019;129:e324–9.
10. Wang B, He P, Liu X, Wu Z, Xu B. Complications of unilateral biportal endoscopic spinal surgery for lumbar spinal stenosis: a systematic review of the literature and meta-analysis of single-arm studies. Orthop Surg. 2022;15(1):3–15.
11. Lee SY, Shin DA, Yi S, Ha Y, Kim KN, Lee CK. Overview and prevention of complications during biportal endoscopic lumbar spine surgery. J Minim Invasive Spine Surg Tech. 2023;8(2):145–52.

15 Full Endoscopic Interlaminar Decompression

Hyun Jin Ma

Abstract

Uniportal full-endoscopic spine surgery is a highly advanced minimally invasive technique that provides exceptional flexibility in addressing various spinal pathologies with precision. Through the use of thin and elongated instruments, it facilitates targeted neural decompression while effectively preserving paraspinal muscles, stabilizing ligaments, and critical bony structures. This approach not only minimizes iatrogenic damage but also significantly reduces postoperative pain, accelerates recovery times, and allows for earlier patient mobilization and discharge. By minimizing surgical trauma and optimizing outcomes, uniportal full-endoscopic surgery has become a key advancement in modern spine surgery. This chapter examines the clinical advantages, technical aspects, and practical applications of this surgical approach.

Keywords

Full endoscopy · Uniportal endoscopy · Lumbar stenosis · Minimally invasive spine surgery

15.1 Introduction

Every surgeon strives to fully address the patient's pathology while minimizing damage to surrounding healthy tissues. Over the generations, minimally invasive approaches have been prioritized, leading to the development of the endoscope. In the field of spinal endoscopy, a major milestone was the introduction of percutaneous posterolateral endoscopic lumbar disc decompression by Kambin in 1983. Since then, not only has the endoscope itself evolved but also various instruments such as high-speed drills, lasers, working cannulas, radiofrequency probes, different types of Kerrison punches, and chisels designed for endoscopic use have been developed. These advancements have significantly expanded the indications for endoscopic surgery. Initially limited to treating soft disc herniation and annuloplasty, endoscopic techniques are now applicable to spinal stenosis involving hard components such as hard discs or ossified ligamentum flavum. Endoscopic approaches have even been extended to spinal fusion procedures. More recently, efforts have been made to incorporate advanced technologies such as navigation and robotic systems into endoscopic surgeries, enhancing accuracy and reducing procedural complexity [1, 2]. Uniportal full-endoscopic surgery, in particular, offers remarkable flexibility due to its thin and elongated instruments, allowing access to nearly all spinal lesions regardless

H. J. Ma (✉)
Department of Neurosurgery, Daegu Wooridul Spine Hospital, Daegu, Korea (Republic of)
e-mail: srevolution@hanmail.net

S.-H. Lee et al. (eds.), *Ligament Reconstruction for Spine*,
https://doi.org/10.1007/978-981-95-3971-0_15

of the approach angle or distance. Moreover, compared to open surgery, it minimizes damage to paraspinal muscles, ligaments, and bony structures, enabling early patient recovery [3–6]. The smaller incision, minimized tissue damage, and continuous fluid irrigation of the surgical site contribute to the low infection rate, facilitate easier wound care, and promote quicker hospital discharge [7]. The minimal invasiveness of such surgeries serves as an advantage even in elderly patients [8]. This chapter will explore the surgical techniques that leverage the advantages and unique characteristics of uniportal full-endoscopic surgery, illustrating its effectiveness through clinical case applications.

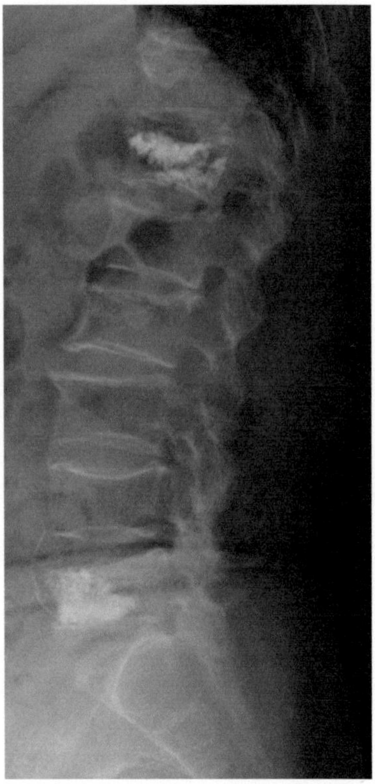

Fig. 15.1 The X-ray showed vertebroplasty that had been performed at T12 and L5, with no definite instability observed at L4-

15.2 Presentation of the Patient

15.2.1 Case 1

The patient is a 72-year-old woman who presented with an 8-year history of low back pain and bilateral leg claudication, with exacerbated severe left leg pain starting 2 weeks prior to presentation. A plain radiograph showed no definite instability (Fig. 15.1). Magnetic resonance imaging (MRI) of the lumbar spine revealed L4-5 stenosis accompanied by bilateral lateral recess stenosis (Fig. 15.2). MR myelogram showed a total signal block at L4-5 (Fig. 15.3). A uniportal full-endoscopic unilateral approach for bilateral decompression was performed at L4-5. Postoperative MRI confirmed that the central stenosis and bilateral lateral recess stenosis were successfully decompressed (Fig. 15.4). The patient was discharged on postoperative day 2.

15.2.2 Case 2

The patient was a 64-year-old male who presented with a 3-year history of low back pain and bilateral claudication, with worsening left leg pain over the past 2 months. MRI revealed central canal stenosis at L3-4 and L4-5, along with a left central disc herniation at L4-5 (Fig. 15.5). MR myelography showed a total signal block at L3-4-5 (Fig. 15.6). As the signal block was nearly continuous, hemilaminectomy at L4 was planned. Uniportal full endoscopic unilateral approach for bilateral decompression was performed at the L3-4-5 levels. Since this involved two levels, the procedure was performed through a single incision. Intraoperative C-arm imaging confirmed work being performed at both the L3-4 and L4-5 levels (Fig. 15.7). Postoperative MRI demonstrated decompression of the thecal sac and removal of the disc at L4-5 (Fig. 15.8). The patient was discharged on postoperative day 2.

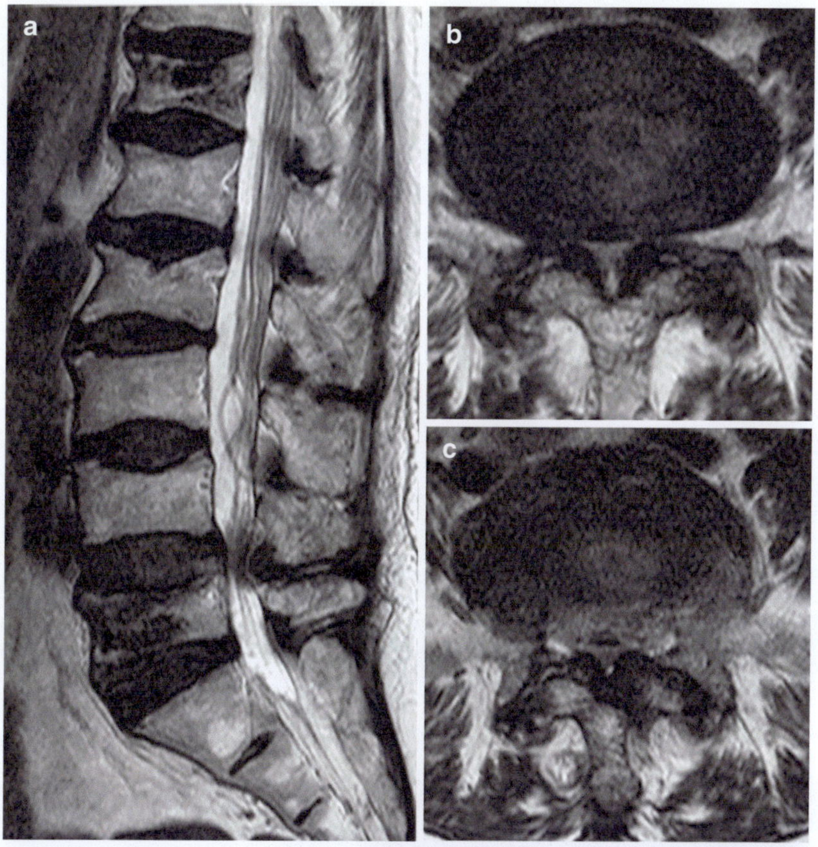

Fig. 15.2 Preoperative MRI. (**a**) Sagittal MRI showed L4-5 stenosis. (**b**) Axial MRI showed central canal stenosis. (**c**) Axial MRI showed bilateral lateral recess stenosis

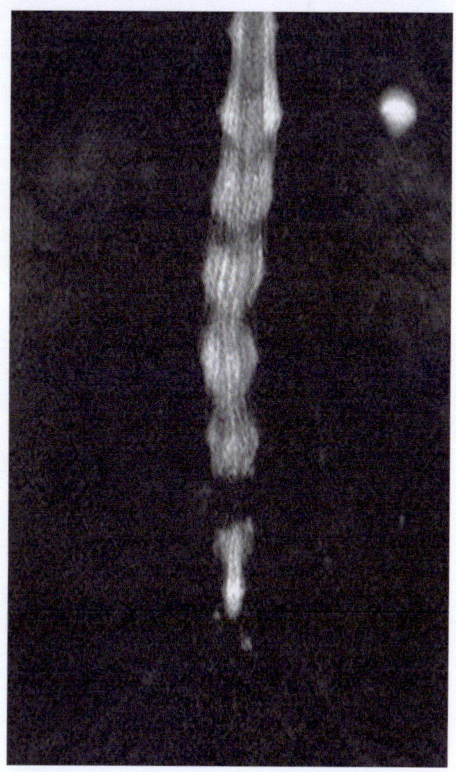

Fig. 15.3 The MR myelogram showed a total signal block at L4-5

Fig. 15.4 Postoperative MRI. (**a**) Sagittal MRI showed the decompressed L4-5 level. (**b**) Axial MRI showed the central stenosis decompressed, with the thecal sac expanded. (**c**) Axial MRI showed the bilateral lateral recesses decompressed

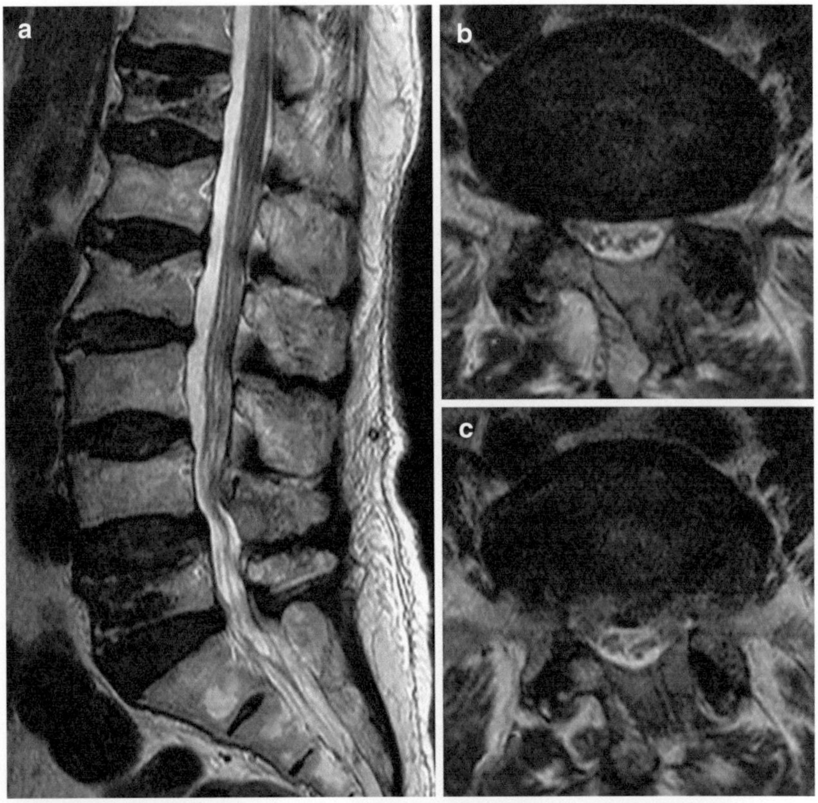

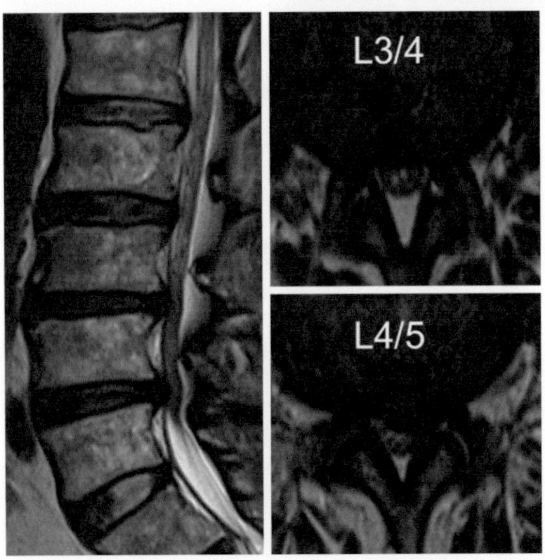

Fig. 15.5 The preoperative MRI showed central canal stenosis at L3-4-5 and a left central ruptured disc herniation at L4-5

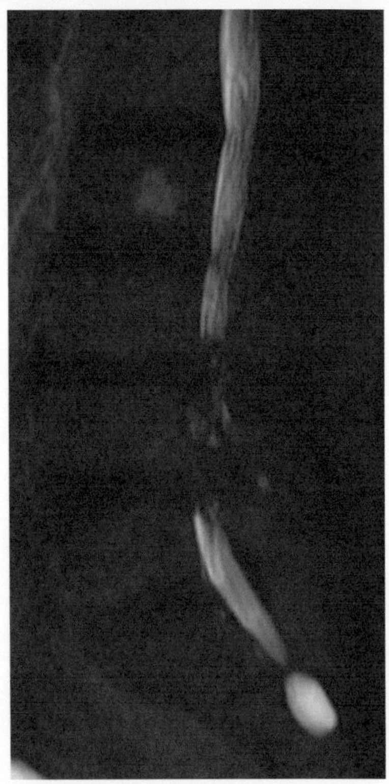

Fig. 15.6 The MR myelogram showed an almost continuous total signal block at L3-4-5

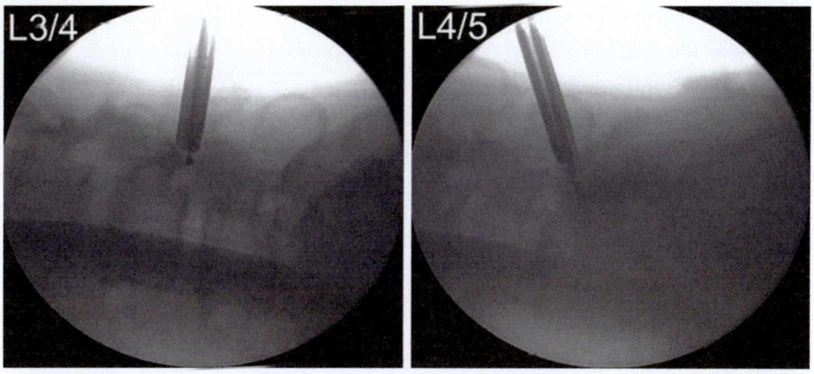

Fig. 15.7 The intraoperative C-arm image showed the endoscope covering both the L3-4 and L4-5 levels by adjusting its angle from a single incision point

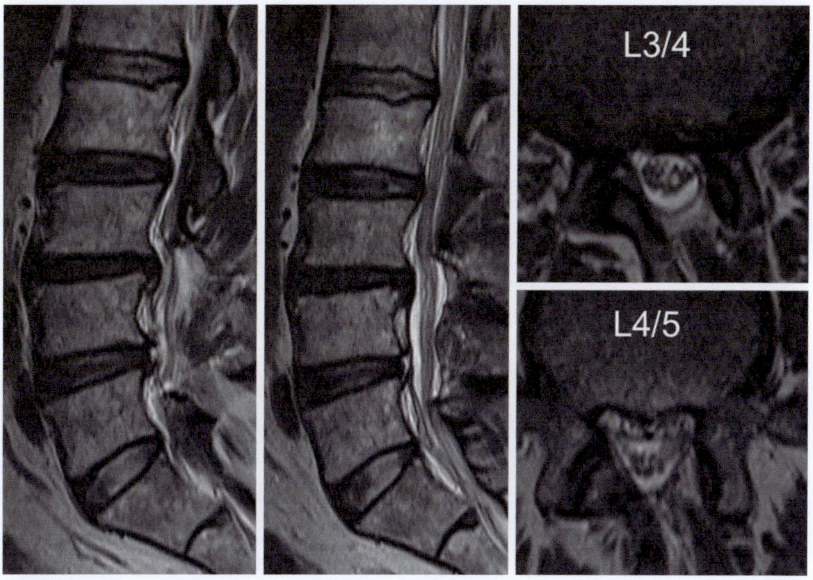

Fig. 15.8 The postoperative MRI showed the restored thecal sac after the removal of stenosis and the disc

15.3 Preoperative Planning

15.3.1 Indications

For patients who do not respond to conservative treatment or those with progressive paralysis,

- Spinal stenosis
- Lateral recess stenosis
- Foraminal stenosis
- Disc herniation (hard or soft)

15.3.2 Contraindications

- Severe spinal instability
- Tumor
- Infection
- Significant kyphosis
- Significant scoliosis

15.3.3 Imaging Assessment

- *MRI*: This is the most fundamental and essential imaging study for evaluating lumbar stenosis. It allows for the accurate identification of the location and severity of central canal stenosis, as well as the detection of associated foraminal stenosis and disc herniation.
- *CT*: Computed tomography is useful for assessing calcified lesions and determining the location and extent of spinal stenosis.

- *L-spine X-ray*: This imaging modality helps assess the presence and severity of spinal instability and kyphosis.
- *MR Myelography*: MR myelography is valuable for determining whether there is nerve compression. When combined with MRI, it aids in delineating the extent of the surgical field.
- *NCV-EMG*: Nerve conduction velocity and electromyography are used to assess radiculopathy and to confirm the presence of potential concomitant myelopathy.
- *Root Selective Block*: This procedure allows for a detailed assessment of radiculopathy, aiding in determining the surgical range.

15.3.4 Equipment (Fig. 15.9)

- 150-mm working length, dual irrigation channels, 15° optical angle, and 4.7-mm outer diameter with 7.3-mm working channel endoscope (iLESSYS Pro, Joimax, Inc.).
- Serial dilators

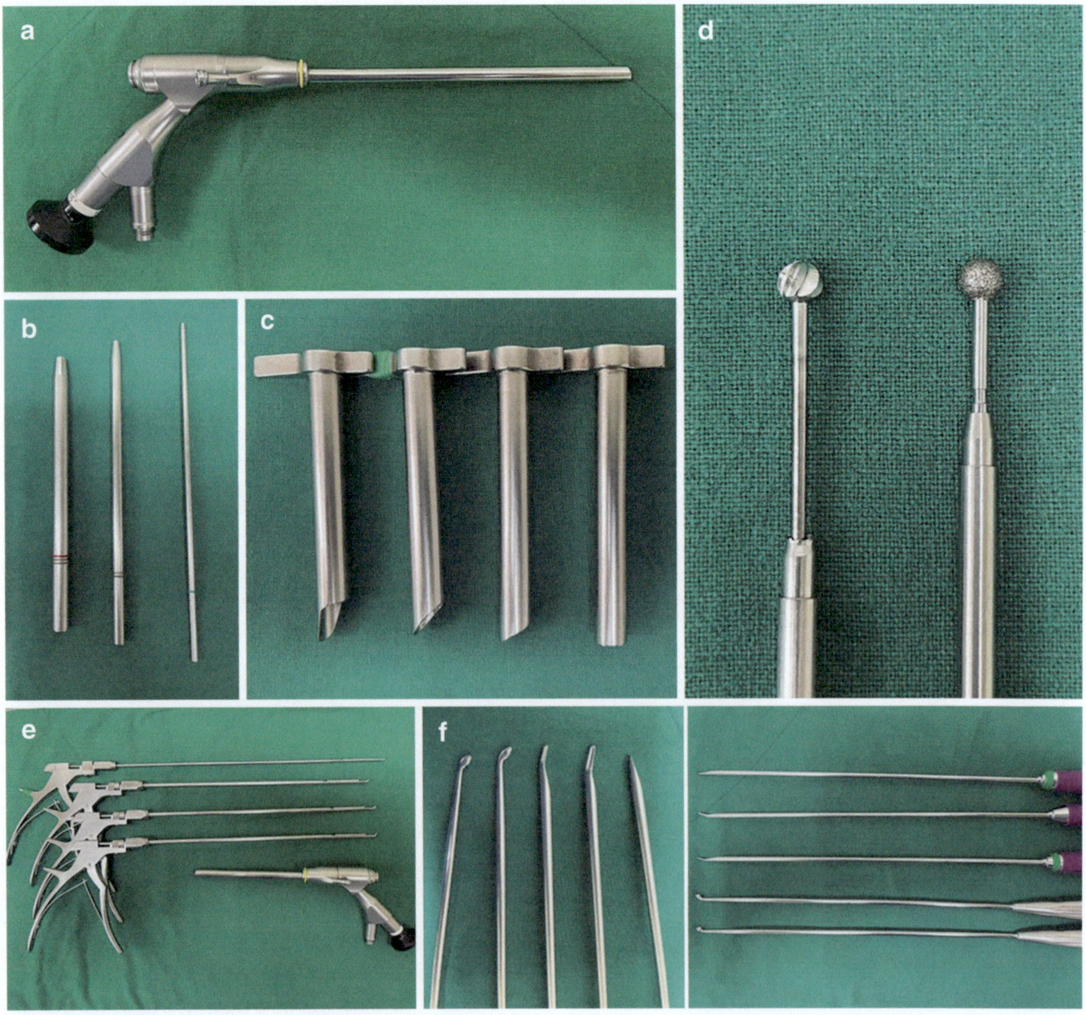

Fig. 15.9 Various instruments. (**a**) Endoscope. (**b**) Serial dilators. (**c**) Working tubes with various tip shapes. (**d**) Burr tips of different types. (**e**) Endoscopic Kerrison punches in various lengths and sizes. (**f**) Endoscopic probe, curettes, and chisel

- Working tube of various shape
- High-speed drill of various shape
- Endoscopic punch, probe, curette, chisel
- Radiofrequency probe
- *C-arm*: The uniportal endoscope significantly magnifies the smallest areas, so a C-arm is necessary to accurately confirm orientation during surgery
- *Fluid Irrigation Pump*: Endoscopic surgery is a water-based procedure, and the pump facilitates clear visualization by washing away surgical debris and blood. Occasionally, increasing the pressure helps identify the focus of massive bleeding.

15.4 Surgical Steps

15.4.1 Patient Position and Anesthesia

This surgery can be performed with the patient positioned prone on a Wilson frame, using various anesthesia methods such as general, epidural, or local anesthesia. Proper positioning adjustments are required based on the patient's body morphology. The surgery was carried out in a uniportal full endoscopic approach.

15.4.2 Skin Incision

Using the C-arm lateral view, confirm the surgical level and the location of the lesion. Palpate the spinous process and make a single small skin incision of 9 mm as close as possible to the lateral side of the spinous process. If the incision is made too caudal, the angle of the punch will become too horizontal, making it difficult to work on the upper lamina. Therefore, determine the incision site while considering the angle required for the instruments.

15.4.3 Working Tube and Endoscope Insertion

Through the skin incision, the obturator is inserted over the ipsilateral spinolaminar junction, and a working tube is advanced along the obturator. The obturator is then removed, and the endoscope is inserted into the working tube. We used a 150-mm working length endoscope with two irrigation channels, a 7.3-mm outer diameter and a 4.7-mm working channel (iLESSYS Pro, Joimax, Inc., Irvine, CA, USA) (Fig. 15.10).

15.4.4 Ipsilateral Decompression

After landing on the spinolaminar junction area of the cranial lamina, the soft tissue is cleared. Carefully identify and clean the point where the caudal edge of the lamina meets the spinous process, where the angle changes sharply. The change in angle can be palpated with a probe. Perform a laminectomy cranially using a drill. Since the inner layer of the ligamentum flavum is broadly and strongly attached to the cranial lamina, the laminectomy should proceed sufficiently until the ligamentum flavum detaches cranially. For patients with bony stenosis, additional bone

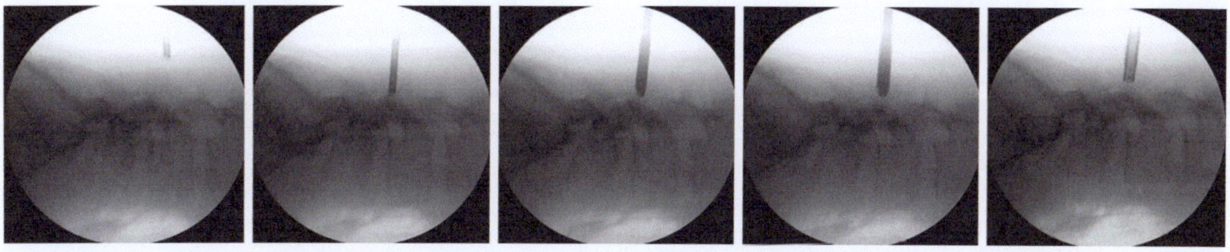

Fig. 15.10 The intraoperative C-arm images show the process from level check to endoscope insertion. From left to right: the level is checked; a thin obturator is inserted considering the surgical site and angle; a thicker obturator is inserted; a working tube is inserted; the obturator is removed, and the endoscope is inserted into the working tube

work should be performed as calculated preoperatively. For patients requiring bilateral decompression, ensure the landmark is established by confirming the detachment point of the ligamentum flavum medially. Proceed caudally with the laminectomy, taking care as the ligamentum flavum is thinly attached to the caudal lamina. Identify where the ligamentum flavum detaches medially and follow the curve of the lamina's upper margin craniolaterally until reaching the lateral recess. Use a punch or a probe to safely isolate the ligamentum flavum by observing the detached area. For patients with accompanying lateral recess stenosis, caution is necessary when inserting the punch near the lateral recess. First, detach the disc, thecal sac, and traversing root to make them movable. Then, position the punch opening laterally to decompress the lateral recess without nerve injury. Palpate the medial margin of the pedicle of the caudal vertebra to use it as a landmark for determining the extent of bone resection.

15.4.5 Contralateral Decompression

During ipsilateral surgery, the medial detachment point of the ligamentum flavum is identified and used as the center for contralateral flavectomy. For cranial laminectomy, the ventral lamina is removed using a drill while leaving the ligamentum flavum intact as a protector. In the caudal area, since the ligamentum flavum is weakly attached, extra caution is required when using the drill. Following the lateral trajectory leads to the contralateral lateral recess. Care must also be taken when inserting the punch into the lateral recess. If there is severe lateral recess stenosis, similar to the ipsilateral side, the neural components should be released to make them movable. Then, the punch should be directed laterally to ensure safe decompression (Fig. 15.11). In endoscopic surgery, central dural folding is often observed, likely caused by fluid irrigation from the endoscope and the dura's connective tissue (Fig. 15.12) [9, 10]. The folded thecal sac may resemble part of the ligamentum flavum, increasing the risk of incidental dural tears. Therefore, if epidural fat is present, the punch should be inserted above the fat layer. If the fat is absent, the ligamentum flavum and thecal sac must be clearly separated before inserting the punch. If bone work is performed bilaterally first, the ligamentum flavum can be removed en bloc. When bilateral decompression is properly

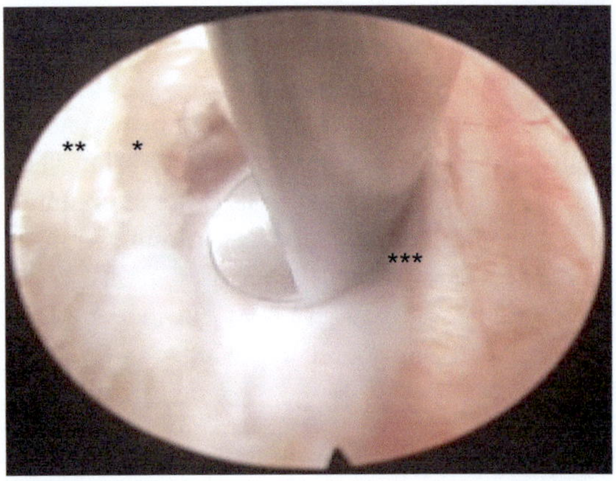

Fig. 15.11 The image shows the use of a punch in the contralateral lateral recess. The mouth of the punch is directed laterally, with the thecal sac and root released and safely positioned dorsally to the punch. The asterisk (*) indicates the superior articular process. The double asterisks (**) indicate the inferior articular process. The triple (***) asterisks indicate the traversing root, which has been released and medially displaced

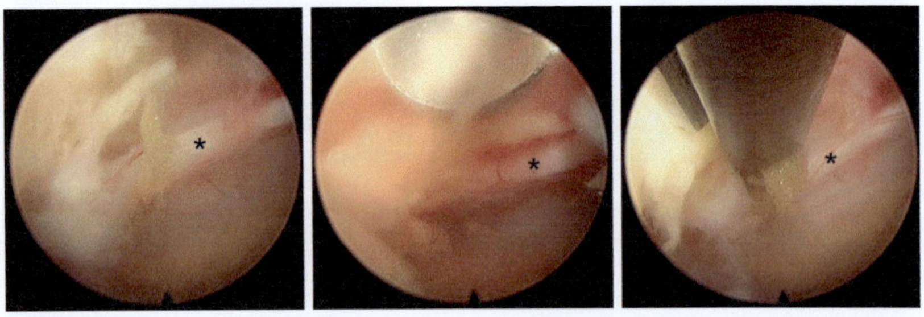

Fig. 15.12 The endoscopic view shows the use of a punch while avoiding the central dural folding. The asterisk (*) indicates the central dural folding

achieved, the thecal sac can be observed freely fluttering due to pulsation and irrigation fluid.

15.4.6 Drainage and Closure

A drain was inserted at the surgical site, and a subcutaneous tunnel was created to exit the drain at a different location from the incision. The skin was closed with two subcutaneous sutures and skin bond.

15.5 Commentary

Uniportal full-endoscopic spine surgery represents a transformative advancement in the field of minimally invasive spinal procedures. By leveraging the precise visualization and targeted decompression afforded by advanced endoscopic tools, this approach offers significant advantages over traditional open and even other minimally invasive techniques. Key benefits include minimized tissue disruption, reduced postoperative pain, shorter recovery periods, and earlier mobilization, all of which contribute to improved patient satisfaction and outcomes. The smaller incision, minimized tissue damage, and continuous fluid irrigation of the surgical site further enhance these benefits, resulting in lower infection rates, easier wound care, and quicker hospital discharge. These attributes make this approach particularly advantageous for elderly patients, who often face increased risks with traditional open surgery. As technological advancements such as navigation and robotic integration continue to evolve, the potential for greater accuracy and expanded indications for endoscopic spine surgery will further solidify its role in modern spinal care. However, it is essential to recognize that endoscopic surgery demands a steep learning curve, and its success heavily relies on the surgeon's expertise and familiarity with the nuances of endoscopic instruments and anatomy. In conclusion, uniportal full-endoscopic surgery is one of the most promising options in minimally invasive spine surgery, combining technical precision with superior clinical outcomes. Its adoption in spinal care will continue to grow as surgeons refine their skills and new technologies further enhance procedural capabilities.

References

1. Schmidt BT, Chen KT, Kim J, Brooks NP. Applications of navigation in full-endoscopic spine surgery. Eur Spine J. 2024;33(2):429–37. https://doi.org/10.1007/s00586-023-07918-8.
2. Heo DH, Ha Y, Yi S, Chung H. The future of minimally invasive spine surgery. Neurol India. 2022;70(Supplement):S104–s7. https://doi.org/10.4103/0028-3886.360930.
3. Komp M, Hahn P, Oezdemir S, Giannakopoulos A, Heikenfeld R, Kasch R, et al. Bilateral spinal decompression of lumbar central stenosis with the full-endoscopic interlaminar versus microsurgical laminotomy technique: a prospective, randomized, controlled study. Pain Physician. 2015;18(1):61–70.
4. Gadjradj PS, Rubinstein SM, Peul WC, Depauw PR, Vleggeert-Lankamp CL, Seiger A, et al. Full endoscopic versus open discectomy for sciatica: randomised controlled non-inferiority trial. BMJ. 2022;376:e065846. https://doi.org/10.1136/bmj-2021-065846.
5. Hasan S, Härtl R, Hofstetter CP. The benefit zone of full-endoscopic spine surgery. J Spine Surg. 2019;5(Suppl 1):S41–s56. https://doi.org/10.21037/jss.2019.04.19.
6. Ahn Y. Current techniques of endoscopic decompression in spine surgery. Ann Transl Med. 2019;7(Suppl 5):S169. https://doi.org/10.21037/atm.2019.07.98.
7. Mahan MA, Prasse T, Kim RB, Sivakanthan S, Kelly KA, Kashlan ON, et al. Full-endoscopic spine surgery diminishes surgical site infections - a propensity score-matched analysis. Spine J. 2023;23(5):695–702. https://doi.org/10.1016/j.spinee.2023.01.009.
8. Leyendecker J, Prasse T, Rückels P, Köster M, Rumswinkel L, Schunk V, et al. Full-endoscopic spine-surgery in the elderly and patients with comorbidities. Sci Rep. 2024;14(1):29188. https://doi.org/10.1038/s41598-024-80235-2.
9. Kim JE, Choi DJ, Park EJ. Risk factors and options of management for an incidental dural tear in biportal endoscopic spine surgery. Asian Spine J. 2020;14(6):790–800. https://doi.org/10.31616/asj.2019.0297.
10. Stevens DS, Balkany AD. Appearance of plica mediana dorsalis during epidurography. Pain Physician. 2006;9(3):268–70.

Part III

Recently Expanded Clinical Indications of the Ligament Reconstruction

Multilevel Lumbar Spinal Stenosis

16

Han Joong Keum

Abstract

Lumbar spinal stenosis is the narrowing of the spinal canal by surrounding bone and soft tissues, which compromises neural structures. Multilevel lumbar stenoses are encountered much more frequently, driven by aging population and increased surveillance with imaging modalities. Extensive laminectomy and facetectomy often provide sufficient decompression, but the mechanical integrity can be severely impaired, especially in multilevel decompression surgery. Patients who underwent multilevel decompressive laminectomy had more complications and may require additional arthrodesis. Ligament reconstruction using interspinous ligaments can be useful in stabilization of the spine after multilevel decompression of spinal stenosis.

Keywords

Lumbar spinal stenosis · Ligament reconstruction · Interspinous ligament Multilevel stenosis · Lumbar stabilization

16.1 Introduction

Lumbar spinal stenosis is the narrowing of the spinal canal by surrounding bone and soft tissues, which compromises neural structures. Symptoms range from numbness and fatigue to pain in the low back, buttock, and/or legs and disability, particularly in the older population [1]. Intermittent neurogenic claudication, which is defined as uni- or bilateral radicular pain during walking or standing that is relieved by sitting down or flexing the lumbar spine, is the most important feature of lumbar spinal stenosis as it limits patients' walking ability and causes a major impact on their quality of life. Lumbar stenosis can be a result of multiple factors, such as intervertebral disc protrusion, loss of intervertebral space height, hypertrophy of joint capsules and ligaments, and osteophytes. Radiographic evidence of spinal stenosis on magnetic resonance imaging (MRI) are highly prevalent among those older than 60 years of age and can be as high as 80% in a specific populations [2]. The prevalence estimates of lumbar spinal stenosis with a clinical diagnostic criterion ranged from 25% to 39% [3]. Multilevel lumbar stenoses are encountered much more frequently, driven by aging population and increased surveillance with imaging modalities.

H. J. Keum (✉)
Department of Neurosurgery, Cheongdam Wooridul Spine Hospital, Seoul, Korea (Republic of)
e-mail: hanj@wooridul.co.kr

S.-H. Lee et al. (eds.), *Ligament Reconstruction for Spine*,
https://doi.org/10.1007/978-981-95-3971-0_16

16.2 Surgical Treatment of Multilevel Spinal Stenosis

Surgical treatment of lumbar spinal stenosis can be divided into some form of decompression alone or decompression combined with arthrodesis. The main objective in the operative treatment of spinal stenosis is to provide adequate decompression without compromising the stability of the lumbar spine. Surgeons must decide whether to provide selective solutions to limited symptomatic levels or more inclusive treatments to address all levels of significant stenosis. Advancement of less invasive options such as endoscopic decompressions has enabled more frequent use of focal neural decompression in one to two levels, but decompression by laminectomy is still more favorably used in multilevel stenosis [4]. Extensive laminectomy and facetectomy often provide sufficient decompression, but the mechanical integrity can be severely impaired. The extent of the surgical procedure did worsen the outcome of surgical treatment [5]. In addition, patients who underwent multilevel decompressive laminectomy had more complications and may require arthrodesis in the follow-up period [6]. To provide additional stability after decompression, interspinous ligament devices has been used with favorable outcomes [7, 8]. Stability of the motion segment could be obtained by applying soft ligaments around the spinous processes to give some additional power. This was based on biomechanical studies in which devices similar to the interspinous ligamentous devices had a stabilizing effect in flexion, extension, and lateral bending of spinal motion segments [9]. Ligament reconstruction using interspinous ligaments can be useful in stabilization of the spine after multilevel decompression of spinal stenosis.

16.3 Surgical Procedure

A midline skin incision was made and muscle dissection was done and retracted laterally, exposing both laminae. Bilateral minimal laminotomy, preserving the facets, was performed with a high-speed drill, and the ligamentum flavum and ventral portion of the interspinous ligament were removed. After full decompression of the neural tissue, the operating table was positioned to provide lumbar extension. The artificial ligament (SH ligament) was applied around the upper and lower spinous processes of the decompressed levels and tied with non-absorbable sutures. Ligaments should be tightly tied with the spine in lordosis to conserve the proper curvature (Fig. 16.1).

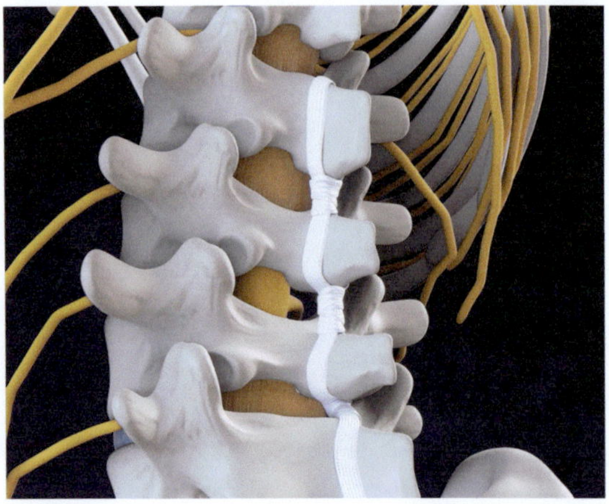

Fig. 16.1 Ligament reconstruction using artificial ligament (SH ligament) in multiple levels

16.4 Case Illustration

An 83–year-old female patient presented with severe back pain, bilateral leg radiating pain and weakness, neurogenic intermittent claudication, and walking difficulty for several years, which had been gradually deteriorating. Several years of conservative treatment, which included medication and pain block, did not improve her symptoms. On magnetic resonance (MR) imaging, central spinal stenosis was seen at multiple levels from the L1/2 to L4/5 levels with relatively preserved disc height. The patient underwent central decompression and ligament reconstruction from the L1/2 to L4/5 levels. Postoperative MR images showed complete decompression of the L1/2 to L4/5 levels. Symptoms were relieved after the operation and no complications were seen during and after the surgery (Fig. 16.2a–c).

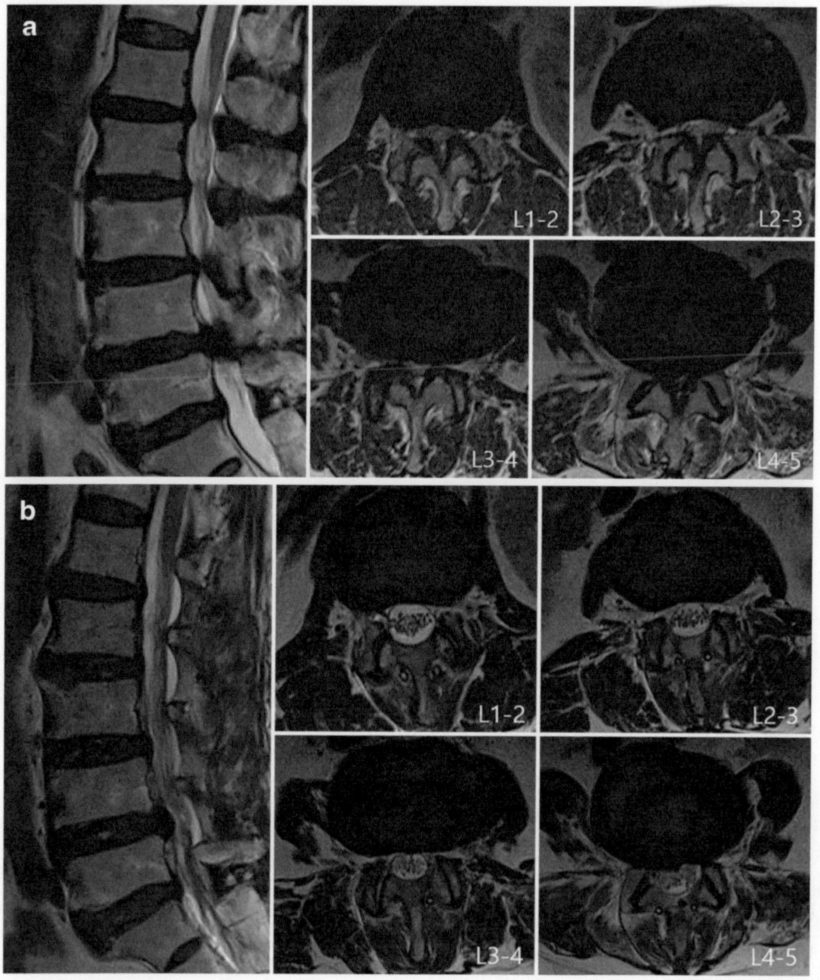

Fig. 16.2 Multilevel spinous stenosis from the L1/2 to L4/5 levels. (**a**) Preoperative T2-weighted sagittal and axial MR image. (**b**) Postoperative T2-weighted sagittal and axial MR image. (**c**) Postoperative x-ray showing placement of artificial ligaments

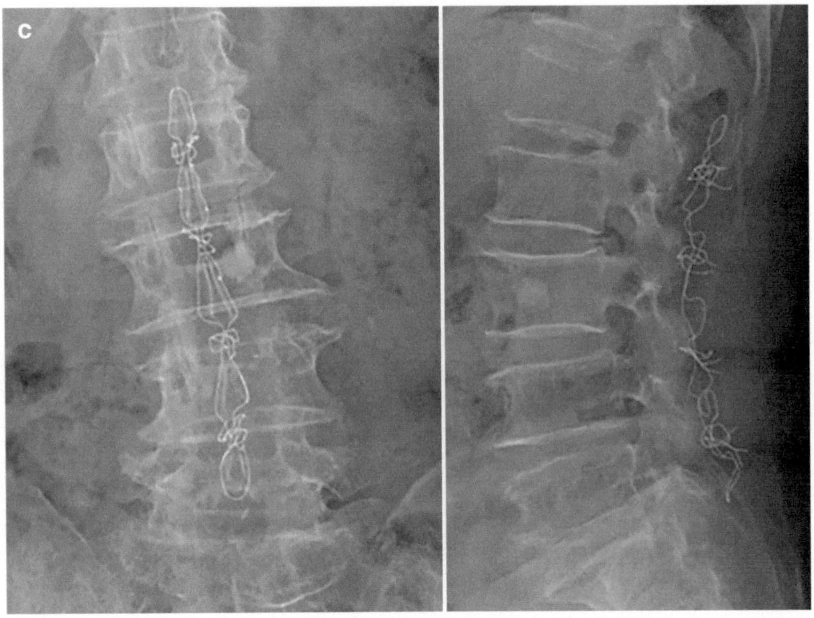

Fig. 16.2 (continued)

16.5 Summary

Multilevel lumbar stenoses are encountered much more frequently with the aging population and the advancement of imaging modalities. Surgical treatment of multilevel lumbar stenosis can be challenging because of injury to the mechanical integrity of the spine after extensive decompression. Ligament reconstruction using artificial interspinous ligaments is a useful option in stabilization of the spine after multilevel decompression of spinal stenosis without arthrodesis.

References

1. Katz JN, Harris MB. Clinical practice. Lumbar spinal stenosis. N Engl J Med. 2008;358:818–25.
2. Ishimoto Y, Yoshimura N, Muraki S, Yamada H, Nagata K, Hashizume H, Takiguchi N, Minamide A, Oka H, Kawaguchi H, Nakamura K, Akune T, Yoshida M. Associations between radiographic lumbar spinal stenosis and clinical symptoms in the general population: the Wakayama Spine Study. Osteoarthr Cartil. 2013;21:783–8.
3. Jensen RK, Jensen TS, Koes B, Hartvigsen J. Prevalence lumbar spinal stenosis in general and clinical populations: a systematic review and meta-analysis. Eur Spine J. 2020;29(9):2143–63.
4. Murata S, Nagata K, Iwasaki H, Hashizume H, Minamide A, Nakagawa Y, Tsutsui S, Takami M, Ishimoto Y, Teraguchi M, Iwahashi H, Murakami K, Taiji R, Kozaki T, Kitano Y, Yoshida M, Yamada H. Long-term outcomes after selective microendoscopic laminotomy for multilevel lumbar spinal stenosis with and without remaining radiographic stenosis: a 10-year follow-up study. Spine Surg Relat Res. 2022;6(5):488–96.
5. Grabias S. Current concepts review: the treatment of spinal stenosis. J Bone Joint Surg Am. 1980;62:308–13.
6. Adilay U, Guclu B. Comparison of single-level and multilevel decompressive laminectomy for multilevel lumbar spinal stenosis. World Neurosurg. 2018;111:E235–40.
7. Hong SW, Lee HY, Kim KH, Lee SH. Interspinous ligamentoplasty in the treatment of degenerative spondylolisthesis: midterm clinical results. J Neurosurg Spine. 2010;13(1):27–35.
8. Shim CS, Lee SH, Park SH, Whang JH. Soft stabilization with an artificial intervertebral ligament in grade 1 degenerative spondylolisthesis:comparison with instrumented posterior lumbar interbody fusion. SAS J. 2007;1(3):118–24.
9. Voydeville G, Diop A, Lavaste F, Girard F, Hardy P. Experimental lumbar instability and artificial ligament. Eur J Orthop Surg Traumatol. 2000;10:167–76.

Spinal Stenosis at Lumbosacral Junction

17

Pratyush Shahi and Sang-Ha Shin

Abstract

Soft stabilization with ligament reconstruction leads to excellent outcomes in patients with spinal stenosis. However, it can be challenging to perform ligament reconstruction for the L5-S1 spinal level. Unlike spinous processes of the lumbar vertebra, the S1 spinous process is often short and fused. As such, there is a lack of a bony docking point caudally for the longitudinal ligament. To bypass this issue, we utilize the technique of "spinous-sacrum plasty" for ligament reconstruction at the lumbosacral junction. In this technique, a high-speed diamond burr is used to create a hole in the median sacral crest bilaterally. After confirmation of bone plasty and continuity of the passageway across both sides, the needle with attached longitudinal ligament is passed through the hole. Adequate tension in the ligament is checked and ligament reconstruction is performed. This technique is safe and effective for soft stabilization of the lumbosacral junction. However, caution should be exercised not to injure the dura during this procedure.

Keywords

Lumbosacral · L5-S1 · Spinous-sacrum plasty Median sacral crest · Ligament reconstruction

17.1 Introduction

Soft stabilization with ligament reconstruction has been shown to result in excellent outcomes in patients with spinal stenosis [1–4]. It helps in restoring the degenerated interspinous ligament, which is crucial in preventing back pain after surgery. It also prevents iatrogenic instability by minimizing injury to the facet joints. Ligament reconstruction has also been shown to be associated with favorable outcomes in multilevel stenosis. Spinal stenosis is commonly seen at the lumbosacral junction. However, performing ligament reconstruction for the L5-S1 level can be difficult because of lack of a bony docking point for the longitudinal ligament caudally. In this chapter, we describe the technique of "spinous-sacrum plasty," which can be utilized to perform ligament reconstruction for spinal stenosis at the lumbosacral junction.

P. Shahi
Department of Orthopedics, Cheongdam Wooridul Spine Hospital, Seoul, Korea (Republic of)

S.-H. Shin (✉)
Department of Neurosurgery, Cheongdam Wooridul Spine Hospital, Seoul, Korea (Republic of)
e-mail: burrhoer@wooridul.co.kr

S.-H. Lee et al. (eds.), *Ligament Reconstruction for Spine*,
https://doi.org/10.1007/978-981-95-3971-0_17

17.2 Relevant Anatomy of Lumbosacral Junction

The L5-S1 level is a transitional segment between the lumbar spine and sacrum. It is an important spinal segment as it contributes significantly to the motion and lordosis of the lumbar spine. It is the most caudal motion segment of the spine and supports the entire upper body. The orientation of the sacrum also determines spinopelvic alignment (pelvic incidence, pelvic tilt, and sacral slope) and global alignment. The S1 vertebra has various anatomical differences compared to lumbar vertebra. The spinous process is shorter in length, lamina is relatively thin, dorsal surface and thecal sac are convex [5]. There is also a higher prevalence of spina bifida and other morphological variances [6]. Including the L5-S1 segment in soft stabilization surgery can be challenging as there is a lack of inferior bony docking point for the longitudinal ligament. The S1 spinous process is often small (<15 mm), fused, and has inadequate tension force within the soft tissues nearby [7]. Therefore, unlike spinous processes of the lumbar vertebra, it can fail to provide a strong docking point for the longitudinal ligament.

17.3 Spinous-Sacrum Plasty Technique

To bypass the issue of ligament docking and enable inclusion of L5-S1 segment in ligament reconstruction surgery, we utilize the "spinous-sacrum plasty" technique. It involves making a hole in the median sacral crest and passing the longitudinal ligament through the hole for a firm inferior docking point.

17.3.1 Surgical Steps

Figure 17.1 shows the location of the planned hole in the median sacral crest on preoperative sagittal CT and lateral X-ray. Intraoperatively, the length of the S1 spinous process is first checked (Fig. 17.2a, b). A 3 mm/5 mm high-speed diamond burr is used to drill a hole at the junction of the median sacral crest and S1 lamina bilaterally (Fig. 17.2c–f). Once the hole is created, a neurosurgical patty is used to protect the dura (Fig. 17.3). Curette and long probe are used to check the bone plasty and continuity of the created passageway across both sides (Fig. 17.4). The length and depth are checked (Fig. 17.5).

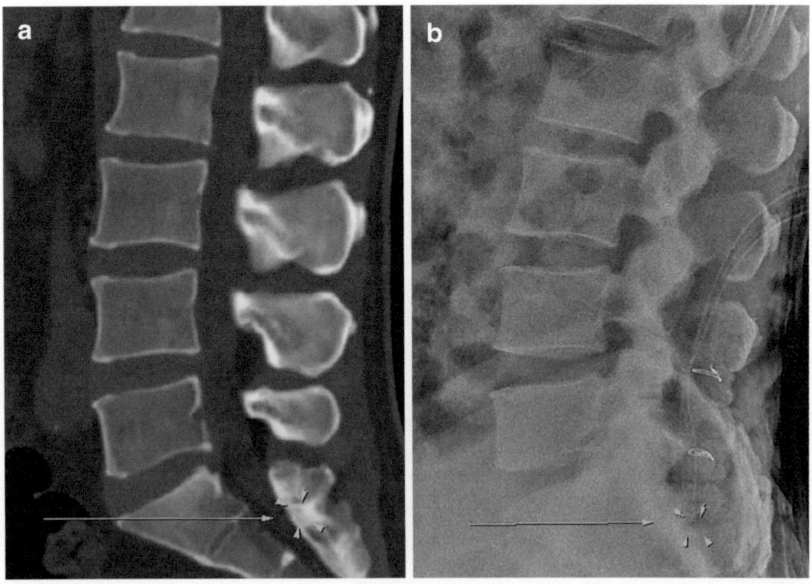

Fig. 17.1 Location of the planned hole in the median sacral crest on preoperative sagittal CT (**a**) and lateral X-ray (**b**)

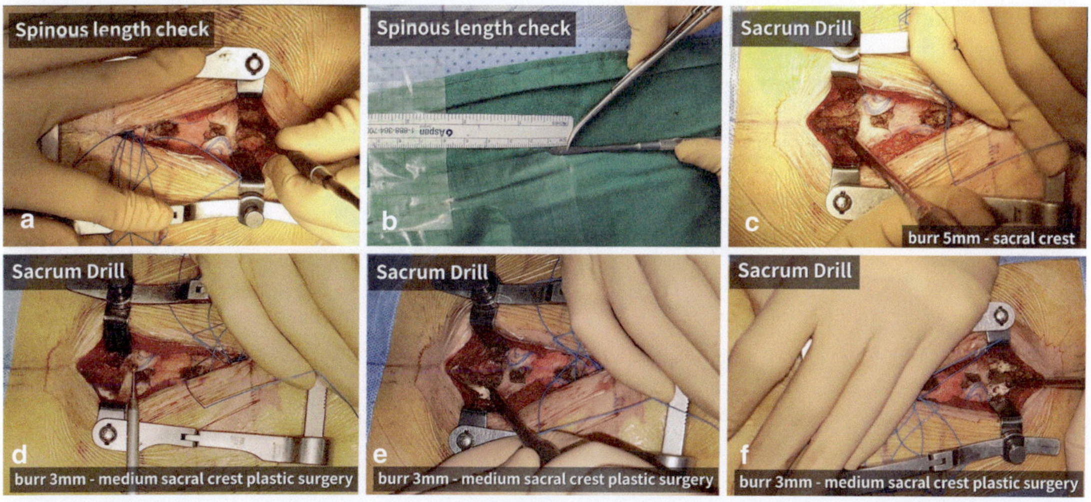

Fig. 17.2 (**a, b**) Length of the S1 spinous process is checked; (**c–f**) A 3 mm/5 mm high-speed diamond burr is used to drill a hole at the junction of the median sacral crest and S1 lamina bilaterally

Fig. 17.3 (**a–d**) Neurosurgical patty is used to protect the dura

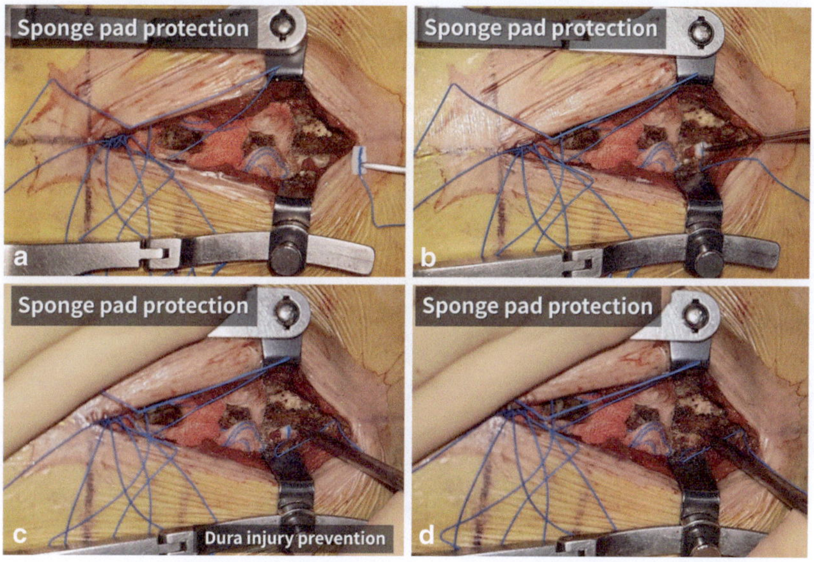

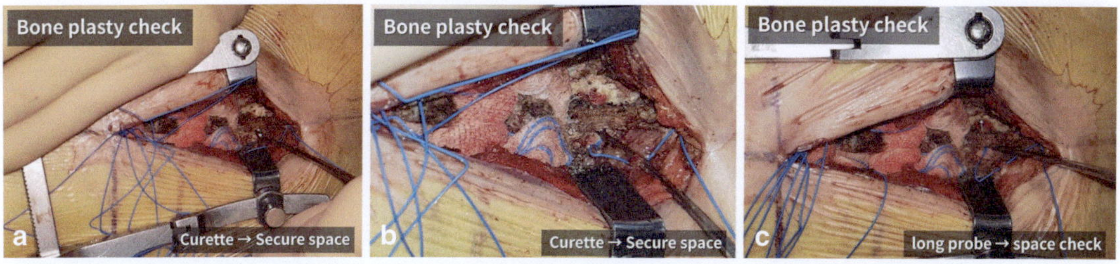

Fig. 17.4 (**a–c**) Curette and long probe are used to check the bone plasty and continuity of the created passageway across both sides

The needle and attached longitudinal ligament are then passed through the hole (Fig. 17.6a–c). Adequate tension is confirmed by pulling on the ligament (Fig. 17.6d, e). Ligament reconstruction is then performed by inserting the longitudinal and horizontal ligaments (Fig. 17.6f–j).

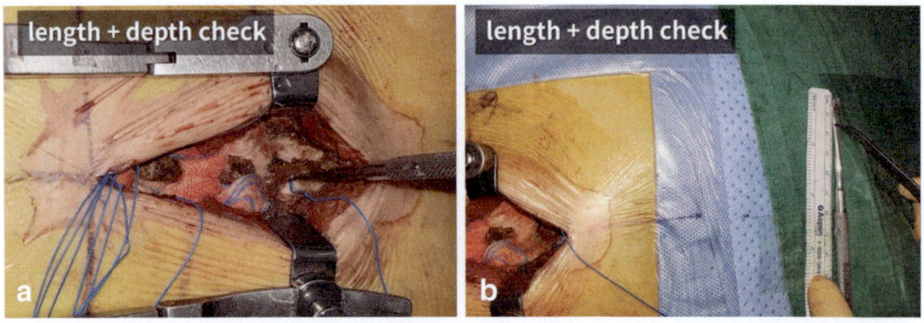

Fig. 17.5 (**a**, **b**) Length and depth are checked

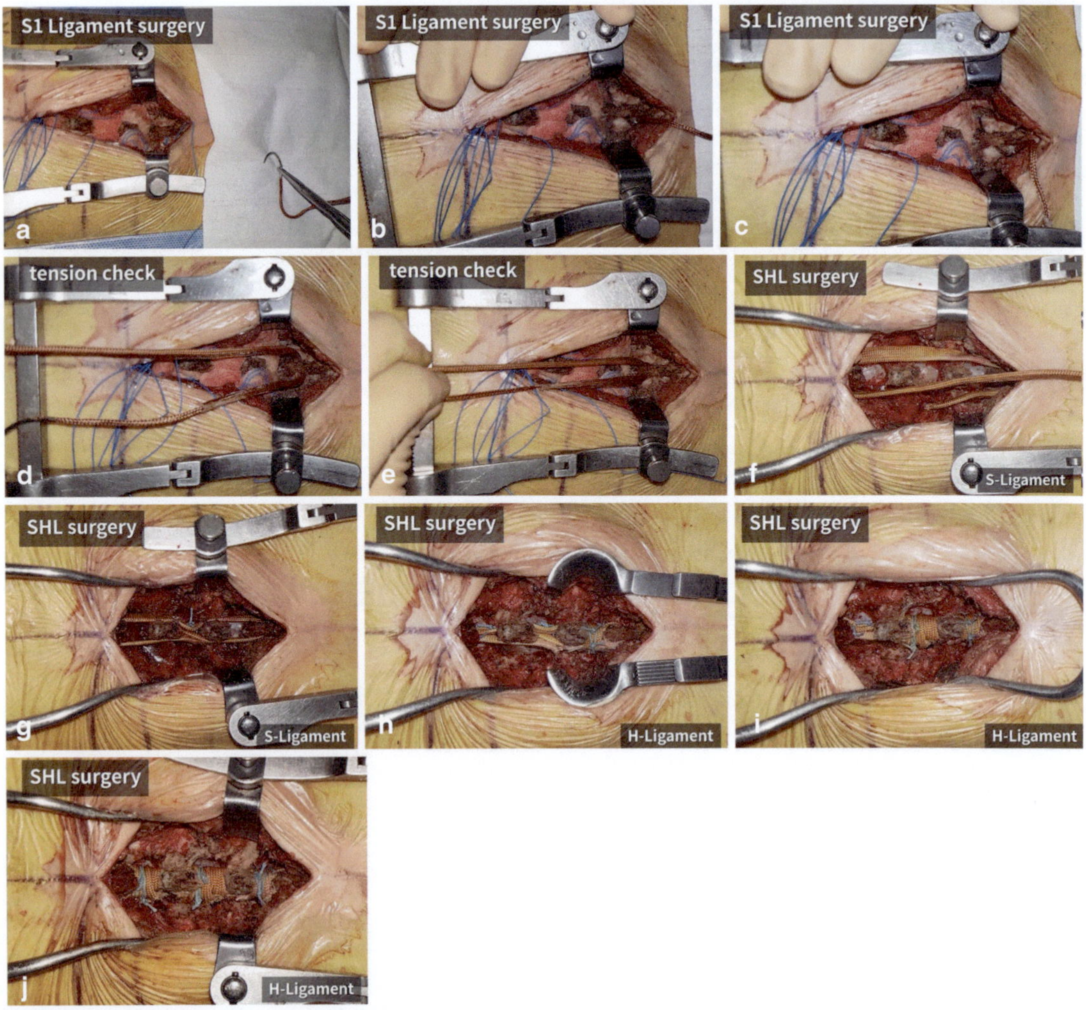

Fig. 17.6 (**a**–**c**) Needle and attached longitudinal ligament are passed through the hole; (**d**, **e**) Adequate tension is confirmed by pulling on the ligament; (**f**–**j**) Ligament reconstruction is then performed by inserting the longitudinal and horizontal ligaments

17.3.2 Pearls and Pitfalls

The thecal sac is convex in the sacral region. Caution should be exercised not to injure the dura especially while passing the needle. The dura should be protected with a neurosurgical patty. The bone mineral density of the patient should also be assessed. The ligament is tied under tension. In case of osteoporosis, a fracture of the median sacral crest at the point of bone plasty can occur leading to failure of ligament reconstruction.

17.4 Summary

Spinal stenosis is commonly seen at the lumbosacral junction. Given a short and fused spinous process, S1 often lacks a bony docking point for the longitudinal ligament. Spinous-sacrum plasty technique can be utilized to create a hole in the median sacral crest through which the ligament can be passed and tied. This technique enables soft stabilization with ligament reconstruction for the L5-S1 level.

References

1. Lee SH, Enes M, Hoogland T. Soft stabilization with interspinous artificial ligament for mildly unstable lumbar spinal stenosis: a multicenter comparison. Arch Orthop Trauma Surg. 2010;130(11):1335–41. https://doi.org/10.1007/s00402-009-1031-5. Epub 2010 Jan 5.
2. Lee SH, Lee JH, Hong SW, Chung SE, Yoo SH, Lee HY. Spinopelvic alignment after interspinous soft stabilization with a tension band system in grade 1 degenerative lumbar spondylolisthesis. Spine (Phila Pa 1976). 2010;35(15):E691–701. https://doi.org/10.1097/BRS.0b013e3181d2607e.
3. Shim CS, Lee SH, Park SH, Whang JH. Soft stabilization with an artificial intervertebral ligament in grade I degenerative spondylolisthesis: comparison with instrumented posterior lumbar interbody fusion. SAS J. 2007;1(3):118–24. https://doi.org/10.1016/SASJ-2006-0006-RR. PMID: 25802588; PMCID: PMC4365580.
4. Lee SH, Lee JH, Hong SW, Shim CS, Chung SE, Yoo SH, Lee HY. Factors affecting clinical outcomes in treating patients with grade 1 degenerative spondylolisthesis using interspinous soft stabilization with a tension band system: a minimum 5-year follow-up. Spine (Phila Pa 1976). 2012;37(7):563–72. https://doi.org/10.1097/BRS.0b013e31821c0b97.
5. Hashmi SS, Seifert KD, Massoud TF. Thoracic and lumbosacral spine anatomy. Neuroimaging Clin N Am. 2022;32(4):889–902. https://doi.org/10.1016/j.nic.2022.07.024.
6. Matson DM, Maccormick LM, Sembrano JN, Polly DW. Sacral dysmorphism and lumbosacral transitional vertebrae (LSTV) review. Int J Spine Surg. 2020;14(Suppl 1):14–9. https://doi.org/10.14444/6075. PMID: 32123653; PMCID: PMC7041668.
7. Wang T, Fielding LC, Parikh A, Kothari M, Alamin T. Sacral spinous processes: a morphologic classification and biomechanical characterization of strength. Spine J. 2015;15(12):2544–51. https://doi.org/10.1016/j.spinee.2015.08.058. Epub 2015 Sep 4.

18 Usefulness of Ligament Reconstruction to Prevent Adjacent Segment Disease Following Lumbar Fusion Surgery

Dong-Ju Yun

Abstract

In this case series, we evaluated the potential of ligament reconstruction combined with open midline decompression following lumbar fusion surgery to mitigate adjacent segment disease (ASD). The focus is on its capacity to reduce mechanical stress on adjacent segments and support spinal biomechanics. This retrospective case series included 32 patients with a mean follow-up of 19 months. Radiological ASD was observed in 4 cases (12.5%), while no ASD was detected in 28 cases (87.5%). Among the cases of ASD, none required reoperation, and only 1 patient underwent additional surgery. Postoperative clinical outcomes showed significant improvement. Facet arthrodesis was identified in 7 cases (21.9%), and cortical calcification around the facet joint was noted in 5 cases (15.6%). Ligament reconstruction and open midline decompression provide dynamic stabilization by reducing hypermobility and mechanical stress on adjacent segments, which may help to mitigate the risk of adjacent segment disease (ASD) following lumbar fusion surgery. This case series demonstrated a lower-than-expected incidence of radiological ASD and favorable clinical outcomes, suggesting that ligament reconstruction could serve as an effective motion-preserving alternative to traditional fusion, particularly for patients with high ASD risk.

Keywords

Reconstructive surgical procedures · Decompression · Mechanical stress · Spinal fusion · Ligaments/surgery

18.1 Introduction

Lumbar fusion surgery is considered as the gold standard for treating various lumbar degenerative diseases, such as spondylolisthesis, spinal stenosis, and disc herniation. This technique stabilizes the affected segments, thereby reducing pain and preventing further degeneration [1]. Nevertheless, lumbar fusion surgery is often associated with various complications, including pseudarthrosis, non-union, implant failure, and adjacent segment degeneration (ASD) [2]. ASD involves acceler-

Supplementary Information The online version contains supplementary material available at https://doi.org/10.1007/978-981-95-3971-0_18.

D.-J. Yun (✉)
Department of Neurosurgery, Busan Wooridul Spine Hospital, Busan, Korea (Republic of)
e-mail: djyunns@wooridul.co.kr

S.-H. Lee et al. (eds.), *Ligament Reconstruction for Spine*,
https://doi.org/10.1007/978-981-95-3971-0_18

ated degeneration of spinal segments adjacent to the fused levels, often resulting in conditions such as disc herniation, facet-joint arthritis, or instability, which cause back pain or radiculopathy [3].

ASD pathophysiology is attributed to the biomechanical changes induced by fusion. By eliminating motion at the fused segment, fusion surgery redirects mechanical stress to adjacent, unfused segments, causing these sections to undergo accelerated degenerative changes [4, 5]. Numerous studies have described ASD, which often leads to unfavorable clinical outcomes and occasionally necessitates additional fusion surgery [6].

To reduce ASD incidence, various dynamic stabilization systems have been developed, all of which incorporate motion-preserving technologies [7]. As an alternative to traditional fusion surgery, ligament reconstruction has emerged as a soft stabilization technique that aims to provide dynamic support, while preserving segmental mobility [8, 9]. Interspinous-based ligament reconstruction is designed to stabilize the spine by limiting abnormal motion, particularly flexion, while allowing controlled mobility. This technique reduces the stress at adjacent segments by distributing axial loading and controlling excessive flexion and extension [8, 9].

In this study, we investigated the usefulness of ligament reconstruction and open midline decompression in preventing post-lumbar fusion surgery-related ASD. We particularly focused on its potential to alleviate the mechanical stress on segments adjacent to the fused region and preserve spinal biomechanics over the long-term.

18.2 Materials and Methods

18.2.1 Study Design

This retrospective analysis was conducted from August 2016 to April 2023. The study included patients who underwent lumbar fusion surgery along with ligament reconstruction and open midline decompression at the level above the fusion site, at our institution. This study was approved by the institutional ethics committee.

18.2.2 Inclusion Criteria

We included patients who underwent lumbar fusion surgery with concurrent ligament reconstruction and open midline decompression at the level superior to the fusion site, performed by a single surgeon. All superior levels were diagnosed with spinal stenosis and had Grade I of lower spondylolisthesis. Patients who had a follow-up period of 12 months or longer were included, provided that lumbar spine computed tomography (CT) and X-ray imaging were performed at the time of their visits.

18.2.3 Exclusion Criteria

Patients were excluded if they had been followed-up for less than 12 months or if lumbar spine CT and X-ray imaging were not performed at the time of visits. Additionally, patients with Grade II or higher spondylolisthesis, severe foraminal stenosis, or significant instability were excluded, as fusion surgery was indicated in these cases.

18.2.4 Patient Demographics and Clinical Data

Forty-two patients were initially enrolled in the study, of whom 32 eventually met the inclusion criteria and were thus included in the final analysis. Data collected included demographic characteristics (age, sex, body mass index), preoperative and postoperative clinical symptoms, surgical details, and radiological assessments.

18.2.5 Radiological Evaluation and Definition of ASD

ASD was defined radiologically based on several criteria: disc-height reduction >20%, slippage distance >3 mm, osteophytes >3 mm, and segmental motion instability >15 degrees.

The segmental range of motion (ROM) during flexion and extension was assessed using lateral dynamic radiographs. Segmental ROM was determined by calculating the difference in Cobb angles between the superior and inferior endplates of the most cephalad and caudal segments during flexion and extension. A ROM ≤3° during flexion and extension was defined as immobility.

A facet gap was defined as the measurable distance between the superior articular process and the inferior articular process within the facet joint. This distance reflects the separation, or gap, within the joint space, and an increase in this measurement may indicate changes in joint morphology or degeneration.

Facet arthrodesis was characterized by the obliteration of facet-joint space and the presence of continuous cortical calcification bridging the superior and inferior articular processes, as observed on postoperative CT scans.

Imaging assessments included preoperative and postoperative CT scans and lateral dynamic X-ray imaging. Images were reviewed by two neurosurgeons to evaluate degenerative changes in adjacent segments.

18.2.6 Surgical Technique

After inducing general anesthesia, each patient was placed in a prone position, with support pillows placed under the trunk to preserve lumbar lordosis. A midline skin incision was made over the targeted lumbar interspinous space, exposing the lower half of the upper spinous process and the upper half of the lower spinous process.

Once exposed, bilateral laminotomy and ligamentum flavectomy were performed, with minimal facet resection, to preserve stability, while decompressing the neural elements. The hypertrophied ligamentum flavum was removed as extensively as possible to relieve pressure on the spinal canal.

An artificial ligament (Ligament Vertebral de Renfort; Cousin Biotech, Wervicq-Sud, France) was then used in ligament reconstruction. The ligament was anchored in a figure-of-eight pattern, spanning the interspinous spaces above and below the target level. Before tightening the ligament with a contractor device, the regional lordotic angle of the lumbar spine was set by changing the angle of the operating table. Subsequently, 2-0 nylon sutures were placed in three places near the center of the figure-of-eight knot to maintain firm stability and to prevent excessive extension of the spine. This technique was designed to provide controlled dynamic stabilization, thereby reducing biomechanical stress on the adjacent segments, while maintaining some degree of mobility (Fig. 18.1, Video 18.1) [10].

18.2.7 Follow-Up

Clinical evaluations and imaging studies were routinely performed at 1 month and 12 months postoperatively, as well as at the patient's final follow-up visit. Postoperative outcomes were monitored using standardized clinical questionnaires and radiological evaluations to assess ASD incidence and other degenerative changes.

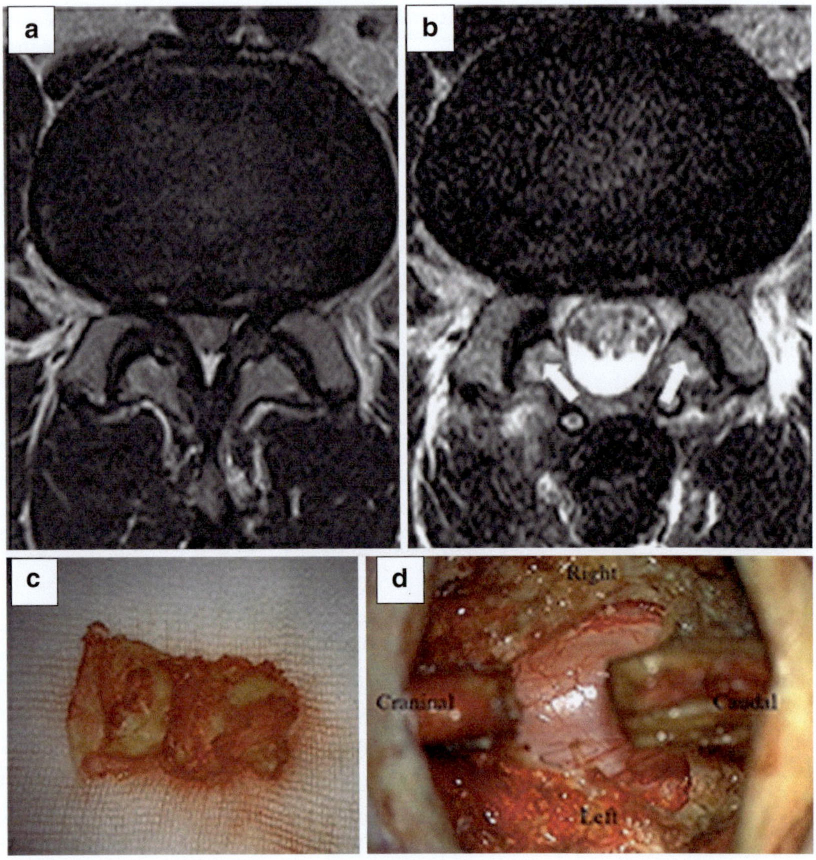

Fig. 18.1 (**a**) Preoperative axial magnetic resonance (MR) image showing central spinal stenosis at the L4/5 level. (**b**) Postoperative axial MR image confirming central decompression. The facet joints are largely preserved, with only minimal resection of the facet and lamina, resulting in minimal damage to the joint (white arrows). (**c**) The excised ligamentum flavum. (**d**) Intraoperative photograph showing decompression after the removal of the ligamentum flavum

18.3 Results

18.3.1 Patient Demographics and Clinical Characteristics

The study finally included 32 patients, comprising 18 males and 14 females, with a mean age of 63.5 ± 6.9 years. Characteristics of the patients and their clinical evaluation details are presented in Table 18.1. Mean VAS scores improved from preoperatively to postoperatively (Table 18.1, Fig. 18.2).

Table 18.1 Demographic and clinical data of patients

Characteristics	Value
No. of patients	32
Sex	
Male	18
Female	14
Mean age (years)	63.5 ± 6.9
Smoking (%)	6 (18.8)
DM (%)	3 (9.4)
Weight (kg)	71.25 ± 8.63
Height (m)	1.66 ± 0.08
BMI (kg/m^2)	26.01 ± 4.56
Mean clinical follow-up period (months)	19.56 ± 11.75
Mean time to last CT evaluation (months)	18.94 ± 11.60
Preoperative VAS	
Back	5.94 ± 2.08
Leg	8.41 ± 1.14
Postoperative VAS	
Back	1.59 ± 0.61
Leg	1.84 ± 0.91

DM diabetes mellitus, *BMI* body mass index, *VAS* Visual Analog Scale, *CT* computed tomography

18.3.2 Radiological Data

Radiological outcomes and fusion details are summarized in Table 18.2. Among the fusion techniques employed, anterior lumbar interbody fusion was performed in 28 cases, transforaminal lumbar interbody fusion in three cases, and oblique lumbar interbody fusion in one case.

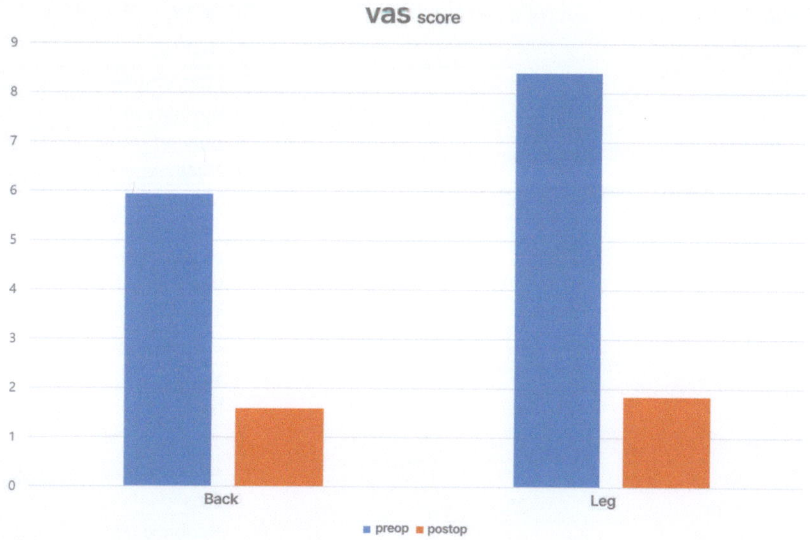

Fig. 18.2 Pre- and postoperative Visual Analogue Scale scores

Most patients (65.6%) underwent single-level fusion surgery, while the remaining 34.4% underwent two-level fusion. Fusion levels predominantly included L4/5 and L5/S1. Ligament reconstruction was implemented at a single level in 78.1% and at two levels in 21.9% of patients. Spondylolisthesis at preoperative evaluation was present in 31 patients, with anterior spondylolisthesis found in 25 cases, posterior spondylolisthesis in 6 cases, and no spondylolisthesis in 1 patient. Mean preoperative slip length was 3.76 ± 2.10 mm, which changed to 4.11 ± 2.01 mm postoperatively, with an average slip length change of 0.35 ± 1.54 mm (Table 18.2).

Table 18.2 Radiologic data of patients 1

Type of Fusion	
ALIF	28
TLIF	3
OLIF	1
Bridged level	
1-level	21
2-level	11
Fusion level	
L3/4	0
L4/5	21
L5/S1	22
Ligament Reconstruction	
1-level	25
2-level	7
Spondylolisthesis (no.)	
Anterior	25
Posterior	6
No	1
Slip length (mm)	
Preoperative	3.76 ± 2.10
Postoperative	4.11 ± 2.01
Slip length change (mm)	
Mean ± standard deviation	0.35 ± 1.54 (−2.6 to 6.3)

ALIF anterior lumbar interbody fusion, *OLIF* oblique lumbar interbody fusion, *TLIF* transforaminal lumbar interbody fusion

Global lumbar lordosis improved from 32.84 ± 10.56 degrees preoperatively to 37.31 ± 13.28 degrees postoperatively. Segmental ROM at the fused segments demonstrated a mean of 4.25 ± 6.25 degrees (range: −11 to 25 degrees). Following ligament reconstruction, 56.25% of fused segments were classified as immobile, while the remaining 43.75% retained some degree of mobility.

Facet arthrodesis was present in 21.9% of cases. The interfacet gap showed an increase in 5 patients, preservation in 17 patients, and a reduction in 9 patients. Cortical calcification was observed in 15.6% of patients (Table 18.3).

During the follow-up period, 12.5% (four patients) developed radiological evidence of ASD, while 87.5% (28 patients) did not show any signs of ASD. During the follow-up period, one patient (3.1%) underwent reoperation due to ASD, while the remaining 31 patients (96.9%) did not require additional surgery (Table 18.4).

Table 18.3 Radiologic data of patients 2

Global LL	
Preoperative	32.84 ± 10.56
Postoperative	37.31 ± 13.28
Segmental range of motion in degrees	
Mean ± standard deviation	4.25 ± 6.25 (−11 to 25)
Immobile (%)	
Yes	18 (56.25)
No	14 (43.75)
Facet arthrodesis (%)	
Yes	7 (21.9)
No	25 (78.1)
Gap of facet (%)	
Increased (+)	5 (15.6)
Preserved (=)	17 (53)
Reduced (−)	9 (28)
Cortical calcification (%)	
Yes	5 (15.6)
No	27 (84.4)

Table 18.4 Radiologic data of patients 3

Adjacent segment disease (%)	
Present	4 (12.5)
absent	28 (87.5)
Reoperation (%)	
yes	1 (3.1)
no	31 (96.9)

18.3.3 Case Presentation

Representative cases from this study are illustrated in Figs. 18.3, 18.4, 18.5, and 18.6. Detailed descriptions of each case, including their preoperative and postoperative findings, surgical techniques, and outcomes, are provided within the respective figure legends.

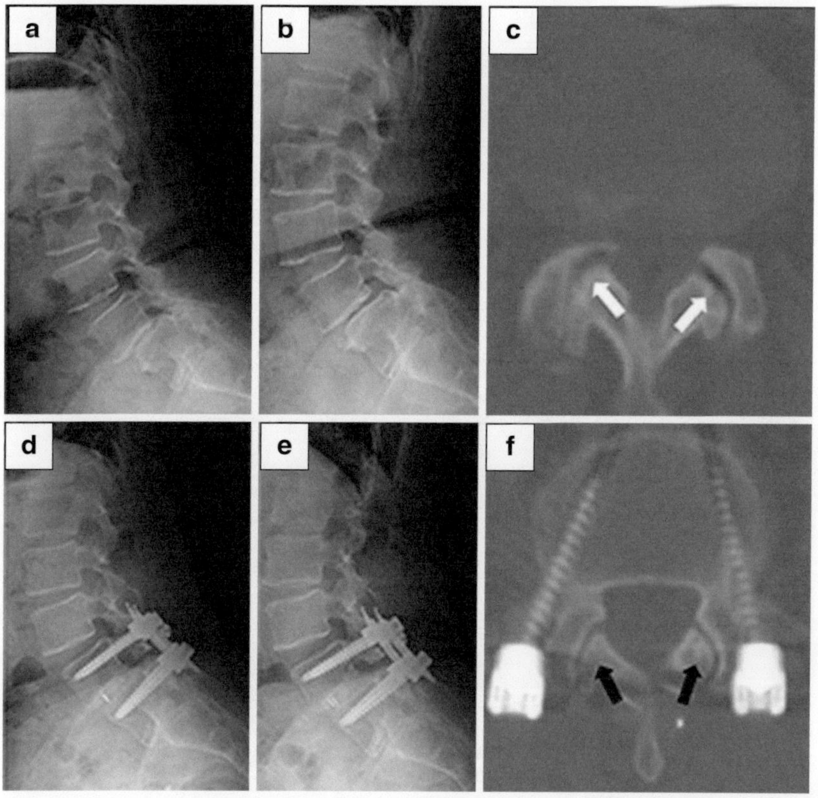

Fig. 18.3 This case involves a 61-year-old female patient. (**a**, **b**, and **c**) Preoperative flexion and extension X-ray images and a computed tomography (CT) scan, respectively. (**d**, **e**, and **f**) Postoperative findings at 41 months. (**a**, **b**, **d**, **e**) (**a**) and (**b**) are preoperative X-rays. In (**d**) and (**e**), postoperative X-ray images, ligament reconstruction is observed at the L3/4 level following L4/5 fusion surgery. At 41 months postoperatively, no progression of spondylolisthesis is seen at the L3/4 level, and the disc space remains preserved. (**c**, **f**) (**c**) is a preoperative CT scan at the L3/4 level, showing vacuum phenomena within the bilateral facet joints and widening of the left facet joint (white arrows). In the CT scan obtained 41 months postoperatively, the vacuum phenomena are no longer observed in the bilateral facet joints at the same level, and the widening of the facet joint has decreased (black arrows)

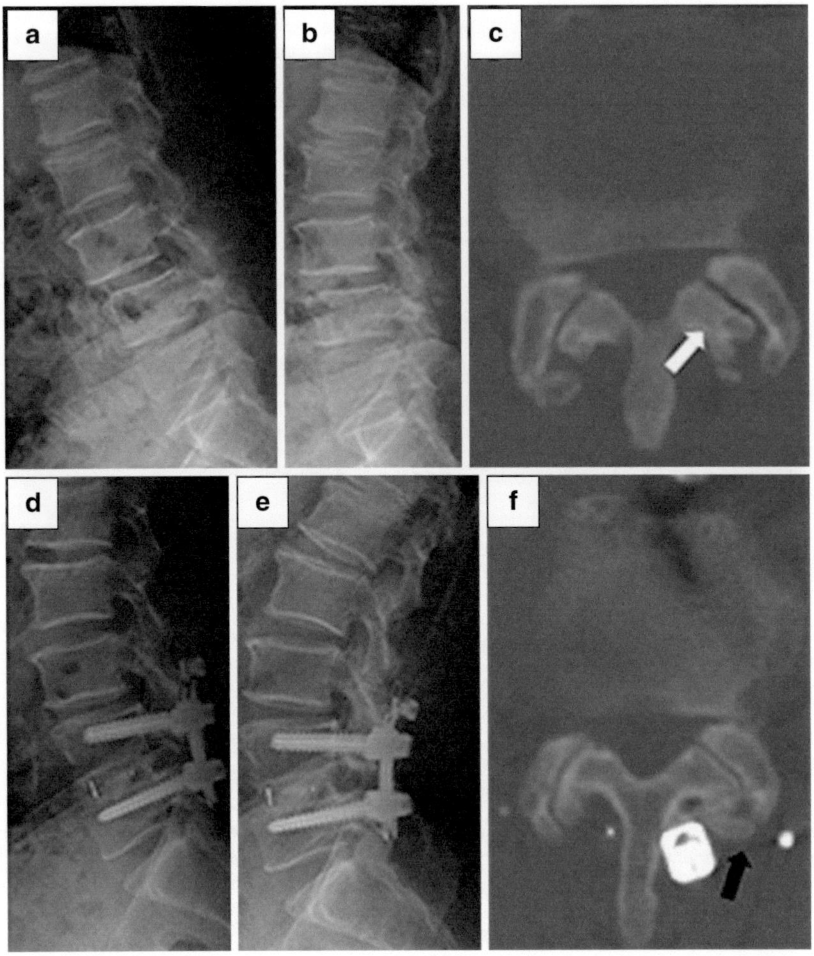

Fig. 18.4 This case involves a 62-year-old male patient. (**a**, **b**, and **c**) represent preoperative flexion and extension X-ray images and a computed tomography (CT) scan, respectively. (**d**, **e**, and **f**) depict postoperative findings at 63 months. (**a**, **b**, **d**, **e**) (**a**) and (**b**) are preoperative X-ray images. In (**d**) and (**e**), postoperative X-rays, ligament reconstruction is observed at the L3/4 level following L4/5 fusion surgery. At 63-months postoperatively, no progression of spondylolisthesis is observed at the L3/4 level, and the disc space remains preserved. (**c**, **f**) Image (**c**) is a preoperative CT scan at the L3/4 level, showing a vacuum phenomenon and widening of the left facet joint (white arrow). In the CT scan obtained at 63 months postoperatively, the vacuum phenomenon is no longer observed at the same level, and the widening of the left facet joint has decreased. Additionally, cortical calcification is noted (black arrow)

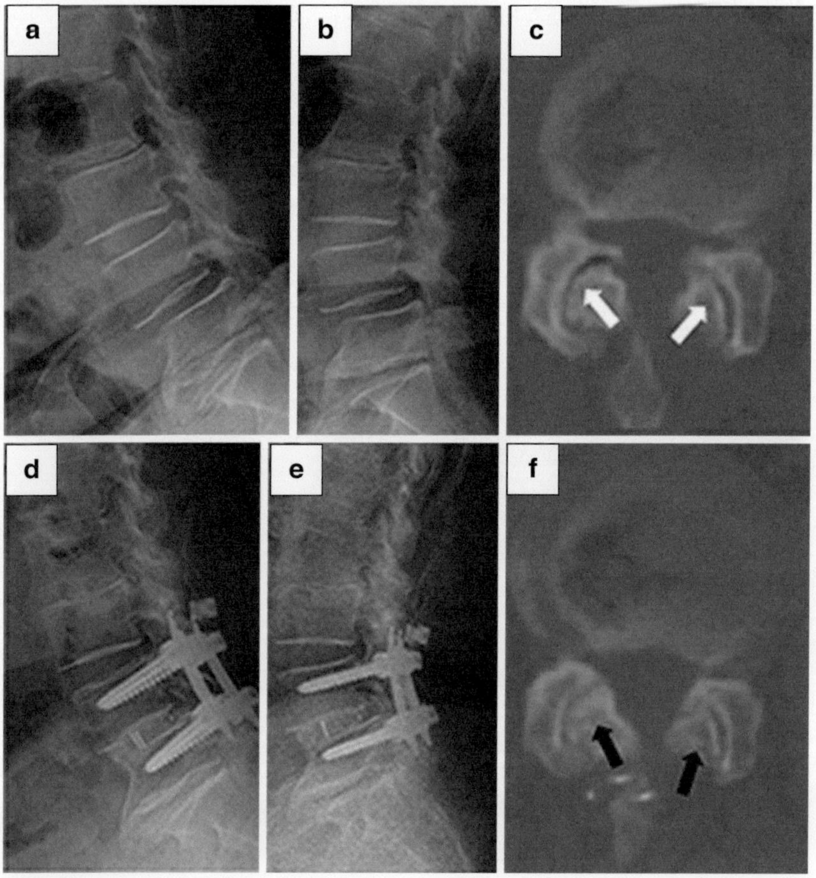

Fig. 18.5 The case of a 74-year-old female patient. (**a**, **b**, and **c**) represent preoperative flexion and extension X-ray images and a computed tomography (CT) scan, respectively, while (**d**, **e**, and **f**) depict postoperative findings at 39 months. In (**d**) and (**e**), postoperative X-ray images, ligament reconstruction is observed at the L3/4 level following L4/5 fusion surgery. At 39-months postoperatively, no progression of spondylolisthesis is observed at the L3/4 level, and the disc space remains preserved. (**d**, **e**) (**c**) is a preoperative CT scan at the L3/4 level, showing a vacuum phenomenon and widening of the right facet joint (white arrow). In the CT scan obtained at 39-months postoperatively, the vacuum phenomenon is no longerobserved at the same level, and the widening of the right facet joint has decreased (**f**) (black arrow)

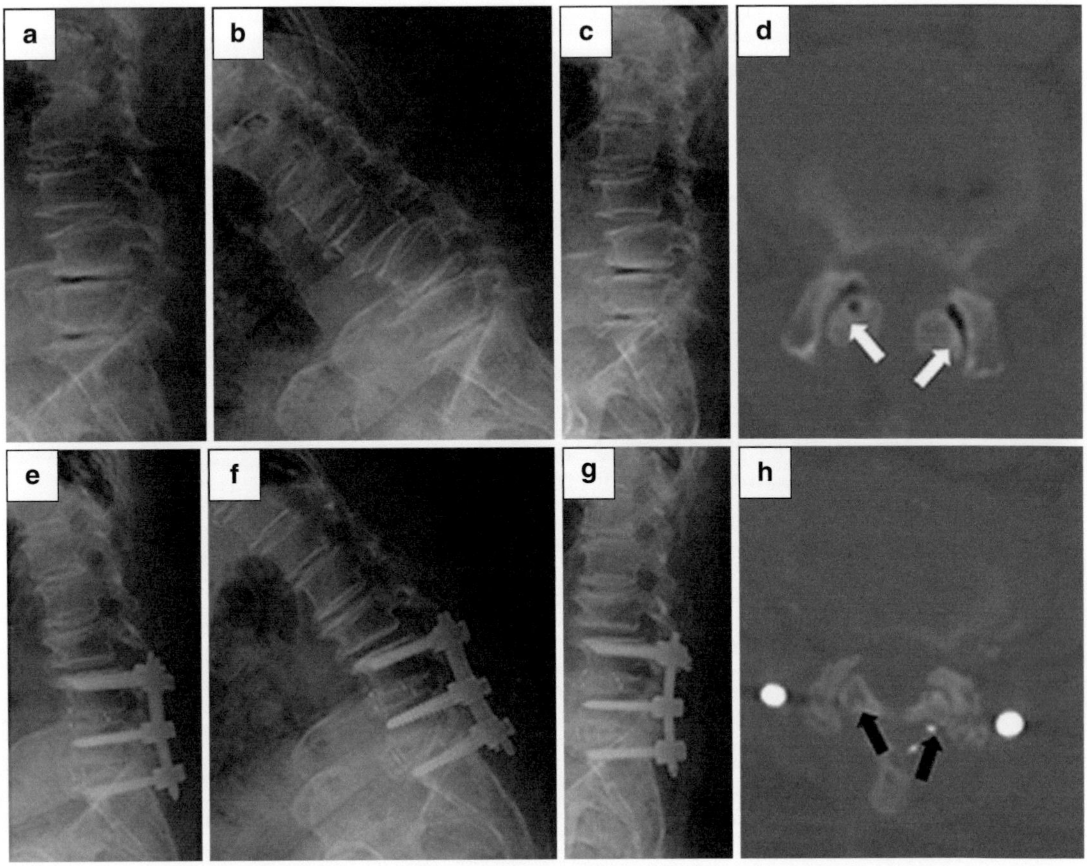

Fig. 18.6 The case of a 64-year-old female patient. (**a**, **b**, **c**, and **d**) Preoperative simple lateral, flexion, and extension X-ray images, along with a computed tomography (CT) scan, respectively. (**e–h**) depict postoperative findings at 44 months. (**a–c**) are preoperative X-ray images. In (**e–g**), postoperative X-rays, ligament reconstruction is observed at the L3/4 level following L4/5 and L5/S1 fusion surgery. At 44-months postoperatively, no progression of spondylolisthesis is observed at the ligament reconstruction level. However, sagittal imbalance has progressed, resulting in reduced lumbar lordosis. Additionally, angular instability at the ligament reconstruction level has increased, leading to an elevated segmental range of motion, confirming the development of ASD. (**d**) is a preoperative CT scan at the L3/4 level, showing vacuum phenomena and widening of the bilateral facet joints (white arrows). In the CT scan obtained at 44-months postoperatively, the vacuum phenomena are no longer observed at the same level, and the widening of the bilateral facet joints has decreased. Additionally, cortical calcification is noted (**h**) (black arrows). ASD: adjacent segment disease

18.4 Discussion

This study demonstrated the long-term clinical and radiological outcomes of lumbar fusion surgery combined with ligament reconstruction and open midline decompression at the superior level, which has not been reported previously. Among the 32 patients included in the study, with a mean follow-up period of 19 months, the majority showed favorable clinical outcomes. Radiological outcomes revealed the occurrence of radiological ASD in 4 cases (12.5%), while no ASD was observed in 28 cases (87.5%). Among the patients with ASD, none required reoperation, and among the entire cohort, only one patient underwent additional surgery.

The incidence of ASD after lumbar fusion surgery, based on radiological criteria alone, has been reported to vary widely, ranging from 8% to 100%. Symptomatic ASD, however, has been reported to have an incidence ranging from 5% to 36% [3]. In this study, the incidence of ASD was lower than that previously reported.

Ligament reconstruction is intended to stabilize the motion segment in flexion and extension by achieving segmental lumbar lordosis, to limit abnormal rotatory motion with its posterior tightening tension, and to diminish pathological movement by locking the facet joints [10]. The ability of this system to stabilize the vertebrae has been demonstrated in several cadaveric biomechanical tests [11]. The use of interspinous-based ligamentoplasty has shown potential in mitigating ASD by preserving the biomechanical integrity of the spine. Clinical studies have indicated that ligament reconstruction offers a balance between stability and mobility, theoretically preventing hypermobility and stress concentration that contribute to ASD [8–10].

The facet arthrodesis observed on CT scans, along with the reduction in the gap of the facet-joint capsule following ligament reconstruction and open midline decompression, may contribute to spinal stabilization. In the present study, facet arthrodesis was identified in 7 cases (21.9%) on CT scans performed at 1 year after ligament reconstruction and open midline decompression. Additionally, the gap in the facet-joint capsule remained unchanged in 17 cases (53%) and decreased in 9 cases (28%). New ossification around the facet joint, observed as cortical calcification, was noted in 5 cases (15.6%).

The surgical approach employed during open midline decompression minimizes damage to the facet joints, ensuring their postoperative integrity. Decompression was performed using undercutting from the contralateral side, with a drill used carefully around the facet joint, which likely reduced joint damage. During surgery, drilling causes partial heating and coagulation of the medial side of the facet-joint capsule. Although this can open a portion of the capsule, use of ligament reconstruction ensures stabilization of the facet joint, which may allow partial rehydration of the minimally affected facet joint (Video 18.1).

Additionally, the surgeon utilized bipolar cauterization along the facet-joint capsule after decompression. This technique is thought to aid in facet-joint remodeling, contributing to improved postoperative outcomes and spinal stability. These findings suggest that a combination of meticulous decompression techniques and ligament reconstruction provides an effective strategy for preserving and stabilizing facet joints (Video 18.1).

Minimizing facet-joint damage during surgery is crucial for maintaining spinal stability. Lener et al. reported that the extent of facet-joint injury during surgery significantly influenced postoperative ROM [12]. Similarly, Zhong et al. found that decompression at an adjacent level is a significant risk factor for ASD development following various interbody fusion approaches [13]. Maragkos et al. also reported that decompression outside the fusion construct was associated with a significant increase in the incidence of ASD following surgical treatment [14]. These findings suggest that decompression surgery at levels adjacent to a fused region can increase the risk of ASD, highlighting the importance of minimizing facet-joint damage when possible. In this context, open midline decompression, which preserves facet-joint integrity, may reduce ASD risk. However, the relationship between disc rehydration and facet arthrodesis remains unclear and warrants further investigation in future studies.

Ligament reconstruction and open midline decompression represent a method of dynamic stabilization and constitute motion-preserving technologies. This approach reduces hypermobility and mechanical stresses at adjacent levels. By restoring more natural spinal motion, ligament reconstruction theoretically preserves mobility, rather than eliminating it, thereby minimizing the transfer of forces to superiorly located segments. Specifically, this technique may prevent the abrupt transfer of stress from a rigid construct to neighboring segments, potentially reducing the risk of ASD. By ensuring a "soft landing" of forces on adjacent segments, this approach may reduce the incidence of ASD. Consequently, the application of ligament reconstruction could help mitigate the progression of degenerative processes by decreasing hypermobility and stress at adjacent levels. As such, ligament reconstruction may serve as a valid and safe option for preventing or managing ASD adjacent to instrumented arthrodesis.

18.4.1 Limitations

This study had some limitations. First, this was a retrospective analysis, which inherently introduced potential biases in data collection and interpretation. Second, the sample size was relatively small, with only 32 patients included in the final analysis, which may limit the generalizability of the findings. Third, the follow-up period, while sufficient to observe short- to mid-term outcomes, may not capture the long-term implications of ligament reconstruction on ASD development or overall spinal stability. Fourth, the study lacked a control group, such as patients undergoing traditional fusion without ligament reconstruction, making it difficult to draw definitive conclusions about the comparative efficacy of this approach. Additionally, the study did not fully explore the biomechanical mechanisms underlying the observed outcomes, such as the role of facet-joint remodeling or the relationship between disc rehydration and facet arthrodesis. Finally, while radiological outcomes were assessed, use of more detailed functional and patient-reported outcome measures could provide a more comprehensive evaluation of the clinical benefits of ligament reconstruction. Future prospective, randomized controlled trials with longer follow-up periods and larger cohorts are warranted, to address these limitations and to confirm the efficacy of ligament reconstruction in preventing ASD.

18.5 Conclusion

This study highlighted the potential of ligament reconstruction and open midline decompression as effective techniques for mitigating ASD after lumbar fusion surgery. By preserving segmental mobility and reducing mechanical stress at adjacent levels, ligament reconstruction offers a dynamic stabilization method that may address some of the limitations associated with traditional fusion techniques. Radiological outcomes demonstrated a lower-than-expected incidence of ASD, with favorable clinical results and a minimal need for reoperation, indicating its efficacy and safety in preventing degenerative progression.

Given its advantages, ligament reconstruction represents a promising alternative to traditional fusion, particularly for patients at high ASD risk. Future studies with longer follow-up periods and larger patient populations are needed to validate these findings and to explore the long-term implications of ligament reconstruction on spinal biomechanics and patient outcomes.

References

1. Bydon M, Xu R, Santiago-Dieppa D, et al. Adjacent-segment disease in 511 cases of posterolateral instrumented lumbar arthrodesis: floating fusion versus distal construct including the sacrum. J Neurosurg Spine. 2014;20:380–6.
2. Lee SE, Park SB, Jahng TA, Chung CK, Kim HJ. Clinical experience of the dynamic stabilization system for the degenerative spine disease. J Korean Neurosurg Soc. 2008;43:221–6.
3. Cheh G, Bridwell KH, Lenke LG, et al. Adjacent segment disease followinglumbar/thoracolumbar fusion with pedicle screw instrumentation: a minimum 5-year follow-up. Spine (Phila Pa 1976). 2007;32:2253–7.

4. Jiang S, Li W. Biomechanical study of proximal adjacent segment degeneration after posterior lumbar interbody fusion and fixation: a finite element analysis. J Orthop Surg Res. 2019;14:135.
5. Mesregah MK, Yoshida B, Lashkari N, et al. Demographic, clinical, and operative risk factors associated with postoperative adjacent segment disease in patients undergoing lumbar spine fusions: a systematic review and meta-analysis. Spine J. 2022;22:1038–69.
6. Putzier M, Hoff E, Tohtz S, et al. Dynamic stabilization adjacent to single-level fusion: part II. No clinical benefit for asymptomatic, initially degenerated adjacent segments after 6 years follow-up. Eur Spine J. 2010;19:2181–9.
7. Mashaly H, Paschel EE, Khattar NK, et al. Posterior lumbar dynamic stabilization instead of arthrodesis for symptomatic adjacent-segment degenerative stenosis: description of a novel technique. Neurosurg Focus. 2016;40:E5.
8. Shim CS, Lee SH, Park SH, et al. Soft stabilization with an artificial intervertebral ligament in grade I degenerative spondylolisthesis: comparison with instrumented posterior lumbar interbody fusion. SAS J. 2007;1:118–24.
9. Lee SH, Enes M, Hoogland T. Soft stabilization with interspinous artificial ligament for mildly unstable lumbar spinal stenosis: a multicenter comparison. Arch Orthop Trauma Surg. 2010;130:1335–41.
10. Lee SH, Lee HY, Baek OK, et al. Clinical significance of achieving a flexion limitation with a tension band system in grade 1 degenerative spondylolisthesis: a minimum 5-year follow-up. Spine (Phila Pa 1976). 2015;40:E349–58.
11. Shim CS, Park SW, Lee SH, et al. Biomechanical evaluation of an interspinous stabilizing device, locker. Spine (Phila Pa 1976). 2008;33:E820–7.
12. Lener S, Schmölz W, Abramovic A, et al. The effect of various options for decompression of degenerated lumbar spine motion segments on the range of motion: a biomechanical in vitro study. Eur Spine J. 2023;32:1358–66.
13. Zhong ZM, Deviren V, Tay B, et al. Adjacent segment disease after instrumented fusion for adult lumbar spondylolisthesis: incidence and risk factors. Clin Neurol Neurosurg. 2017;156:29–34.
14. Maragkos GA, Motiei-Langroudi R, Filippidis AS, et al. Factors predictive of adjacent segment disease after lumbar spinal fusion. World Neurosurg. 2020;133:e690–4.

Ligament Reconstruction of Baastrup's Disease

19

YongSoo Choi

Abstract

Bastrop's disease, commonly known as the "kissing spine" syndrome, is a condition characterized by abnormal contact between adjacent spinous processes of the spine, usually in the lumbar region (Farinha et al. Acta Reumatol Port 40:302–303, 2015; Hagner Med Pr 39(1):65–70, 1988; Maes et al. Spine (Phila Pa 1976) 33(7):211–215, 2008; Lamer et al. Pain Physician 11:549–554, 2008; Okada et al. Asian Spine J 8:260–266, 2014). Commonly associated with degenerative changes, anatomical alterations, or postural factors, this syndrome is characterized by localized back pain and restricted motion, particularly during spinal extension (Farinha et al. Acta Reumatol Port 40:302–303, 2015; Hagner Med Pr 39(1):65–70, 1988; Maes et al. Spine (Phila Pa 1976) 33(7):211–215, 2008; Mitra et al. Arch Phys Med Rehabil 88:1353–1356, 2007; Okada et al. Asian Spine J 8:260–266, 2014; Beks Acta Neurochir 100:134–135, 1989). Diagnosis is mainly based on imaging techniques such as X-ray and MRI, which show the approximation of the spinous processes and potential intervertebral bursitis (Hagner Med Pr 39(1):65–70, 1988; Philipp et al. Cureus 8(1):E465, 2016). Management focuses on conservative measures, including physiotherapy, pain management, and lifestyle modifications, with interventions such as corticosteroid injections or radiofrequency ablation considered in persistent cases (Maes et al. Spine (Phila Pa 1976) 33(7):211–215, 2008; Lamer et al. Pain Physician 11:549–554, 2008). Surgical solutions such as resection or spinal fusion are reserved for severe and resistant conditions (Maes et al. Spine (Phila Pa 1976) 33(7):211–215, 2008; Lamer et al. Pain Physician 11:549–554, 2008; Filippiadis et al. Insights Imaging 6:123–128, 2015). Ligament reconstruction surgery is a minimally invasive and effective treatment for Baastrup's disease.

Keywords

Baastrup's disease · Kissing spine · Spinous process · Ligament reconstruction · Interspinous Ligament

Baastrup's disease, also known as "kissing spine syndrome," is a degenerative condition of the spine characterized by abnormal contact between adjacent spinous processes, leading to chronic back pain [1–5]. It commonly affects the lumbar

Y. Choi (✉)
Department of Neurosurgery, Cheongdam Wooridul Spine Hospital, Seoul, Korea (Republic of)
e-mail: yong@wooridul.co.kr

S.-H. Lee et al. (eds.), *Ligament Reconstruction for Spine*,
https://doi.org/10.1007/978-981-95-3971-0_19

spine, particularly between L3 and L4 or L4 and L5, and is associated with repetitive mechanical stress, hyperlordosis, and age-related degenerative changes [1–3, 6, 7]. Patients with Baastrup's disease often experience midline lumbar pain that worsens with extension and improves with flexion (Fig. 19.1a, b) [1, 2, 4, 8]. Diagnosis is typically confirmed through imaging studies such as X-rays, CT scans, or MRI, which reveal enlarged and abutting spinous processes with associated sclerosis or reactive changes [1–3, 6, 9, 10]. Treatment includes conservative measures such as physical therapy, anti-inflammatory medications, and postural correction, while severe cases may require interventional procedures or surgery [1, 2, 4, 5].

Baastrup's disease was first described by Christian Ingerslev Baastrup, a Danish radiologist, in 1933 [1–4, 6, 8, 9, 11]. He observed that patients with chronic back pain often exhibited close approximation and reactive changes in the spinous processes of the lumbar vertebrae. Since then, further studies have elaborated on the pathophysiology and contributing factors, recognizing that mechanical stress, postural abnormalities, and degenerative spinal changes play crucial roles in its development [7, 8, 10]. Over the years, advancements in imaging techniques have enhanced the understanding and diagnosis of this condition.

The spinal column is made up of several vertebrae, each with a bony projection known as the spinous process. These projections provide attachment points for muscles and ligaments. In Baastrup's disease, these processes abnormally approach each other, leading to potential contact and ultimately causing attrition or wear [4, 6, 7].

The primary cause of Baastrup's disease is chronic mechanical stress leading to excessive friction between adjacent spinous processes [1–4, 8, 9]. As individuals age, degenerative changes in the spine, such as intervertebral disc narrowing and facet joint arthritis, can lead to increased contact between spinous processes. Conditions such as hyperlordosis (excessive inward curvature of the lumbar spine) predispose individuals to excessive spinous process contact. Occupational or athletic activities that involve repeated spinal extension and flexion can accelerate degenerative changes [9, 11]. Procedures such as laminectomy, which alter spinal mechanics, may increase the risk of Baastrup's disease. Increased axial loading on the spine can contribute to degenerative changes and excessive spinous process contact [5, 7, 8]. Understanding these contributing factors is crucial for managing and preventing Baastrup's disease, with emphasis on lifestyle modifications and targeted therapies to reduce mechanical stress on the spine.

The primary symptom of Baastrup's disease is chronic low back pain, which is typically localized to the midline of the lumbar spine [1–4, 7]. The severity and nature of the symptoms can vary based on the extent of the disease and individual patient factors. The pain is often localized between the affected spinous processes and may worsen with certain movements. Patients frequently report increased pain when arching their back (lumbar extension), as this increases the contact between adjacent spinous processes [4, 5, 8]. Bending forward (lumbar flexion) often alleviates discomfort by reducing pressure on the spinous processes. Direct pressure over the involved spinous processes may cause significant tenderness [4, 5, 8]. Due to pain and mechanical irritation, patients may experience difficulty with activities that require lumbar extension [4, 5, 8, 10]. In some cases, pain may radiate laterally or to the buttocks, mimicking symptoms of other lumbar spine conditions. Chronic irritation can lead to soft tissue swelling and inflammation around the affected area. Some patients may develop paraspinal muscle spasms, further restricting movement. In advanced cases, there may be bursa formation between the spinous processes, leading to increased swelling and discomfort. If nerve structures are secondarily affected due to associated degenerative changes, patients may experience neuropathic symptoms, such as tingling or numbness. Early recognition of these symptoms can help guide appropriate diagnosis and treatment, preventing progression and improving the patient's quality of life.

The diagnosis of Baastrup's disease is based on a combination of clinical evaluation and imag-

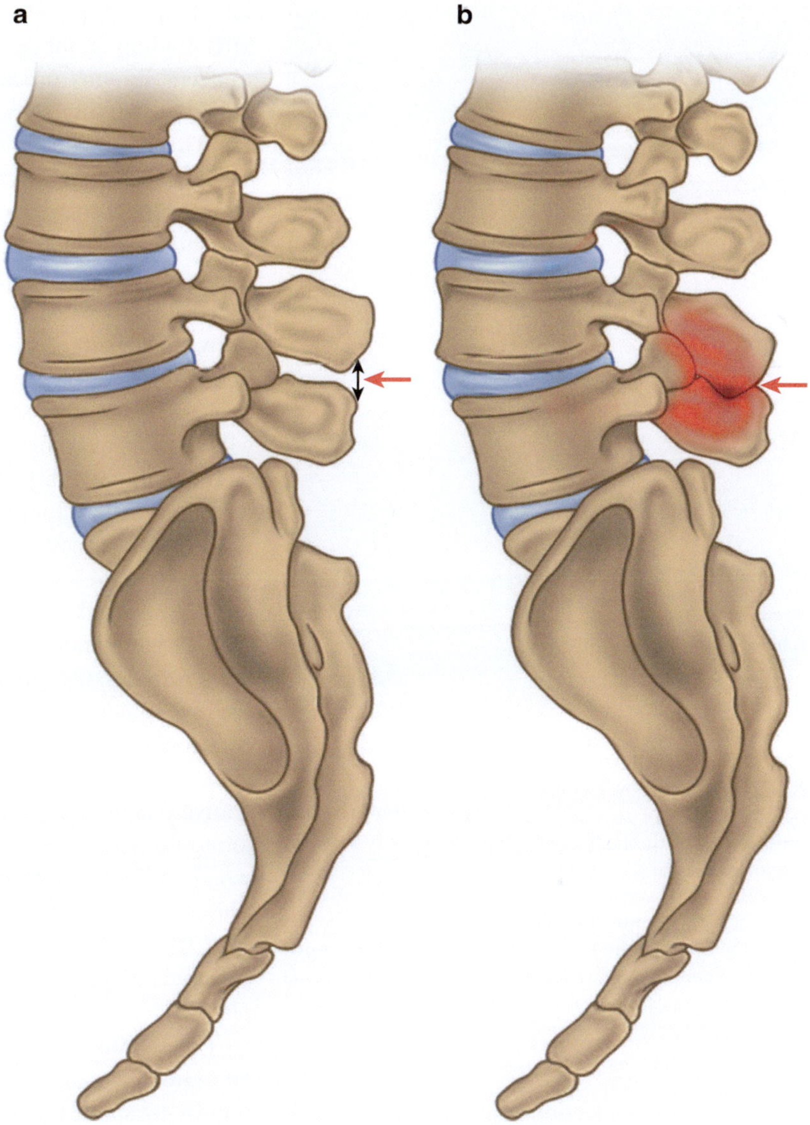

Fig. 19.1 Baastrup's disease, also known as "kissing spine," is a condition that affects the spine, specifically the lumbar region (lower back). It occurs when the spinous processes (the bony protrusions on the back of the vertebrae) of two adjacent vertebrae come into contact with each other (**a**), which can cause pain, inflammation (**b**)

ing studies [3, 6, 9, 11]. Since its symptoms resemble other spinal conditions, a thorough assessment is necessary to confirm the diagnosis and rule out other causes of back pain.

Doctors begin by taking a detailed patient history, focusing on symptoms such as chronic midline low back pain that worsens with lumbar extension and improves with flexion. Patients may also report tenderness in the lower back, especially over the spinous processes. During the physical examination, doctors check for pain on palpation of the lumbar spine and assess spinal mobility. Pain typically worsens when the patient arches their back (extension) and improves when they bend forward (flexion).

To confirm the diagnosis, imaging studies are essential. X-rays can reveal close approximation of the spinous processes, sometimes referred to as the "kissing spine" appearance, along with sclerosis or hypertrophic changes (Fig. 19.2) [1–3, 6, 9, 11]. Magnetic resonance imaging (MRI) provides a more detailed view of soft tissues and can detect inflammation or bursa formation between the affected spinous processes [1, 2, 4, 8, 9]. In some cases, a CT scan is used to assess bony changes more precisely.

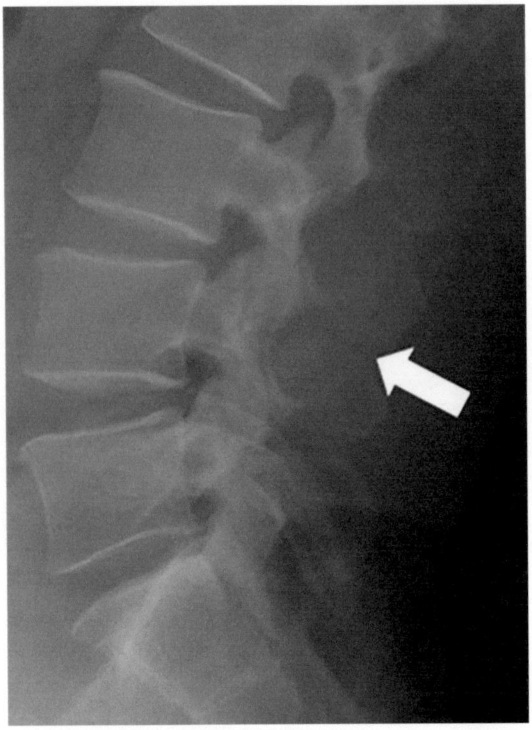

Fig. 19.2 The hallmark sign of Baastrup's disease on an X-ray is the apparent contact or kissing between the spinous processes of two adjacent vertebrae. This is often most noticeable in the lumbar spine, particularly between the lower lumbar vertebrae (L4-L5, L5-S1). The spinous processes of the vertebrae appear unusually close to each other, sometimes touching or almost touching. In some cases, the intervertebral discs (the cushion-like structures between vertebrae) may show signs of degeneration. This disc narrowing can exacerbate the pressure on the spinous processes, contributing to the "kissing" of the vertebrae

A diagnostic injection may be performed to confirm the condition. If injecting a local anesthetic around the affected spinous processes provides significant pain relief, it supports the diagnosis of Baastrup's disease.

Because Baastrup's disease shares symptoms with other spinal disorders such as facet joint syndrome, degenerative disc disease, and spinal stenosis, it is important for healthcare providers to differentiate between these conditions. A thorough evaluation ensures the correct diagnosis and appropriate treatment plan.

Magnetic Resonance Imaging (MRI) is an essential tool for diagnosing Baastrup's disease, as it provides a detailed view of both bone and soft tissue structures. The most characteristic MRI finding is the abnormal approximation of adjacent spinous processes, commonly referred to as the "kissing spine" appearance [1–3, 6, 9, 11]. This occurs due to repetitive friction between the spinous processes, leading to chronic irritation. One key feature seen on MRI is bone marrow edema, which appears as a high signal intensity on T2-weighted and STIR images (Fig. 19.3a, b) [1, 2, 4, 8, 9]. This edema results from constant mechanical stress and inflammation in the affected vertebrae. In some cases, MRI may also show sclerosis of the spinous processes, which indicates chronic degenerative changes. Another important MRI finding is interspinous bursitis, where a fluid-filled bursa forms between the spinous processes due to prolonged friction. This bursa appears as a hyperintense (bright) area on T2-weighted images and may be associated with inflammation of the surrounding soft tissues. Additionally, thickening or degeneration of the interspinous ligament can be observed, which contributes to reduced flexibility and increased pain. MRI also helps identify associated degenerative changes, such as disc degeneration, facet joint arthritis, and paraspinal muscle atrophy, which may coexist with Baastrup's disease. These findings help differentiate Baastrup's disease from other spinal conditions, ensuring an accurate diagnosis and appropriate treatment plan.

The treatment of Baastrup's disease focuses on relieving pain, reducing inflammation, and improving spinal function. The approach depends on the severity of symptoms, ranging from conservative management to interventional procedures or surgery in severe cases. The first line of treatment is conservative therapy, which includes physical therapy, posture correction, and lifestyle modifications. Strengthening the core and back muscles through exercise programs can help stabilize the spine and reduce excessive movement of the spinous processes [7, 9, 10]. Patients are advised to avoid activities that involve excessive lumbar extension, as this can worsen symptoms. Medications such as nonsteroidal anti-inflammatory drugs (NSAIDs) and muscle relaxants are often prescribed to help manage pain and

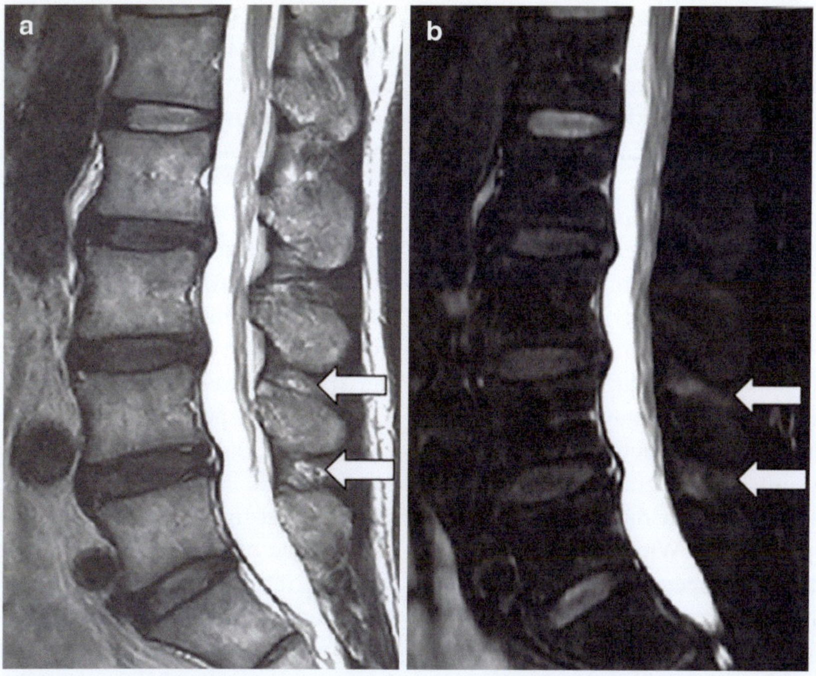

Fig. 19.3 An MRI (Magnetic Resonance Imaging) is a more advanced imaging technique than X-rays and is often used to diagnose Baastrup's disease when more detailed information about the soft tissues, spinal discs, and nerve structures is required (**a**) T2-weighted images: These are particularly useful for detecting disc degeneration, inflammation, and edema in the soft tissues and nerve roots, as well as fluid-filled areas like cysts or areas of nerve compression. (**b**) STIR (Short TI Inversion Recovery): This sequence is useful for highlighting edema and inflammation in the soft tissues, including muscles and ligaments

inflammation. In cases where pain is severe or persistent, local corticosteroid injections may be administered between the affected spinous processes to provide temporary relief. For patients who do not respond to conservative treatments, minimally invasive procedures such as radiofrequency ablation can be considered. This procedure targets the nerves responsible for transmitting pain signals from the affected area, providing longer-lasting relief. In severe cases where conservative and interventional treatments fail, surgical intervention may be necessary. Partial excision of the spinous processes (spinoplasty) is a surgical option that helps reduce friction between the affected vertebrae [5, 6, 8]. In some cases, spinal fusion may be performed if significant instability or other degenerative conditions are present. By following a tailored treatment plan, most patients with Baastrup's disease can experience significant pain relief and improved mobility. Early diagnosis and management are crucial in preventing the progression of the disease and maintaining spinal health [7, 10].

Ligament reconstruction is very effective in treating Baastrup's disease. The pathological interspinous ligament causing the back pain is removed and replaced with an artificial ligament. This can replace fusion surgery for treating Baastrup's disease and overcomes the problem of limited movement of fusion surgery. The artificial ligament prevents the spinous processes from touching each other while maintaining the movement of the lumbar spine. This is an ideal method to remove the lesion and provide normal movement.

The prognosis of Baastrup's disease varies depending on the severity of the condition and the effectiveness of treatment. In many cases, conservative management with physical therapy, posture correction, and pain relief medications can significantly reduce symptoms and improve the patient's quality of life [7, 8]. Patients who adopt lifestyle modifications, such as avoiding excessive lumbar extension and strengthening their core muscles, often experience long-term symptom relief. For individuals who do not respond to conservative treatments, interventional procedures like corticosteroid injections or radiofrequency ablation can provide temporary or prolonged pain relief. However, in some cases, symptoms may return, requiring repeated treatments or adjustments in therapy. In severe or persistent cases, surgical intervention may be necessary. Ligament reconstruction generally have good outcomes, with many patients experiencing significant pain reduction and improved mobility. Overall, the prognosis of Baastrup's disease is favorable when diagnosed early and managed appropriately. While the condition is not life-threatening, it can lead to chronic pain and functional limitations if left untreated. With proper medical care and rehabilitation, most patients can achieve symptom control and maintain an active lifestyle [7, 8].

19.1 Surgical Technique

The patient is in the prone position and a surgical frame is used to flex the lumbar spine. After aseptic surgical site preparation, a longitudinal central incision is made over the relevant lesion. Periosteal dissection is performed while preserving the paraspinous muscles. When the spinous process and interspinous ligament are exposed, the interspinous ligament causing the lesion is removed. In general, when the pathological interspinous ligament is removed, the narrowed interspinous space is changed to be widened (Fig. 19.4). Two artificial ligaments are placed. One is the sagittal ligament, and the other is the horizontal ligament. The sagittal ligament controls flexion and extension movements, and the horizontal ligament maintains the space between the spinous processes and effectively disperses shock. When the spine rotates and makes complex movements, these two artificial ligaments work simultaneously. The sagittal ligament is placed in the interspinous space of the upper segment of the lesion and the interspinous space of the lower segment, and is tightened to maintain elasticity in an oval shape. The horizontal ligament is tied horizontally to the segment of the lesion, and the sagittal ligament is changed into the shape of the number "8" (Fig. 19.5). After the placement is completed, the elasticity of the artificial ligament should be confirmed. Finally, the muscles and skin are sutured. This series of surgical procedures can be completed in a short time, so the surgery can be performed under a short anesthesia period. Short surgical time and anesthesia time greatly help the patient's immediate recovery.

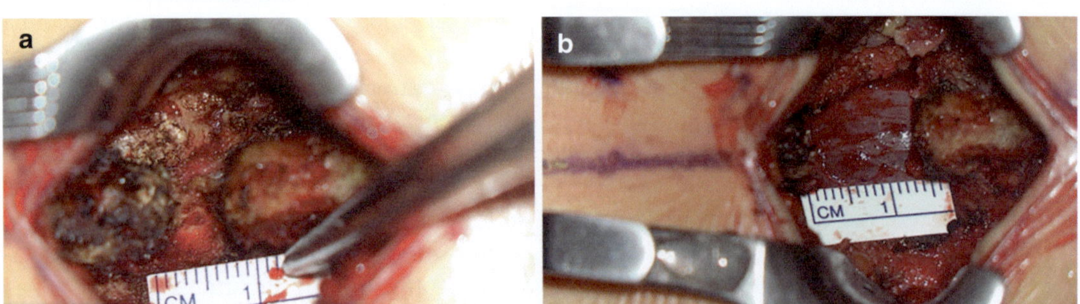

Fig. 19.4 Baastrup's disease is a condition in which the interspinous space narrows. A clearly narrowed interspinous space is confirmed during surgery (**a**). After removing the interspinous ligament and resolving the lesions causing the space narrowing, the interspinous space widens (**b**)

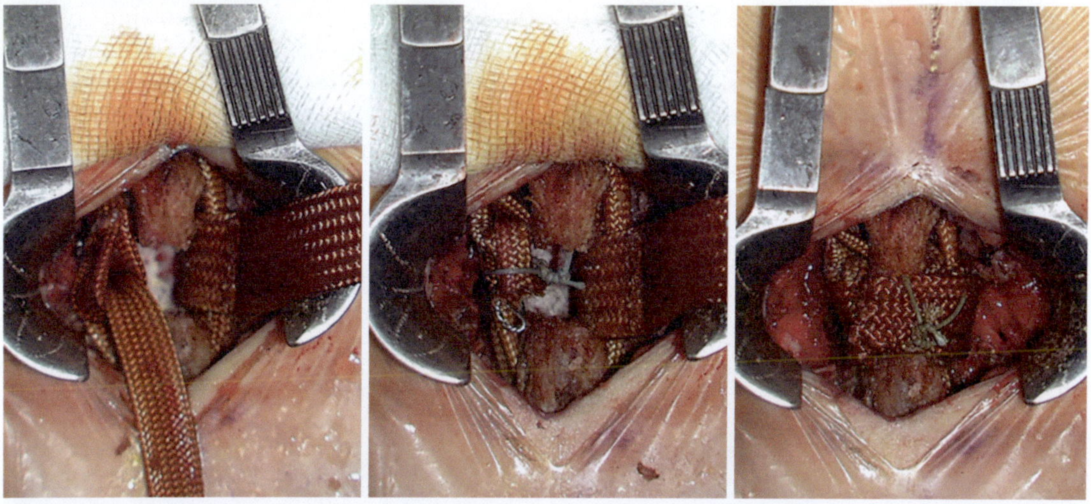

Fig. 19.5 The sagittal ligament is placed in the interspinous space of the upper segment of the lesion and the interspinous space of the lower segment, and is tightened to maintain elasticity in an oval shape. The horizontal ligament is tied horizontally to the segment of the lesion, and the sagittal ligament is changed into the shape of the number "8"

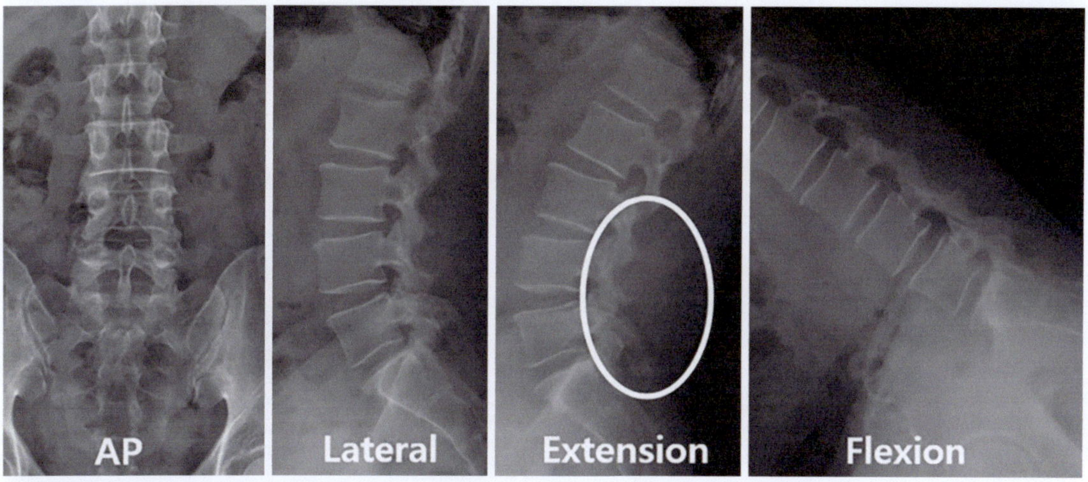

Fig. 19.6 The patient's X-ray showed a decreased interspinous interval between the third, fourth, and fifth lumbar vertebrae, and the spinous processes impinged on each other during extension

19.2 Case Illustration

A 55-year-old male patient complained of back pain that had persisted for more than 5 years. When he bent over and straightened, the back pain was severe. When he walked, the back pain was so severe that he collapsed. The pain was as if he was being hit by an electric shock. There was no evidence of radiating to the legs. He had visited the hospital and undergone tests several times over the past 5 years, but he had not received proper treatment because the lesions, such as intervertebral disc disease and stenosis, were not clear. He received epidural injection therapy, but there was no improvement, and he could barely endure it with strong painkillers. The patient's X-ray showed a decreased interspinous interval between the third, fourth, and fifth lumbar vertebrae, and the spinous processes impinged on each other during extension (Fig. 19.6). On MRI, the interspinous ligament showed high signals in T2W-image and STIR image (Fig. 19.7). The patient's symptoms and imaging findings led to the diagnosis of Baastrup's disease. Because of severe pain that did not improve with conservative treatment, ligament reconstruction was performed. The surgical findings clearly showed narrowing of the interspinous space, and the interspinous space was widened after ligament reconstruction (Fig. 19.8). After surgery, the patient's back pain disappeared, and he has not complained of back pain any longer.

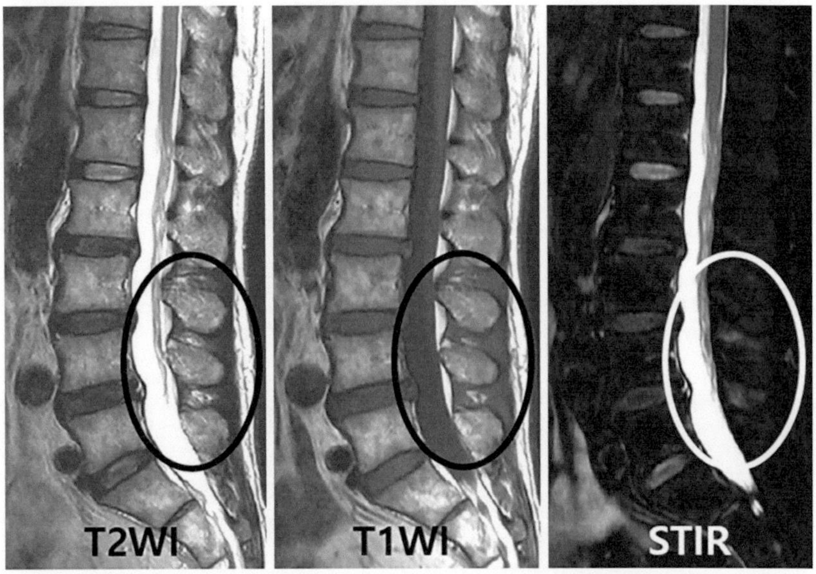

Fig. 19.7 The interspinous ligament showed high signals in T2W-image and STIR image on MRI

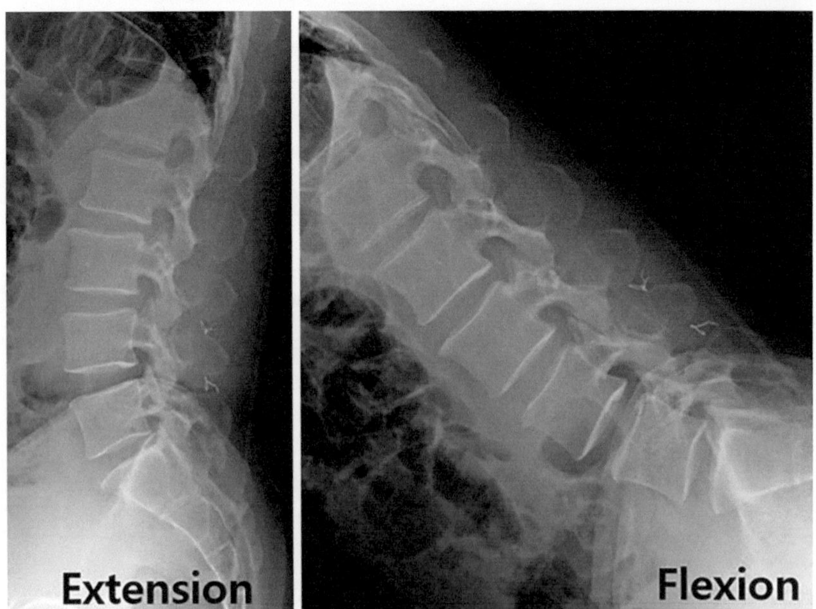

Fig. 19.8 The interspinous space was widened after ligament reconstruction on X-ray

19.3 Summary

In conclusion, while Baastrup's disease can be a source of considerable discomfort, proper management through a multidisciplinary approach holds promise for improving quality of life and functional outcomes for those affected. Baastrup's disease that does not respond to conservative treatment is treated surgically. Ligament reconstruction is performed with minimal invasion to overcome the disadvantages of fusion surgery and treat interspinous ligament lesions while maintaining normal movement.

References

1. Farinha F, Raínho C, Cunha I, Barcelos A. Baastrup's disease: a POORLY recognized cause of back pain. Acta Reumatol Port. 2015;40:302–3.
2. Hagner W. Baastrup 's disease of the lumpar segment of the spine among drivers of heavy motor vehicles. Med Pr. 1988;39(1):65–70.
3. Maes R, Morrison WB, Parker L, Schweitzer M, Carrino J. LUMBAR InterSpinous Bursitis (Baastrup Disease) in a symptomatic population: prevalence on magnetic resonance imaging. Spine (Phila Pa 1976). 2008;33(7):211–5.
4. Lamer TJ, Tiede JM, Fenton DS. Fluoroscopgy-guided injections to trade "kissing spine" disease. Pain Physician. 2008;11:549–54. [PUBMED] [Google School].
5. Okada K, Ohtori S, Inoue G, et al. InterSpinous ligocaine and steroid injections for the management of baastrup's disease: a case series. Asian Spine J. 2014;8:260–6.
6. Mitra R, Ghazi U, Kirpalani D, Cheng I. Interspinous ligament steroid injections for the management of Baastrup's disease: a case report. Arch Phys Med Rehabil. 2007;88:1353–6. [PUBMED] [Google School].
7. Beks JW. Kissing spines: fact or fancy? Acta Neurochir. 1989;100:134–5.
8. Alonso F, et al. Baastrup's disease: a comprehensive review of the EXTANT literature. World Neurosurg. 2017;101:331–4.
9. Filippiadis DK, Mazioti A, Argentos S, Anselmetti G, Papakonstantinou O, Kelekis N, Kelekis AW. Baastrup's disease (kissing spines syndrome): a pictorial review. Insights Imaging. 2015;6:123–8.
10. Okada K, et al. Interspinous ligocaine and steroid injections for the management of baastrup's disease: a case series. Asian Spine J. 2014;8(3):260–6. https://doi.org/10.4184/asj.2014.8.3.2.
11. Philipp LR, Baum GRR, Grossberg JA, Ahmad F. Baastrup's disease: an offen missed etiology for back pain. Cureus. 2016;8(1):E465.

Ligament Reconstruction with Spondylolysis Repair

20

YongSoo Choi

Abstract

Spondylolysis is a stress fracture of the pars interarticularis, a region of the vertebra located between the superior and inferior articular processes. It commonly occurs in the lumbar spine, particularly in adolescents and young athletes involved in activities that involve repetitive hyperextension and rotation. Symptoms of spondylolysis can range from asymptomatic to lower back pain and discomfort, which may worsen with physical activity. When conservative treatments such as rest, physical therapy, and bracing fail to alleviate symptoms, surgical intervention may be considered. Spondylolysis repair involves procedures like direct pars repair, fusion, or instrumentation to stabilize the affected vertebrae. Early diagnosis and appropriate management are crucial to prevent progression to spondylolisthesis, where one vertebra slips over another. This paper explores the etiology, diagnosis, and management strategies, with an emphasis on surgical repair techniques and outcomes.

Keywords

Spondylolysis · Lumbar Stenosis · Ligament Reconstruction · Spondylolysis Repair Interspinous Ligament

Spondylolysis is a condition characterized by a stress fracture or defect in the pars interarticularis of the vertebra. It is most commonly seen in the lumbar spine, particularly in the lower lumbar vertebrae (Fig. 20.1) [1–6]. The condition can lead to chronic lower back pain, especially in young athletes or individuals who engage in activities involving repetitive hyperextension and rotation of the spine [1–3, 5]. Spondylolysis may be asymptomatic or symptomatic, and if left untreated, it can progress to spondylolisthesis, where one vertebra slips forward over another, potentially causing further instability and pain [1, 2, 5].

The term "spondylolysis" was first described by the French surgeon Paul Broca in 1851, who recognized a defect in the pars interarticularis as the underlying cause of back pain in certain individuals [1, 2, 5–7]. Initially, spondylolysis was thought to be primarily a congenital defect, but over time, it became evident that repetitive stress and mechanical loading could contribute to its development. In the mid-twentieth century, advancements in imaging techniques such as X-rays and later MRI helped in the accurate diagnosis of the condition [1, 7]. This allowed for bet-

Y. Choi (✉)
Department of Neurosurgery, Cheongdam Wooridul Spine Hospital, Seoul, Korea (Republic of)
e-mail: yong@wooridul.co.kr

S.-H. Lee et al. (eds.), *Ligament Reconstruction for Spine*,
https://doi.org/10.1007/978-981-95-3971-0_20

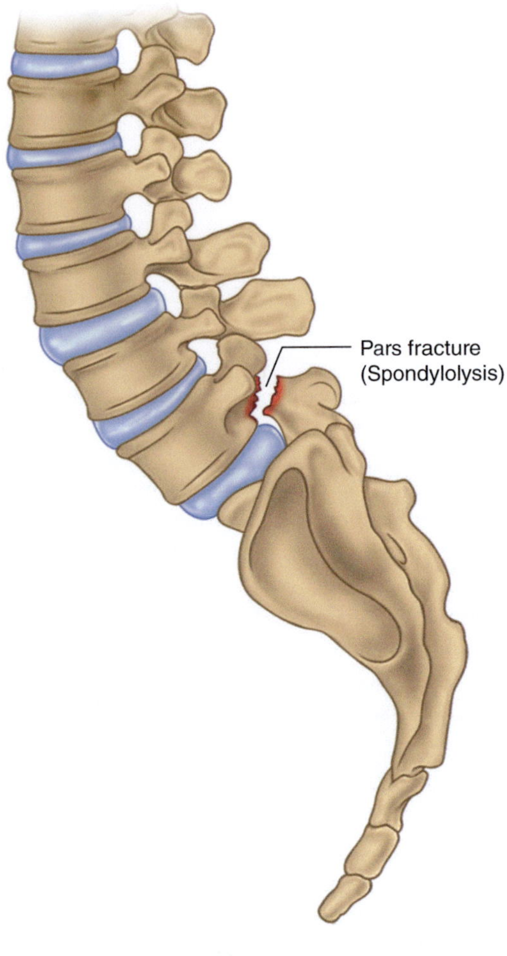

Fig. 20.1 Spondylolysis is a defect or stress fracture in the pars interarticularis, a small bony region of the vertebra that connects the upper and lower facet joints. It most commonly occurs in the lumbar spine, particularly at L5, and is a common cause of lower back pain in adolescents and young athletes

ter understanding of its etiology, progression, and treatment options.

The primary cause of spondylolysis is repetitive mechanical stress on the pars interarticularis, which leads to microfractures and ultimately a stress fracture [1, 2, 4, 7]. This condition is often seen in athletes involved in sports that require repeated hyperextension and rotation of the spine, such as gymnastics, football, and weightlifting. Genetic predisposition, structural anomalies, and high levels of physical activity are considered contributing factors. Additionally, trauma or an acute injury to the lumbar spine can also cause a spondylolysis, though this is less common than stress-related injuries. Other factors such as lumbar lordosis and excessive body weight can further increase the risk of developing spondylolysis [7].

Spondylolysis is most common in adolescents and young adults, particularly athletes who engage in high-risk sports. Studies indicate that it affects 3–6% of the general population, with higher rates in specific sports populations. The condition is more frequently diagnosed in males than females, likely due to the higher incidence of sports participation in young males. In adolescents, spondylolysis is typically seen during periods of rapid growth, and in many cases, it resolves with conservative management. However, in some individuals, the condition can progress and result in spondylolisthesis. The incidence of spondylolysis is higher in certain athletic populations, with rates reaching 25% or more in sports like gymnastics and football [1, 2, 4, 7].

The primary cause of spondylolysis is repetitive stress or overuse of the spine, leading to microfractures in the pars interarticularis, a bony structure connecting the vertebrae. This condition is most commonly seen in athletes who participate in sports that involve frequent hyperextension, rotation, or axial loading of the spine, such as gymnastics, football, weightlifting, and swimming. The constant strain on the lower lumbar spine, particularly in the L5 vertebra, can weaken the pars interarticularis, eventually causing a stress fracture. Other contributing factors include anatomical variations such as a congenital weakness in the pars interarticularis, which may make individuals more susceptible to the condition. Additionally, trauma or a sudden impact, though less common, can also lead to a fracture in this region. Genetic predisposition, age (particularly during periods of rapid growth in adolescence), and excessive lumbar lordosis or poor posture can further increase the risk of developing spondylolysis [1, 2, 5, 7].

The symptoms of spondylolysis can vary depending on the severity of the condition. In many cases, individuals with spondylolysis may be asymptomatic, meaning they experience no noticeable pain or discomfort. However, when symptoms do occur, the most common complaint is lower back pain, particularly in the lumbar region. This pain is often aggravated by physical activity, especially movements that involve bending, twisting, or extending the spine, such as during sports or heavy lifting. In some cases, the pain may worsen with prolonged standing or sitting [1–3, 8].

Other symptoms can include stiffness and muscle tightness in the lower back, which can restrict mobility and flexibility. In more severe cases, if the spondylolysis progresses to spondylolisthesis (vertebral slippage), individuals may experience radiating pain, numbness, or weakness in the legs due to nerve compression. Additionally, some individuals may report difficulty in performing certain movements or sports activities due to discomfort or instability in the spine. The intensity of symptoms can fluctuate, and they may improve with rest or conservative treatments like physical therapy, though they may persist if left untreated [1–3, 6, 7, 9].

The diagnosis of spondylolysis typically begins with a thorough medical history and physical examination. The physician will inquire about the patient's symptoms, including the location, intensity, and duration of pain, as well as any history of repetitive activity or trauma that may have contributed to the condition. The physical examination often includes testing for tenderness in the lower back, particularly over the lumbar spine, and assessing for any signs of nerve involvement, such as weakness or numbness [1, 2, 5, 6].

Imaging studies are essential for confirming the diagnosis of spondylolysis. X-rays are the first-line diagnostic tool and can reveal the presence of a fracture in the pars interarticularis, though early-stage spondylolysis may not always be visible on plain films. If the X-rays are inconclusive, more advanced imaging techniques, such as a CT scan or MRI, may be used. A CT scan is particularly useful in identifying bone fractures and evaluating the extent of the defect, while an MRI can help assess any associated soft tissue damage, such as disc degeneration or nerve compression. In some cases, additional tests like single-photon emission computed tomography (SPECT) scans may be used to detect bone activity and confirm the presence of a stress fracture, especially in early or subtle cases. Once the imaging confirms the presence of a fracture in the pars interarticularis, the diagnosis of spondylolysis is made [1, 2, 5, 6].

The natural course of spondylolysis can vary significantly between individuals, depending on factors such as age, activity level, and the extent of the injury. In many cases, spondylolysis may remain asymptomatic, with the individual not experiencing significant discomfort or limitations in daily activities [1, 6, 7]. When symptoms do occur, they are often localized to the lower back, with pain that may fluctuate in intensity depending on activity levels. In these cases, the condition may improve with conservative management such as rest, physical therapy, and avoiding activities that strain the spine. For some individuals, the stress fracture in the pars interarticularis may heal on its own over time, particularly in younger patients or those who modify their activities [6, 7]. However, if the stress fracture does not heal or if repetitive strain continues, there is a risk of progression to spondylolisthesis, where one vertebra shifts forward over another. This can result in increased spinal instability, nerve compression, and potentially more severe pain, leading to the need for more aggressive treatment, such as surgery [1, 6]. Overall, the natural progression of spondylolysis can range from complete recovery with conservative measures to chronic pain and potential complications if left untreated. Early detection and appropriate management are key factors in achieving a positive outcome and preventing long-term disability [1, 5, 6].

Lumbar stenosis accompanied by spondylolysis is a condition where both narrowing of the spinal canal (lumbar stenosis) and a stress fracture in the pars interarticularis (spondylolysis) occur together, often leading to increased back pain and neurological symptoms. Lumbar stenosis involves the narrowing of the spaces within the spine, which can put pressure on the spinal cord and nerve roots, causing symptoms such as leg pain, numbness, weakness, and difficulty walking [1, 4, 6]. When spondylolysis is present, particularly if it progresses to spondylolisthesis (slippage of a vertebra), it can exacerbate the effects of lumbar stenosis by further destabilizing the spine and increasing pressure on the nerve structures. In this combined condition, the typical symptoms of lumbar stenosis—such as pain that radiates into the legs, cramping, and weakness—are often worsened by the mechanical instability caused by the spondylolysis. The instability of the spine due to the pars defect can lead to abnormal movement of the vertebrae, potentially aggravating the stenosis and making it more difficult for the individual to find relief. Treatment for this combined condition generally focuses on managing both the mechanical instability (often with bracing, physical therapy, or surgery) and the nerve compression (typically with medications, physical therapy, or surgical decompression). Early intervention is crucial to prevent further deterioration and to improve long-term outcomes for individuals suffering from both lumbar stenosis and spondylolysis [2, 6].

The treatment of spondylolysis primarily depends on the severity of the condition and the symptoms experienced by the individual. In many cases, conservative management is effective, especially for mild to moderate cases. The first-line treatment often includes rest and activity modification, which involves avoiding activities that exacerbate pain or put strain on the lower back. A physical therapy program is typically recommended to strengthen the core and back muscles, improve flexibility, and correct posture to support spinal stability [7]. Nonsteroidal anti-inflammatory drugs (NSAIDs) may be prescribed to manage pain and inflammation, while bracing or the use of lumbar supports can provide additional stabilization and reduce stress on the spine during the healing process. In many cases, individuals with spondylolysis can experience significant improvement with these noninvasive treatments, especially if the condition is caught early [6, 7]. If conservative measures fail to alleviate symptoms, and if the spondylolysis progresses or leads to complications such as spondylolisthesis (vertebral slippage), surgical intervention may be necessary. Surgical options may include procedures such as spinal fusion to stabilize the affected vertebrae, or pars repair, where the fractured pars interarticularis is surgically repaired. In some cases, decompressive surgery may be required if there is associated nerve compression or lumbar stenosis. The goal of surgery is to relieve pain, restore stability, and prevent further progression of the condition. Overall, early diagnosis and appropriate treatment are key to managing spondylolysis and preventing long-term complications [1, 2, 6].

The treatment of lumbar stenosis accompanied by spondylolysis typically requires a multifaceted approach, as both conditions contribute to pain and spinal instability [1, 6]. The treatment plan will vary depending on the severity of symptoms, the degree of stenosis, and the extent of the spondylolysis or spondylolisthesis. For mild cases where symptoms are manageable, conservative measures are often the first step. This includes activity modification to avoid movements that exacerbate pain, physical therapy to strengthen the muscles around the spine, and improve flexibility and posture. Physical therapy aims to stabilize the spine and reduce the strain on the affected areas. Nonsteroidal anti-inflammatory drugs (NSAIDs) or other pain relievers can be used to reduce inflammation and manage discomfort [6, 7]. Additionally, lumbar braces may help stabilize the spine and reduce movement that can worsen symptoms. If there is significant nerve compression or radiculopathy (pain radiating into the legs), epidural steroid injections may be considered. These injections can provide temporary relief by reducing inflammation around the nerve roots, easing pain, and improving mobility, particularly for individuals with lumbar stenosis symptoms like leg pain and numbness. When conservative treatments fail or the symptoms become severe, surgical options may be necessary [2, 6, 7]. Decompressive Laminectomy involves removing portions of the vertebra or disc material that are compressing the spinal cord or nerve roots, thereby relieving symptoms of stenosis. If the spondylolysis has led to vertebral slippage (spondylolisthesis), spinal fusion may be required to stabilize the affected vertebrae. This procedure fuses two or more vertebrae to prevent abnormal movement and alleviate pressure on the nerves. In cases where spondylolysis has not progressed to slippage but remains symptomatic, surgical repair of the pars defect may be considered to restore stability and alleviate pain [1, 4, 6].

There are several pars repair techniques used to treat spondylolysis, depending on the severity of the condition, the location of the fracture, and the patient's overall health (Fig. 20.2). Direct Pars Repair with Internal Fixation involves making a surgical incision to directly access the affected vertebra [9]. The fractured pars interarticularis is then visualized and repaired using screws, rods, or plates to stabilize the vertebra while it heals [8, 10, 11]. Bone grafts, either from the patient (autograft) or a donor (allograft), may also be used to promote bone healing and fill in any gaps in the fracture site [10]. This procedure provides immediate stability and helps to restore the structural integrity of the spine. In some cases, the fractured pars may not heal on its own, requiring the use of a bone graft [10]. The surgeon will place either an autograft (taken from the patient's own body) or an allograft (donor bone tissue) into the fracture site to stimulate bone healing. This may be done in combination with instrumentation, such as screws and rods, to stabilize the vertebra and allow the bone graft to properly integrate with the surrounding tissue. In

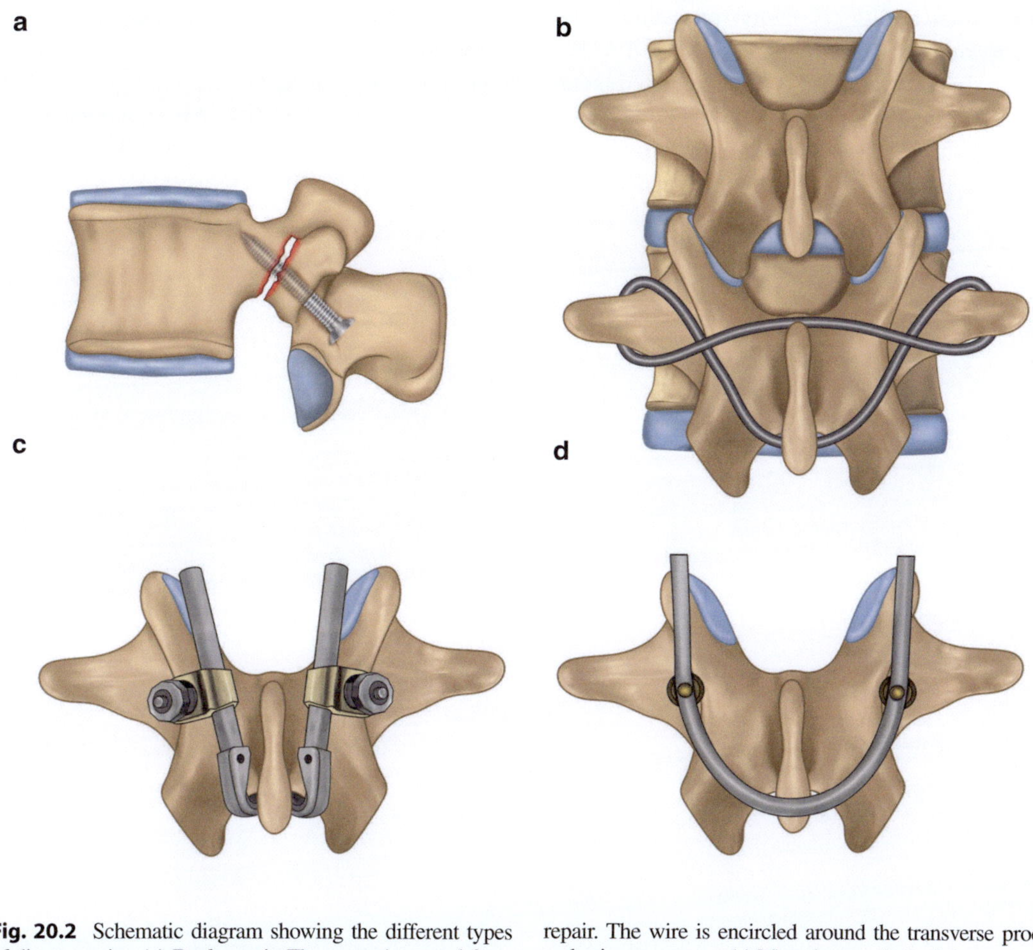

Fig. 20.2 Schematic diagram showing the different types of direct repairs. (**a**) Buck repair. The screw is passed from the lower edge of the lamina across the defect. (**b**) Scott repair. The wire is encircled around the transverse process and spinous process. (**c**) Morscher repair. Pedicle screw with laminar hooks. (**d**) Pedicle screw with a U-shaped rod [8–11]

this approach, smaller incisions are made, and specialized instruments are used to access the affected vertebra. Minimally invasive surgery reduces muscle dissection, minimizes blood loss, and promotes quicker recovery compared to traditional open surgery. The fractured pars is repaired using screws, rods, and bone grafts, with less disruption to surrounding tissues [9, 10]. This technique is particularly advantageous for reducing postoperative pain and shortening recovery time. In pars Repair with compression screw technique, a compression screw is placed across the fractured pars to provide compression at the fracture site, encouraging bone healing. The screw helps stabilize the vertebra without the need for large implants. In some cases, the screw is used in conjunction with a bone graft to further enhance healing. This technique is often less invasive than traditional fusion procedures and can help maintain motion at the affected spinal segment. In cases where there is associated instability, such as in the progression to spondylolisthesis, the surgeon may perform a posterior spinal fusion in conjunction with pars repair. This involves removing damaged or degenerated discs and replacing them with bone grafts, while using screws and rods to stabilize the spine. The goal is to restore alignment and prevent further vertebral slippage, providing both stability and pain relief [8–11].

The Buck's technique for direct pars repair in the treatment of spondylolysis is a method of surgically stabilizing the spine when a fracture in the pars interarticularis (the bone connecting the upper and lower facets of a vertebra) is present (Fig. 20.3) [9]. In this technique, the surgeon directly addresses the fracture by using instrumentation such as screws, rods, or plates to stabilize the vertebra and promote healing of the pars defect. During the procedure, the surgeon makes an incision over the affected area of the spine to access the fractured pars interarticularis [6, 9]. The fracture is then carefully visualized and repaired using screws or other fixation devices, which hold the vertebra in place while the bone heals (Fig. 20.4). Additionally, bone grafts (either from the patient's own body or from a donor) may be placed to help stimulate bone growth and further support the repair. The key aspect of the Buck's

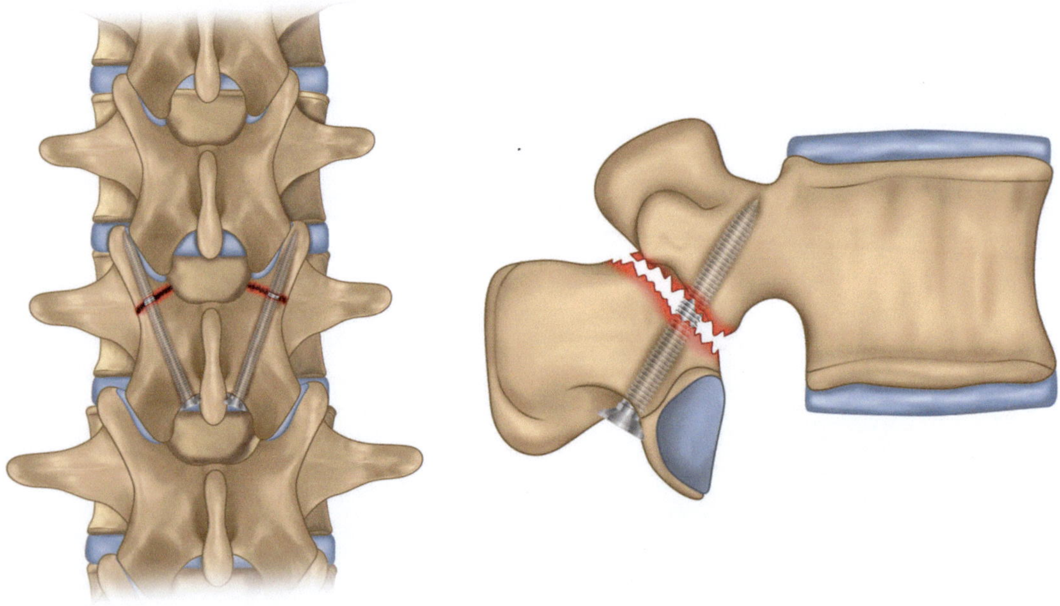

Fig. 20.3 Buck's technique is a direct repair method for treating spondylolysis by stabilizing the pars interarticularis defect without fusing the motion segment

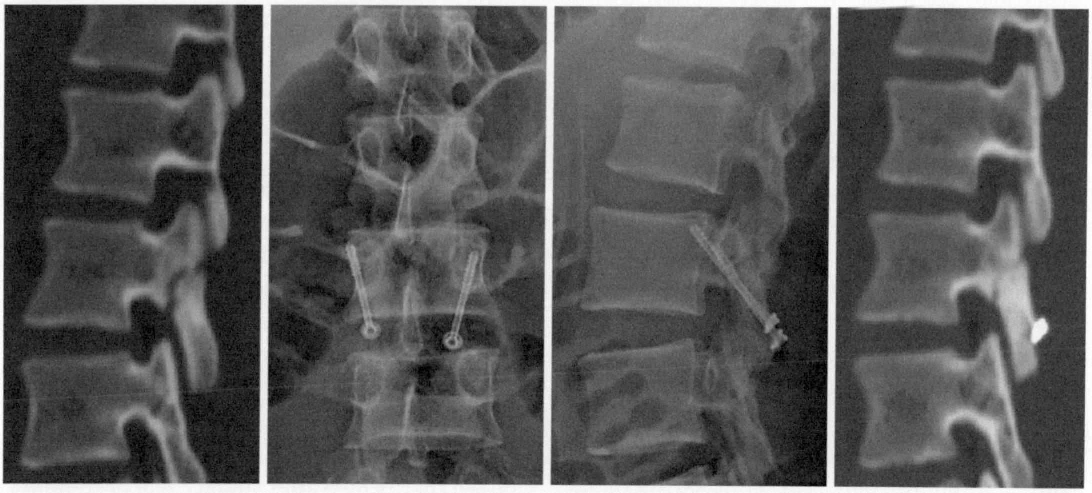

Fig. 20.4 Six months after spondylolysis repair, CT images show fusion of the defective pars interarticularis

technique in direct pars repair is its focus on restoring the structural integrity of the affected vertebra while preserving motion. Unlike spinal fusion, which permanently fuses the vertebrae, this technique aims to stabilize the fractured area without sacrificing flexibility. By repairing the pars interarticularis directly, the Buck's technique seeks to eliminate the instability that results from the fracture, alleviate pain caused by the defect, and prevent further complications such as vertebral slippage (spondylolisthesis). This surgical approach typically offers a good outcome, especially in patients with isolated pars fractures and minimal degeneration of the spinal segments. However, it requires careful surgical technique to ensure that the fractured area heals properly and that surrounding structures are not damaged. Each of these techniques aims to restore the structural integrity of the spine, promote healing of the fractured pars, and alleviate pain caused by spondylolysis. The choice of technique depends on the specific characteristics of the injury and the patient's needs [9].

Most spine surgeons consider interbody fusion and pedicle screw fixation as the primary surgical treatment when spinal stenosis is accompanied by spondylolysis. However, the use of the above-mentioned spondylolysis repair and ligament reconstruction techniques provides an option for treatment without spinal interbody fusion and posterior pedicle screw fixation. After central decompression is performed to resolve spinal stenosis, ligament reconstruction is selected as an effective and minimally invasive treatment. If spondylolysis is present, the artificial ligament placed on the spinous process is difficult to maintain because the spinous process, including lamina, is separated from the pas interarticularis and is floating. In order for ligament reconstruction to be performed, the spinous process must be fixed and not floating, and this is possible with spondylolysis repair. Spondylolysis repair tightens the pars interarticularis, thereby firmly fixing the spinous processes. Spondylolisthesis due to spondylolysis can also be reduced and instability changed to stability through spondylolysis repair and ligament reconstruction. Therefore, the combination of spondylolysis repair and ligament reconstruction is one option for treating spondylolysis and spinal stenosis. This method is less invasive than interbody fusion and pedicle screw fixation, and can eliminate the disadvantages and complications of fusion. This technique accelerates patient recovery and improves quality of life.

20.1 Surgical Technique

The patient undergoes a thorough clinical evaluation, imaging studies (X-ray, CT, MRI), and preoperative counseling. General anesthesia is administered, and the patient is positioned prone on a radiolucent table with appropriate padding to protect pressure points. Fluoroscopic guidance or portable simple radiography is set up to confirm the level of the defect intraoperatively. A midline or paramedian skin incision is made over the affected lumbar level (most commonly L5). The paraspinal muscles (erector spinae and multifidus) are dissected subperiosteally and retracted laterally to expose the lamina and pars interarticularis. Care is taken to avoid excessive muscle damage to minimize postoperative pain and enhance recovery. The fibrous or sclerotic tissue within the defect is carefully debrided using a curette or burr. The bone edges of the defect are freshened to stimulate healing and increase surface area for fusion. A small cancellous bone graft (harvested from the iliac crest or local bone) may be prepared for placement in the defect. A cortical screw (usually 3.5–4.5 mm in diameter) is inserted into the pedicle of the affected vertebra. A loop of stainless steel wire is placed around the screw and passed across the pars defect. The wire is then tightened to compress the defect, securing the fractured pars interarticularis against the pedicle screw. Alternatively, a tension band or small bone graft may be fixed with a screw instead of the wire loop to enhance stability. Fluoroscopy is used to confirm the proper position of the screw and wire construct. The artificial ligament is placed including the spinous process of the repaired segment. The artificial ligaments use the sagittal ligament and the horizontal ligament to achieve vertical and horizontal stability. The sagittal ligament is formed by the spinous processes of adjacent segments being placed in an oval shape, and is shaped and tied to fit the size. The horizontal ligament is tied in a vertical direction to the sagittal ligament in the space between the spinous processes. Performing spondylolysis repair and ligament reconstruction simultaneously provides a minimally invasive and reliable treatment for spondylolysis and spinal stenosis associated with spondylolysis.

20.2 Case Illustration

20.2.1 Case I

An 83-year-old female patient complained of back pain, radiating pain in both lower extremities, numbness, and neurogenic claudication that had persisted for more than 5 years. Spondylolysis of the fifth lumbar vertebra was confirmed on X-ray, and spinal stenosis of the fourth and fifth lumbar vertebrae and stenosis of the fifth lumbar-sacral foramina were confirmed on MRI (Fig. 20.5). Spondylolysis repair was performed using Buck's technique, and ligament reconstruction was performed after spinal canal decompression surgery through a central approach at L4-5. The patient's symptoms disappeared immediately, and she did not complain of any pain, numbness, or gait difficulty after the surgery. Markers for artificial ligaments and the screws for spondylolysis repair were observed on postoperative X-ray, and decompression of the spinal canal of L4-5 and widening of the intervertebral foramen between L5 and Sacrum were shown on MRI after the surgery (Fig. 20.6).

20.2.2 Case II

A 68-year-old female patient complained of back pain that had persisted for more than 10 years. She could not get up immediately after sitting down because of back pain, and complained of severe back pain while walking. Spondylolisthesis due to spondylolysis of L4-5 was seen on X-ray, and there was no spinal stenosis or intervertebral foraminal stenosis (Fig. 20.7). Repair of spondylolysis using Buck's technique and ligament reconstruction of the affected segment were performed. Spondylolysis repair was performed to fix the pars interarticularis, and ligament reconstruction was performed to reduce the spondylolisthesis and stabilize the segment. After surgery, spondylolysis stabilized and spondylolisthesis was reduced (Fig. 20.8). The patient no longer

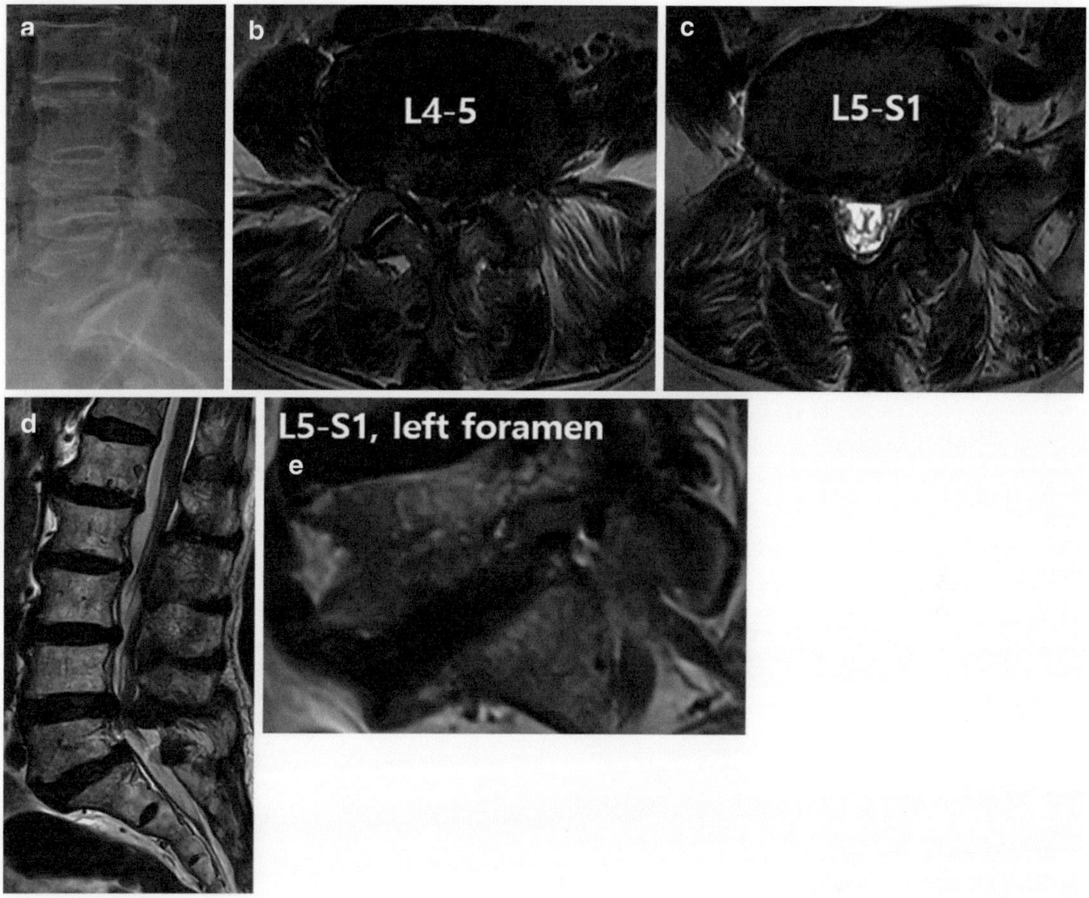

Fig. 20.5 Spondylolysis of the fifth lumbar vertebra was confirmed on X-ray (**a**), and spinal stenosis of the fourth and fifth lumbar vertebrae (**b**, **d**) and stenosis of the fifth lumbar-sacral foramen (**c**, **f**) were confirmed on MRI

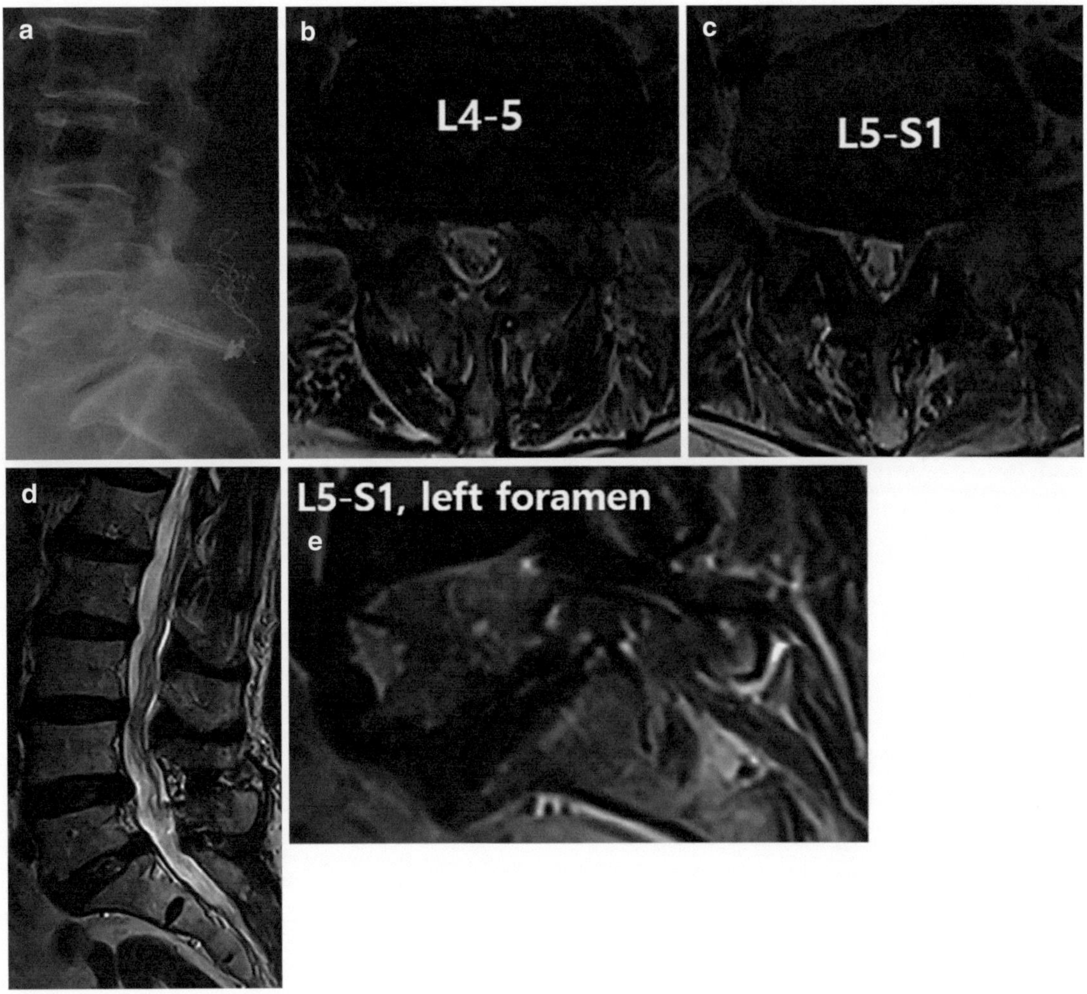

Fig. 20.6 Markers for artificial ligaments and the screws for spondylolysis repair were observed on postoperative X-ray (**a**), and decompression of the spinal canal of L4-5 (**b**, **d**) and widening of the intervertebral foramen between L5 and Sacrum (**c**, **e**) were shown on MRI after the surgery

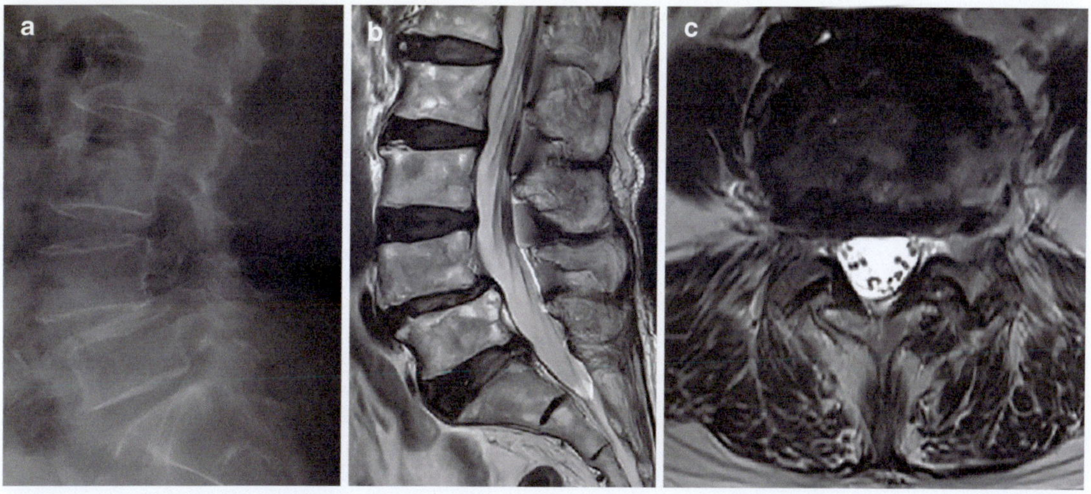

Fig. 20.7 Spondylolisthesis due to spondylolysis of L4-5 (**a**) was seen on X-ray, and there was no spinal stenosis or intervertebral foraminal stenosis (**b**, **c**)

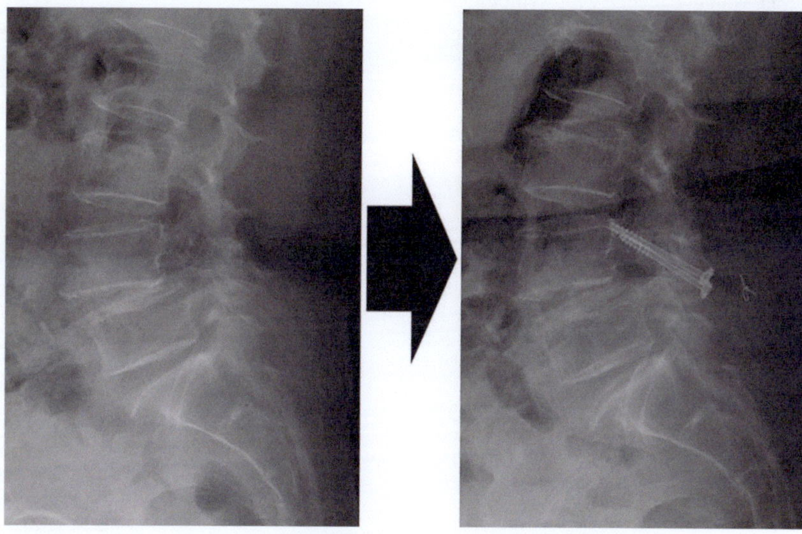

Fig. 20.8 Spondylolysis stabilized and spondylolisthesis was reduced

complained of pain after surgery and was able to lead a normal life. This technique treats both spondylolysis and spondylolisthesis simultaneously, but does not have the movement restrictions that occur when performing interbody fusion surgery. Therefore, this is a method that can treat spondylolysis and spondylolisthesis while maintaining the movement of the lumbar spine.

20.3 Summary

Ligament reconstruction with spondylolysis repair stabilizes the spine without fusion to treat spondylolysis and spinal stenosis with spondylolysis. This method is less invasive than interbody fusion and pedicle screw fixation, and can eliminate the disadvantages and complications of fusion. Ligament reconstruction with spondylolysis repair maintains movement of the spine. Ligament reconstruction with spondylolysis repair is a good option among several ways to treat spondylolysis. This technique accelerates patient recovery and improves quality of life.

References

1. Aoki Y, Takahashi H, Nakajima A. Prevalence of lumbar spondylolysis and spondylolysis in patients with degenerative spinal disease. Sci Rep. 2020;10(1):6739.
2. Grogan JP, Hemminghytt S, Williams AL. Spondylolysis as studied by computed tomography. Radiology. 1982;145(3):737–42.
3. Jin M, Zhang J, Shao H. Percutaneous endoscopic direct repair of patch defects without general anesthesia may be a satisfactory treatment alternative in young patients with symptomatic lumbar spondylolysis: a technical note with a case series. BMC Musculoskelet Disord. 2020;21(1):340.
4. Leone A, Cianfoni A, Cerase A. Lumbar spondylolysis: a review. Skeletal Radiol. 2011;40(6):683–700.
5. Rothman SL, Glenn WV. CT multiplanar reconstruction of 253 cases of lumbar spondylolysis. AJNR Am J Neuroradiol. 1984;5(1):81–90.
6. Tanveer F, Arslan SA, Darain H. Common treatment modalities for lumbar spondylolysis: a systematic review. Medicine(Baltimore). 2021;100(51):e28319.
7. Tawfik S, Phan K, Mobbs RJ. Incidence of pars interarticularis defects in athletes. Glob Spine J. 2020;10(1):89–101.
8. Linhares D, Rodrigues PC, Silva MR. Minimum 10-year follow-up of the V-rod technique in lumbar spondylolysis. Eur Spine J. 2019;28(7):1743–9.
9. Muthiah N, Ozpinar A, Eubanks J. Direct pars repair using cannulated screws in adults: a case series and systematic literature review. World Neurosurg. 2022;163:e263–74.
10. Jamshidi AM, Soldozy S, Levi AD. Percutaneous direct patch repair in young athletes. Neurosurgery. 2023;92(2):263–70.
11. Li DM, Li YC, Jiang W. Application of a novel anatomic hook-rod-pedicle screw system in young patients with lumbar spondylolysis: a pilot study. World J Clin Cases. 2022;10(17):5680–9.

Degenerative Disc Disease

21

Jeong Hoon Choi

Abstract

Degenerative changes of the intervertebral disc are associated with damage of nearby structures, such as ligaments, facet joints, and paraspinal muscles. This leads to functional changes and increases susceptibility to injuries. The causes for pain in the disc degenerative process are complex, and in many cases, structural and mechanical deformations are combined.

The artificial ligament is composed of the sagittal ligament and horizontal ligament; it can be helpful in the treatment of painful spinal disease (instability, foraminal stenosis, and discogenic back pain) caused by degenerative disc disease.

Keywords

Artificial ligament · Disc degeneration · Segmental instability · Foraminal stenosis · Discogenic back pain

J. H. Choi (✉)
Department of Neurosurgery, Cheongdam Wooridul Spine Hospital, Seoul, Korea (Republic of)
e-mail: cjh77@wooridul.co.kr

21.1 Introduction

The intervertebral disc is characterized by a tension-resisting annulus fibrosus and a compression-resisting nucleus pulposus composed largely of proteoglycan. The most important function of the annulus and nucleus is to provide mechanical stability to the disc. Degenerative disc disease in the lumbar spine is a serious health problem.

Degenerative changes of the intervertebral disc are associated with damage of nearby structures, such as ligaments, facet joints, and paraspinal muscles. This leads to functional changes and increases susceptibility to injuries. The causes for pain in the disc degenerative process are complex, and in many cases, structural and mechanical deformations are combined.

In this chapter, we will consider the role that artificial ligament reconstruction as a treatment modality for the instability and foraminal stenosis associated with disc degeneration.

21.1.1 Disc Degeneration and Segmental Instability

The disc degenerative process includes disruption of the collagen fibers, loss of proteoglycan content, loss of water content, and a marked decreased elasticity. Thus, the fibrous annulus structure becomes deformed and torn. These

S.-H. Lee et al. (eds.), *Ligament Reconstruction for Spine*,
https://doi.org/10.1007/978-981-95-3971-0_21

changes lead to a decrease in disc height, which together with changes in all structures of the tripod joint causes instability.

Progression of disc degeneration results in angular and rotatory instability. Such instability usually refers to back pain exacerbated by movement and associated with intersegmental movements that are abnormal or excessive at one or more spinal levels.

The device we used was an interspinous ligament device with interspinous soft anchorage. Although there have been a few clinical results using this ligament or a similar device. We chose this device to provide additional stability after decompression for patients with instability combined with spinal stenosis. Although the problem of the patient with instability is caused by degeneration of the disc and laxity of the facet joint ligaments, we speculated that applying a flexible ligament around the spinous process provided additional stability to the motion segment after decompressive surgery.

This speculation was based on biomechanical studies [1, 2]. Those studies showed that interspinous ligamentous devices had a stabilizing effect in flexion, extension, and lateral bending of spinal motion segments.

The postoperative facet cysts, which were considered complications related to segmental instability in 8.6% of the patients after simple decompression [3].

Considering these aspects, additional stabilization procedures for spinal stability seem to be necessary. The ligament reconstruction system is an effective procedure for treating excessive backward-forward bending and lateral bending. Restriction of angular motion by ligament reconstruction appears to help prevent angular instability after decompressive surgery. Especially in cases of sagittal orientation facet, ligament reconstruction may be a very effective treatment method to prevent flexion instability after decompressive surgery.

21.1.2 Disc Degeneration and Foraminal Narrowing

Several factors contribute to foraminal stenosis. The most common causes include decreased disc height due to disc degeneration, impinging facet joint synovial cysts, facet joint arthropathy, foraminal ligamentum flavum hypertrophy, degenerative or iatrogenic anterolisthesis, and osteophytes of the superior articular process.

As disc height decreases, the vertical distance between the vertebrae also decreases. Degenerative disc disease accelerates osteophyte formation at the foramen and herniation of the nucleus pulposus, which aggravates the foraminal stenosis process. Dynamic instability also promotes facet joint arthropathy, with accompanying osteophyte formation, synovial cyst herniation, joint capsule hypertrophy, and ligamentum flavum hypertrophy. Foraminal stenosis is a dynamic anatomical entity that is exacerbated by lumbar extension, and most patients experience axial low back pain and radiating pain. Foraminal stenosis is stated to be the culprit in 60% of failed back surgeries [4, 5]. Therefore, untreated or ignored foraminal stenosis accounts for a significant proportion of recurrent or residual pain in patients undergoing spine surgery for lumbal spinal stenosis.

The artificial ligament can prevent narrowing of the foramen by filling the interspinous ligament space and preventing foraminal narrowing during extension (Fig. 21.1). Therefore, it can prevent further narrowing of the foramen after decompressive surgery in patients who already have foraminal narrowing, which can prevent back pain occurring after surgery and prevent progression of foraminal stenosis.

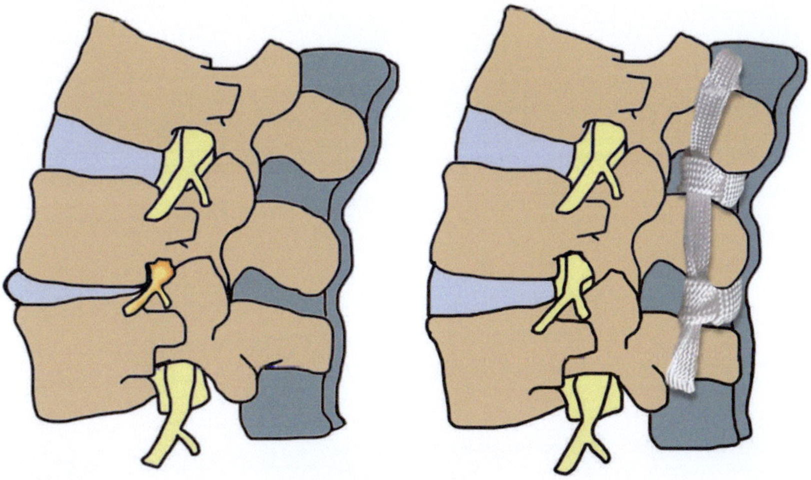

Fig. 21.1 This image shows that by instrumentation of an artificial ligament, the foramen can be widened and the posterior annulus height can be increased, thereby reducing the pain caused by the foramen and posterior annulus

21.1.3 Disc Degeneration and Discogenic Back Pain

Discogenic back pain and axial back pain are terms commonly used to describe back pain associated with disc degeneration without herniation, anatomical deformity, or other alternate clear causes of pain and disability. Disc degeneration is associated with discogenic back pain and is thought to be an important contributing factor. Disc degeneration causes chronic inflammation, neovascularization, neoinnervation, and nociceptive sensitization follows, which ultimately manifests as discogenic pain [6].

Among the various treatment methods for discogenic back pain, there is a method that reduces discogenic back pain by reducing intradiscal pressure.

The artificial ligament that fills the insterspinous ligament space will distribute the pressure within the disc at the instrumentation level because the artificial ligament limits the extension motion and reduces the pressure on the posterior annulus (Fig. 21.1). This can reduce the pressure on the posterior annulus and nucleus in the extension and neutral postition.

21.2 Summary

The artificial ligament is composed of the sagittal ligament and horizontal ligament, so it can completely wrap the spinous process and fill with the interspinous ligament space. Therefore, it reduces the flexion, extension, and some rotation of the index spinal segment. This motion restriction of the artificial ligament can be helpful in the treatment of spinal instability and foraminal stenosis caused by degenerative disc disease, and it can also affect the distribution of intradiscal pressure in patients with discogenic back pain, which will help relieve symptoms.

References

1. Caserta S, La Maida GA, Misaggi B, et al. Elastic stabilization alone or combined with rigid fusion in spinal surgery: a biomechanical study and clinical experience based on 82 cases. Eur Spine J. 2002;11(suppl2):192–197.s.
2. Voydeville G, Diop A, Lavaste F, Girard F, Hardy P. Experimental lumbar instability and artificial ligament. Eur J Orthop Surg Traumatol. 2000;10:167–76.
3. Ikuta K, Tono O, Oga M. Prevalence of clinical features of intraspinal facet cysts after decompression surgery for lumbar spinal stenosis. J Neurosurg Spine. 2009;10:617–22.
4. Yeung A, Gore S. Endoscopic foraminal decompression for failed back surgery syndrome under local anesthesia. Int J Spine Surg. 2014;8(22):22. https://doi.org/10.14444/1022.
5. Lurie JD, Tosteson TD, Tosteson A, et al. Long-term outcomes of lumbar spinal stenosis: eight-year results of the Spine Patient Outcomes Research Trial (SPORT). Spine. 2015;40(2):63–76. https://doi.org/10.1097/brs.0000000000000731.
6. Jha R, Bernstock JD, Chalif JI, Hoffman SE, Gupta S, Guo H, Lu Y. Updates on pathophysiology of discogenic back pain. J Clin Med. 2023;12:6907.

Combination with Laminoplasty for Spinal Tumor

22

Shin-Jae Kim and Sang-Ha Shin

Abstract

This chapter presents a novel hybrid surgical technique that integrates laminoplasty with artificial ligament reconstruction to overcome the limitations of conventional thoracic spinal tumor surgery. Traditional methods often result in compromised stability, chronic pain, and deformities like kyphosis due to the loss of posterior support structures. By restoring the bony integrity through laminoplasty and compensating for absent interspinous and supraspinous ligaments with artificial substitutes, this combined approach enhances spinal stability and alignment. As a result, patients benefit from reduced postoperative complications, minimized pain, and improved functional recovery. Ultimately, this innovative strategy offers a comprehensive, biomechanically sound solution for preserving thoracic spinal integrity and long-term patient quality of life.

Keywords

Thoracic cord tumor · Laminoplasty · Ligament reconstruction · Hybrid surgery · Total laminectomy

S.-J. Kim · S.-H. Shin (✉)
Department of Neurosurgery, Cheongdam Wooridul Spine Hospital, Seoul, Korea (Republic of)
e-mail: burrhoer@wooridul.co.kr

22.1 Introduction

Thoracic spinal tumors present complex surgical challenges due to the intricate anatomy of the region and the critical need to maintain spinal stability while achieving complete tumor resection [1, 2]. Among the available surgical strategies, total laminectomy often provides better visualization and improved access for complete removal of the lesion compared to partial laminectomies [3, 4]. However, this approach is not without significant drawbacks. One of the primary concerns is the weakening of the posterior spinal elements in the thoracic region, which relies heavily on its posterior structures—including the lamina, interspinous ligament, and supraspinous ligament—for stability against flexion and axial loads [5, 6]. While the lamina can be reconstructed through laminoplasty, the interspinous and supraspinous ligaments are frequently removed and left unreconstructed, creating a structural void that compromises thoracic spinal integrity [4].

The absence of these ligamentous supports has several deleterious consequences:

22.1.1 Increased Flexion Instability

The interspinous and supraspinous ligaments serve as key stabilizers against excessive flexion by limiting the separation of adjacent spinous

S.-H. Lee et al. (eds.), *Ligament Reconstruction for Spine*,
https://doi.org/10.1007/978-981-95-3971-0_22

processes [7]. Without these ligaments, the thoracic spine becomes more susceptible to abnormal flexion movements, elevating stress on intervertebral discs and facet joints and potentially leading to instability [8, 9].

22.1.2 Postoperative Kyphosis

Kyphotic deformities are well-documented complications following thoracic spine surgeries, especially when posterior ligamentous structures are not restored [4]. The loss of ligamentous tension can precipitate the progressive collapse of the posterior column, resulting in a kyphotic curve that not only alters spinal alignment but also exacerbates mechanical pain and reduces the patient's mobility and overall quality of life [10].

22.1.3 Chronic Pain and Functional Impairment

The lack of posterior ligamentous support may lead to abnormal load distribution across the thoracic spine, contributing to persistent postoperative pain [11, 12]. This is particularly challenging in the thoracic region, where the interplay between the spine, rib cage, and surrounding musculature is complex. Consequently, patients may experience prolonged discomfort, reduced functionality, and a diminished quality of life.

22.1.4 Impact on Long-Term Recovery

Failing to reconstruct these critical ligaments can adversely influence the long-term recovery trajectory. Although the initial surgical goal focuses on complete tumor resection and neural decompression, ignoring the long-term biomechanical consequences of ligament deficiency can lead to recurrent symptoms and the potential need for revision surgeries [13].

These challenges highlight the limitations of traditional thoracic spinal tumor surgeries and underscore the necessity for innovative solutions. Laminoplasty alone, despite its effectiveness in reconstructing the bony lamina, does not replicate the functional integrity once provided by the interspinous and supraspinous ligaments [14]. This gap presents an opportunity for a hybrid approach that combines laminoplasty with artificial ligament reconstruction, thereby restoring posterior stability more comprehensively and potentially improving patient outcomes [15].

This chapter introduces and explores this hybrid surgical technique, detailing its methodology, biomechanical advantages, and potential to redefine postoperative care in thoracic spinal tumor management. By bridging the gap left by conventional approaches, this combined strategy represents a significant advancement in spinal surgery, aiming to enhance both immediate surgical success and long-term patient well-being.

22.2 Presentation of the Patient

A 65-year-old male patient presented with worsening lower back and leg pain that began approximately 8 months ago. He reported pain and numbness radiating to the front and back of both legs, extending below the knees. He was unable to walk without a cane due to weakness in his legs and exhibited an unsteady gait, frequently losing balance. The patient also experienced diminished perianal sensation and bowel and bladder dysfunction, requiring a laxative dose more than three times the usual prescription. His medical history included a diagnosis of diabetes and liver cirrhosis 4 years ago and a right total knee arthroplasty performed 6 months ago. On physical examination, the patient exhibited a severe limping gait and was unable to perform both heel and toe walking. Paraesthesia was noted. Muscle strength evaluation revealed generalized weakness in the lower extremities: ankle dorsiflexion G3/3, ankle plantarflexion G2/3, knee extension/flexion G3/4, and hip extension/flexion G4/4. Enhanced MRI image shows well enhancing intradural extramedullary (IDEM) mass at T12-L1 level, 1.2 × 1.2 × 2 cm, R/O neurogenic tumor (Fig. 22.1).

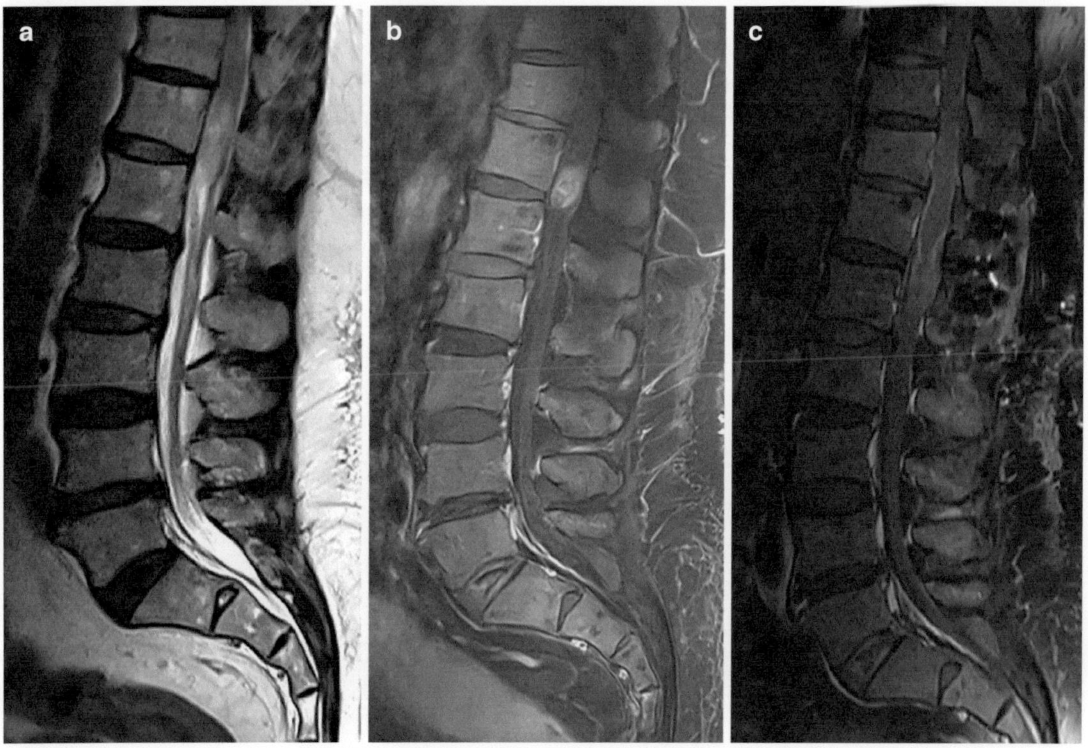

Fig. 22.1 Sagittal image of MRI (**a**) T2 image shows intradural mass at T12-L1 level. (**b**) Enhance T1 image shows well enhancing intradural extramedullary (IDEM) mass at T12-L1 level, 1.2 × 1.2 × 2 cm, R/O neurogenic tumor. (**c**) Postoperative enhance image shows well removed tumor

22.3 Preoperative Planning

Radiologic evaluation revealed an intradural extramedullary mass at the T12-L1 level, suspected to be a schwannoma. Due to significant neurological deficits caused by nerve compression from the mass effect, surgical treatment was planned. The surgical plan included laminectomy and tumor removal at the T12-L1 level. To ensure adequate surgical visualization and minimize the risk of nerve traction injury, a total laminectomy at T12 was planned. Postoperatively, to preserve the posterior structures at the surgical site, T12 laminoplasty using a titanium plate was proposed. Additionally, to reconstruct the supraspinous structures above and below the surgical site, artificial ligament reconstruction was planned for the T11-12 and T12-L1 levels.

22.4 Surgical Steps (Illustration, Photos, Videos)

22.4.1 Preoperative Planning and Imaging

Utilize MRI and CT scans preoperatively to delineate the tumor boundaries and assess its involvement with surrounding structures, including the spinal cord, nerve roots, and posterior elements. Plan the incision to ensure adequate exposure for total laminectomy while preserving as much of the normal anatomy as possible.

22.4.2 Patient Positioning and Exposure

Position the patient in the prone position on a radiolucent table. Ensure proper padding to protect pressure points and maintain optimal alignment of the thoracic spine. Make a posterior midline incision extending beyond the tumor boundaries identified on imaging. The incision should allow sufficient exposure to perform the laminectomy without tension on the soft tissues. Elevate the paraspinal muscles subperiosteally to expose the laminae and surrounding structures (Fig. 22.2a).

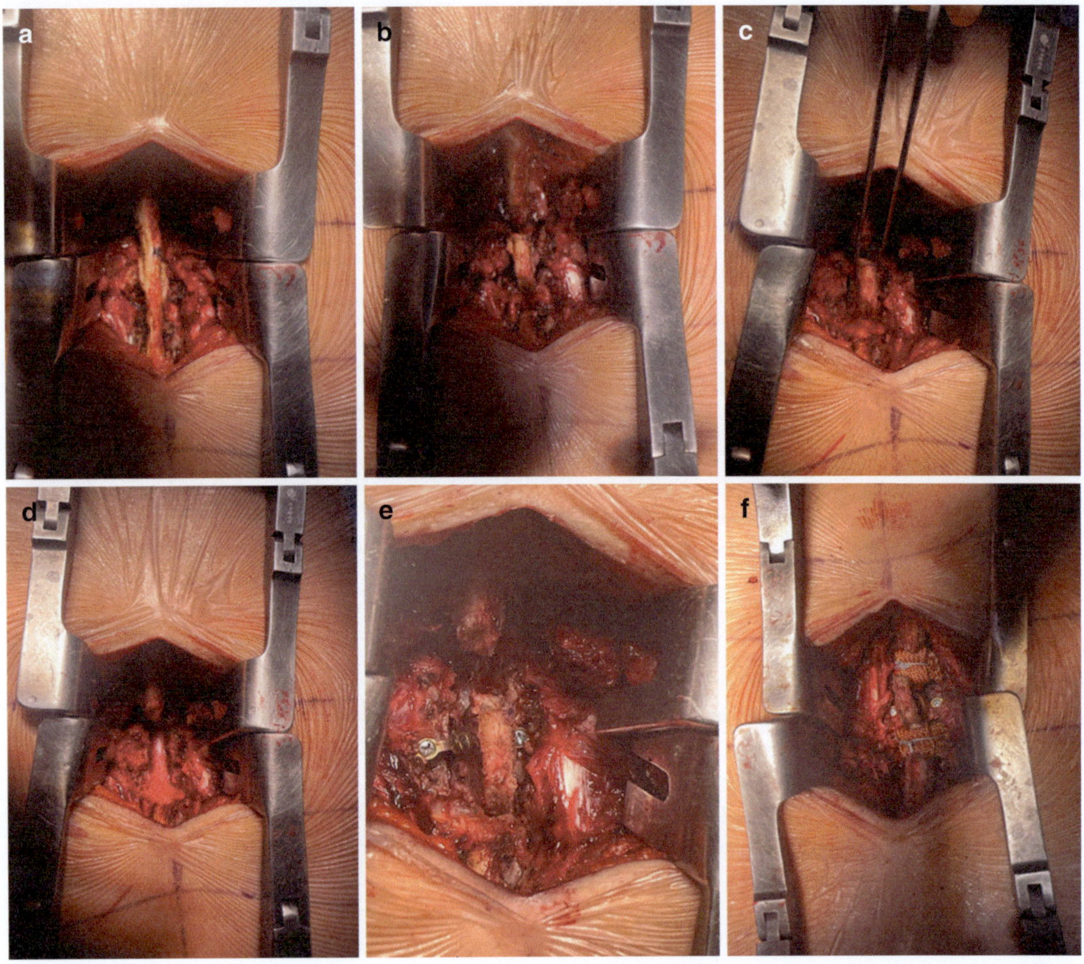

Fig. 22.2 Process of total laminectomy, laminoplasty, and ligament reconstruction (**a**) Bilateral dissection of the paraspinal muscles was performed, and retractors were applied to fully expose the T11-12-L1 spinous processes. (**b**) The T11-12 and T12-L1 supraspinous and interspinous ligaments were removed. (**c**) A high-speed drill was used to perform bilateral laminectomy. (**d**) T12 lamina was completely removed. (**e**) The excised T12 lamina was reattached and secured using titanium screws and a miniplate. (**f**) Ligament reconstruction with artificial ligaments was performed at the T11-12 and T12-L1 levels

22.4.3 Total Laminectomy

Supraspinous and interspinous ligaments were removed using bovie and ronguer. Preserve the spinous processes and laminae in as close to their original shape as possible, as these will be used for reconstruction (Fig. 22.2b). Pay careful attention to preserving the integrity of the surrounding bone and minimize unnecessary resection to maintain the spine's biomechanical properties (Fig. 22.2c). Perform a total laminectomy to achieve complete tumor resection. Use high-speed burrs and Kerrison rongeurs to remove the laminae (Fig. 22.2d). Ensure complete decompression of the neural elements by removing any compressive tumor mass and hypertrophic ligamentum flavum.

22.4.4 Laminoplasty

Reconstruct the excised laminae using titanium plates and screws (Fig. 22.2e). Carefully reattach the laminae to their original position to restore the posterior bony structure. Ensure alignment of the laminae to avoid undue stress on the reconstructed area. Utilize fluoroscopy to confirm proper placement of the implants.

22.4.5 Artificial Ligament Reconstruction

Prepare artificial ligaments tailored to the thoracic spine. Given the narrower interlaminar space in the thoracic region compared to the lumbar spine, thin and flexible artificial ligaments should be selected. Secure the artificial ligament to the spinous processes of the vertebrae above and below the laminoplasty site using suture anchors or screws (Fig. 22.2f). Bind the ligament more narrowly than in lumbar ligament reconstruction to accommodate the thoracic anatomy while ensuring adequate tension to mimic natural ligament function. Confirm the tensioning of the artificial ligament to avoid over-tightening, which could restrict spinal motion or cause discomfort.

22.4.6 Final Inspection and Closure

Carefully inspect the reconstructed laminoplasty and ligament areas to ensure stability. Check for any movement of the implants or ligaments under physiological stress. Use fluoroscopy to verify the structural integrity and alignment of the reconstructed posterior column. Achieve meticulous hemostasis, and close the surgical site in layers to protect the implants and minimize soft tissue disruption.

22.4.7 Postoperative Considerations

Postsurgical imaging (e.g., CT or X-ray) should be performed to confirm that the laminoplasty and artificial ligament reconstruction are intact and appropriately positioned. Patients should be monitored closely for any signs of instability, pain, or complications related to the reconstructed structures. This detailed technique ensures that the tumor is fully resected while preserving and reconstructing the posterior thoracic structure to enhance spinal stability and support optimal patient recovery (Fig. 22.3).

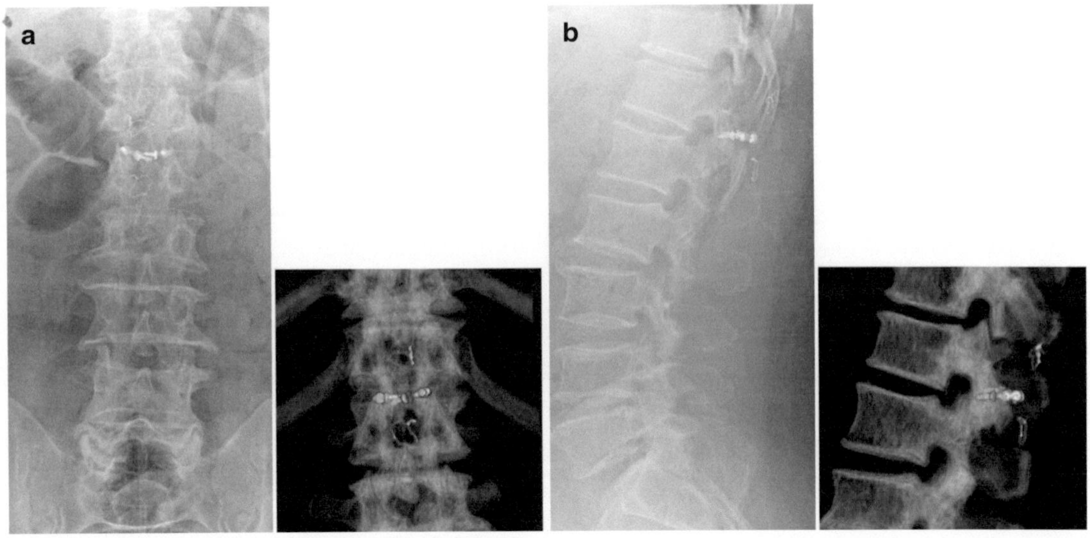

Fig. 22.3 Postoperative X-ray (**a**) AP view (**b**) Lateral view

22.5 Commentary

The hybrid surgical technique that combines laminoplasty with artificial ligament reconstruction represents a significant innovation in managing thoracic spinal tumors. Traditional laminoplasty is well recognized for restoring posterior bony structures after total laminectomy [4, 16]. By reattaching excised laminae using titanium plates and screws, this approach reestablishes spinal stability and reduces the risk of dural adhesions to the surrounding musculature [3, 16]. However, laminoplasty alone does not address the critical biomechanical roles of the interspinous and supraspinous ligaments—structures essential for maintaining thoracic spine stability, controlling flexion, and distributing axial loads [8, 17]. The absence of these ligaments after total laminectomy has been associated with postoperative kyphosis, chronic pain, and functional impairment [7, 17].

The hybrid approach described in this chapter integrates artificial ligament reconstruction into the laminoplasty procedure, thus bridging the gap left by traditional methods. By employing artificial ligaments to restore the interspinous and supraspinous regions, the technique replicates the natural biomechanical properties of the posterior ligamentous complex [15, 18]. Unlike lumbar ligament reconstructions, this thoracic adaptation accounts for the narrower interlaminar space by utilizing thinner, more flexible ligaments that ensure appropriate tensioning and structural integrity without impinging on the spinal cord or adjacent tissues [15, 19].

The potential benefits of this hybrid approach are multifaceted:

22.5.1 Enhanced Stability

By simultaneously addressing both bony and ligamentous deficiencies, this technique provides a more comprehensive restoration of the posterior column. This added stability minimizes the risk of kyphotic deformity and helps maintain proper spinal alignment during the healing process [15, 19].

22.5.2 Improved Recovery and Reduced Pain

Recreating the biomechanical function of the interspinous and supraspinous ligaments promotes even load distribution and alleviates stress on adjacent spinal segments. As a result, patients may experience reduced postoperative pain and a more favorable recovery trajectory [17, 20].

22.5.3 Long-Term Functional Outcomes

Restoring both bony and ligamentous structures can mitigate chronic pain, support normal biomechanics, and preserve mobility. By maintaining natural spinal alignment and load-bearing capacity, the hybrid approach fosters sustained functional improvement and reduces the likelihood of additional interventions [7, 20].

22.5.4 Adaptability for Complex Cases

In complex tumor cases requiring extensive laminectomy and large resections, the dual restoration of structural integrity and ligamentous support provides a robust framework for recovery. Even in scenarios of significant disruption, the hybrid approach offers the necessary stability for satisfactory long-term results [4, 18]. While this technique demands technical expertise and meticulous surgical planning, early clinical data and preliminary reports suggest that patients undergoing this hybrid procedure experience less postoperative pain, fewer complications, and improved functional recovery compared to laminoplasty alone [15, 16]. As such, this novel strategy addresses longstanding limitations in spinal tumor surgery and may set a new standard for thoracic spinal reconstruction.

In conclusion, the integration of laminoplasty with artificial ligament reconstruction represents a paradigm shift in thoracic spinal tumor management. By targeting both bony and ligamentous deficits, this comprehensive approach holds the potential to significantly enhance patient outcomes and redefine the benchmarks of spinal surgery innovation.

References

1. Sandalcioglu IE, Gasser T, Asgari S, Lazorisak A, Engelhorn T, Egelhof T, et al. Functional outcome after surgical treatment of intramedullary spinal cord tumors: experience with 78 patients. Spinal Cord. 2005;43(1):34–41. Chi JH, Gokaslan ZL. Spine tumors: surgical management and outcomes. Spine (Phila Pa 1976). 2006;31(11 Suppl):S54–S61.
2. Ahn DK, Park HS, Choi DJ, Kim KS, Kim TW, Park SY. Surgical treatment for spinal intradural extramedullary tumors. Clin Orthop Surg. 2009;1(3):165–72.
3. Shah S, Kutka M, Lees K, Abson C, Hadaki M, Cooke D, et al. Management of metastatic spinal cord compression in secondary care: a practice reflection from Medway Maritime Hospital, Kent, UK. J Pers Med. 2021;11(2):110.
4. Byvaltsev VA, Polkin RA, Kalinin AA, Kravtsov MA, Belykh EG, Shepelev VA, et al. Laminoplasty versus laminectomy in the treatment of primary spinal cord tumors in adult patients: a systematic review and meta-analysis of observational studies. Asian Spine J. 2023;17(3):595–609.
5. Panjabi MM. Biomechanical evaluation of spinal fixation devices: I. A conceptual framework. Spine (Phila Pa 1976). 1988;13(10):1129–34.
6. White AA, Panjabi MM. Clinical biomechanics of the spine. 2nd ed. Philadelphia: Lippincott Williams & Wilkins; 1990.
7. Adams MA, Roughley PJ. What is intervertebral disc degeneration, and what causes it? Spine (Phila Pa 1976). 2006;31(18):2151–61.
8. Kim HJ, Chun HJ, Kang KT, et al. The biomechanical influence of the facet joint orientation and the facet tropism in the lumbar spine. Spine J. 2013;13(10):1301–8.
9. Chou WY, Hsu CJ, Chang WN, et al. Adjacent segment degeneration after lumbar spinal posterolateral fusion with instrumentation in elderly patients. Arch Orthop Trauma Surg. 2002;122(1):39–43.
10. Glassman SD, Bridwell KH, Dimar JR, et al. The impact of positive sagittal balance in adult spinal deformity. Spine (Phila Pa 1976). 2005;30(18):2024–9.
11. Weinstein JN, Lurie JD, Olson PR, et al. United States' trends and regional variations in lumbar spine surgery: 1992–2003. Spine (Phila Pa 1976). 2006;31(23):2707–14.
12. Chotai S, Zuckerman SL, Parker SL, Stonko D, Wick J, Hale A, et al. Surgical resection of intradural extramedullary spinal tumors: patient-reported outcomes and minimum clinically important difference. Spine J. 2016;16(10 Suppl):S217.
13. Hu SS. Internal fixation in the osteoporotic spine. Spine (Phila Pa 1976). 1997;22(24 Suppl):43S–8S.

14. Galgano MA, Fridley JS, Gokaslan ZL. Instrumented fusion after spinal cord tumor resection. In: Arnautović KI, Gokaslan ZL, editors. Spinal cord tumors. Cham: Springer; 2019. p. 457–66.
15. Stoll TM, Dubois G, Schwarzenbach O. The dynamic neutralization system for the spine: a multicenter study of a novel non-fusion system. Eur Spine J. 2002;11(Suppl 2):S170–8.
16. Sun S, Li Y, Wang X, Lu G, She L, Yan Z, et al. Safety and efficacy of laminoplasty versus laminectomy in the treatment of spinal cord tumors: a systematic review and meta-analysis. World Neurosurg. 2019;125:136–45.
17. Panjabi MM. The stabilizing system of the spine. Part II. Neutral zone and instability hypothesis. J Spinal Disord. 1992;5(4):390–6.
18. Gao K, Chen S, Wang L, et al. Anterior cruciate ligament reconstruction with LARS artificial ligament: a multicenter study with 3- to 5-year follow-up. Arthroscopy. 2010;26(4):515–23.
19. Cakir B, Richter M. Dynamic stabilization of the lumbar spine. Curr Orthop. 2007;21(4):270–7.
20. Schnake KJ, Schaeren S, Jeanneret B. Dynamic stabilization in addition to decompression for lumbar spinal stenosis with degenerative spondylolisthesis. Spine. 2006;31(7):442–9.

Palliative Surgery for Adult Spinal Deformity

23

Jeong woo Kwun and Junseok Bae

Abstract

Corrective surgery for adult spinal deformity (ASD) patients is often difficult to pursue due to the high risks associated with advanced age, osteoporosis, or multiple comorbidities and complications. For such patients, palliative surgical approaches, including decompression and soft stabilization, offer a viable alternative. Techniques like Open Midline Decompression and SH Lee Ligament Reconstruction focus on alleviating symptoms, preserving motion, and minimizing complications. These methods have shown improvements in pain relief, functionality, and long-term stability, and can provide an effective treatment option for patients unable to undergo traditional corrective surgeries.

Keyword

Adult spinal deformity · Artificial ligament
Decompression · Dynamic stabilization
Ligament reconstruction

J. w. Kwun · J. Bae (✉)
Department of Neurosurgery, Cheongdam Wooridul Spine Hospital, Seoul, Korea (Republic of)

23.1 Introduction

Adult spinal deformity (ASD) represents a complex spectrum of spinal pathologies that significantly impact patients' quality of life. ASD encompasses conditions such as scoliosis, kyphosis, and sagittal plane imbalance, which are often accompanied by chronic pain, functional impairment, and neurological symptoms [1]. The prevalence of ASD ranges from 2% to 32% in the general population, with rates as high as 68% reported in individuals over 60 years old [2]. With the increasing aging population, the prevalence of ASD is rising, making it a critical focus for spine surgeons and healthcare providers.

23.1.1 Pain Mechanisms in ASD

Pain is a prevalent and multifaceted symptom in adult spinal deformity (ASD), stemming from various structural and neurological sources. Proper understanding and differentiation of these pain mechanisms are essential for tailored management strategies.

23.1.1.1 Pain Due to Spinal Instability

Spinal instability in ASD results from the degeneration of intervertebral discs, facet joints, and

S.-H. Lee et al. (eds.), *Ligament Reconstruction for Spine*,
https://doi.org/10.1007/978-981-95-3971-0_23

supporting ligaments. This leads to abnormal motion between vertebrae, causing:

- *Mechanical Back Pain*: Activity-related discomfort localized in the lumbar region, often exacerbated by movement or prolonged standing.
- *Progressive Deformity*: Instability may exacerbate spinal misalignment, compounding pain and functional limitations [3].

23.1.1.2 Pain Due to Spinal Stenosis

Spinal stenosis, a common complication in ASD, involves the narrowing of the spinal canal or foramina, compressing neural structures. Symptoms include:

- *Neurogenic Claudication*: Leg pain, numbness, or weakness triggered by standing or walking, relieved by sitting or forward flexion.
- *Radicular Pain*: Sharp, shooting pain radiating from the lower back into the buttocks and legs, following nerve root pathways.
- *Sensory and Motor Deficits*: Compression-induced numbness, tingling, or weakness in the lower extremities [2].

23.1.1.3 Complex Interactions of Pain Mechanisms

In many ASD patients, instability and stenosis coexist, contributing to a mixed pain presentation. A thorough clinical assessment, supported by imaging studies, is crucial for identifying the dominant pain source.

23.1.2 Risk Factors Associated with Adult Spinal Deformity (ASD)

Adult spinal deformity (ASD) surgery carries significant risks due to the complexity of procedures and the patient demographic often involved. The risks can be categorized into surgical complications, patient-specific risk factors such as advanced age and osteoporosis, and systemic considerations. Below is an integrated summary based on the uploaded documents and references.

23.1.2.1 Surgical Risk Factors

ASD surgeries are associated with high rates of complications due to the nature of the procedures, which often involve multi-level fusion and correction of severe deformities [4–6]:

- *Mechanical Failures*: Implant issues like screw loosening, rod breakage, and proximal junctional kyphosis (PJK) are common, with rates ranging from 15.3% to 17.1%.
- *Neurological Complications*: The incidence of nerve root injury and spinal cord damage ranges from 0.3% to 35.5%, leading to long-term deficits in severe cases.
- *Infection*: Infection rates for ASD surgery can reach 8% for deep infections, exacerbated by long operative times and significant blood loss.
- *Revision Surgeries*: Approximately 10–54% of patients require additional surgeries, often due to pseudoarthrosis or implant-related issues.

23.1.2.2 Patient-Specific Risk Factors

1. *Advanced Age*
   - Older patients, especially those over 69 years, face significantly increased risks of major complications. For every year of age, there is a 23% increased likelihood of complications [4, 5].
   - Common issues in the elderly include frailty, comorbidities, and reduced physiological reserve, which complicate recovery and increase the likelihood of systemic complications such as cardiac and pulmonary issues.
2. *Osteoporosis*
   - Reduced bone mineral density compromises the success of surgical fixation, leading to higher rates of screw loosening, pseudoarthrosis, and adjacent segment disease [5, 6].

23.1.3 Palliative Surgery for ASD

The surgical management of adult spinal deformity (ASD) is associated with significant risks, making it particularly challenging to proceed with surgery in high-risk patients. Advanced age, multiple comorbidities, and osteoporosis further complicate decision-making, as these factors increase the likelihood of perioperative complications and poor outcomes.

For patients with osteoporosis, preoperative optimization to improve bone quality is often required, adding delays and additional complexities to the surgical process. In cases where deformity correction surgery is not feasible or is deemed too risky, palliative surgical approaches can provide an effective alternative.

23.1.3.1 Role of Decompression and Dynamic Stabilization in Palliative Surgery

Decompression combined with dynamic stabilization offers a less invasive alternative for patients unsuitable for extensive fusion surgeries. This approach aims to relieve nerve compression, stabilize spinal segments, and improve functionality without the complications associated with traditional fusion methods. Studies have highlighted the following benefits:

1. *Efficacy in Pain and Functional Improvement*
   - Dynamic stabilization systems, such as the Dynesys system, have shown statistically significant improvements in back and leg pain as measured by the Visual Analog Scale (VAS) and functional disability scores (e.g., Oswestry Disability Index). These outcomes highlight the role of non-fusion techniques in achieving durable symptomatic relief [7].
2. *Reduced Risk of Complications*
   - Dynamic stabilization minimizes the risks of implant-related failures and adjacent segment degeneration compared to rigid fusion. This is particularly beneficial for elderly patients with multiple comorbidities or osteoporosis, where maintaining mobility while ensuring stability is paramount [8].

23.1.3.2 Integration of Open Midline Decompression and SH Lee Ligament Reconstruction

At our institute, innovative techniques such as open midline decompression and SH Lee ligament reconstruction have been developed to enhance the management of ASD in patients for whom traditional fusion surgery carries excessive risk. These procedures offer tailored solutions with the following highlights:

1. *Open Midline Decompression*:
   - This minimally invasive approach alleviates neural compression while preserving spinal stability. The technique reduces operative time, blood loss, and postoperative recovery time compared to traditional laminectomy [9, 10].
2. *SH Lee Ligament Reconstruction*
   - Using an artificial ligament, this method provides soft stabilization post-decompression. The ligament, secured in a figure-eight fashion around the spinous processes, ensures motion preservation while preventing postoperative instability. It is particularly beneficial for patients with mild instability and significant comorbidities [11, 12].

23.1.3.3 Indications for Palliative Surgery

Palliative surgeries are particularly indicated for:

- Elderly patients (>65 years) with multiple comorbidities.
- Those with mild to moderate deformities or spinal stenosis unresponsive to conservative treatments.
- Patients with osteoporosis, where the risks of rigid fusion outweigh the benefits.

By integrating open midline decompression and SH Lee ligament reconstruction, our institute

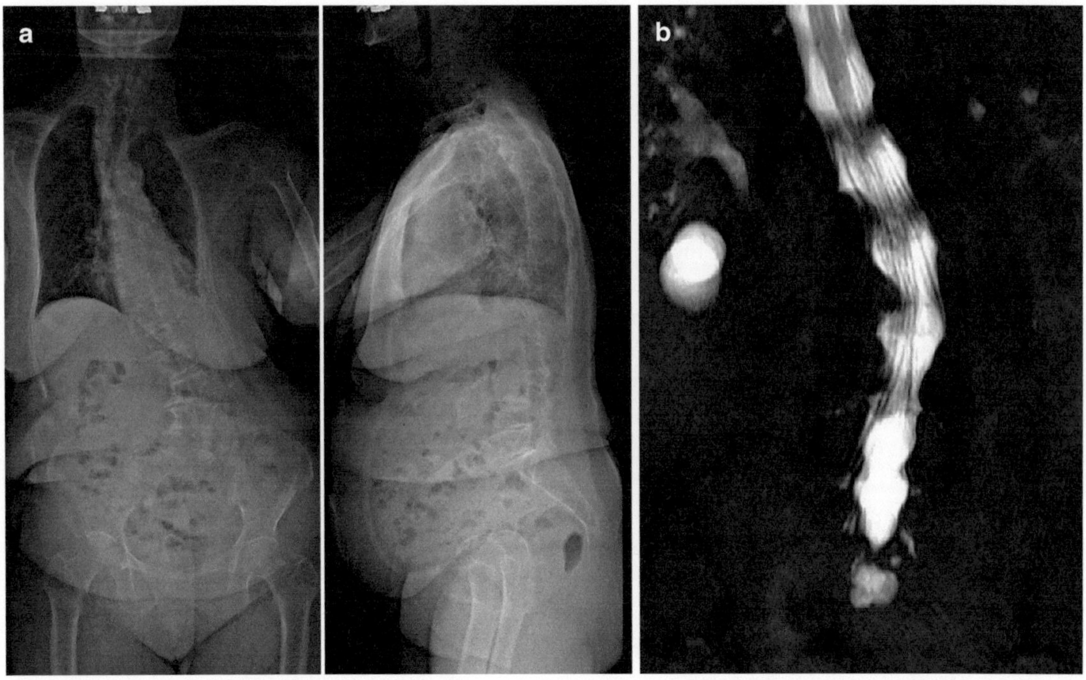

Fig. 23.1 (**a**) The whole spine X-ray shows coronal and sagittal imbalance. (**b**) The myelogram shows partial signal block from L1 to L5, indicating multilevel stenosis

provides a comprehensive palliative surgical approach. These techniques prioritize patient safety while effectively addressing debilitating symptoms, presenting a viable option for palliative surgery in managing high-risk ASD patients.

23.2 Presentation of the Patient

An 84-year-old female patient presented with severe pain in both buttocks, lower back, and thighs, significantly affecting her mobility and daily activities. The patient reported that her symptoms began 30 years ago but had worsened over the past 2–3 months. She was unable to walk effectively, with a neurogenic intermittent claudication (NIC) time of less than 5 minutes. Additionally, she experienced difficulty standing, turning over in bed, and walking straight due to a rightward tilt. Her bone mineral density (BMD) was measured at −3.3, indicating severe osteoporosis. Neurological examination revealed that heel/toe/hoop gait tests were impossible. Preoperative imaging, including whole spine x-ray and MRI Myelogram, demonstrated significant spinal deformity and multilevel stenosis from L1 to L5, with compressed neural elements (Fig. 23.1a, b).

23.3 Preoperative Planning

Given the patient's advanced age, severe osteoporosis, and multilevel stenosis, the treatment was planned in two stages. The first stage focused on symptom relief through palliative surgery, specifically Open Midline Decompression (OMD) and ligament reconstruction at the L1-L5 levels. The second stage was planned to address the underlying deformity through corrective surgery after adequately treating osteoporosis and evaluating the patient's condition.

The primary goals of preoperative planning were to provide immediate relief from pain and functional limitations, minimize surgical risks associated with osteoporosis and advanced age, and stabilize the spine to improve the patient's mobility and quality of life.

23.4 Surgical Steps

The first stage involved Open Midline Decompression (OMD) and ligament reconstruction to alleviate neural compression and stabilize the spine. The procedure began with positioning the patient prone under general anesthesia. A midline incision was made to expose the affected levels from L1 to L5. Hypertrophic ligamentum flavum and bony structures causing stenosis were carefully removed to decompress the neural elements. An SH Lee ligament was used for ligament reconstruction, providing soft stabilization while maintaining motion. The surgical site was then closed in layers, and the patient was monitored for stability and neurological improvement.

Postoperative outcomes were positive, with significant pain relief reported by postoperative day 7 (POD #7). At the 1-year follow-up, the patient demonstrated improved mobility and the ability to walk well, with only minor complaints of heaviness in the lower back. Follow-up X-rays showed no progression of ASD, with spinal alignment and stability well maintained (Fig. 23.2).

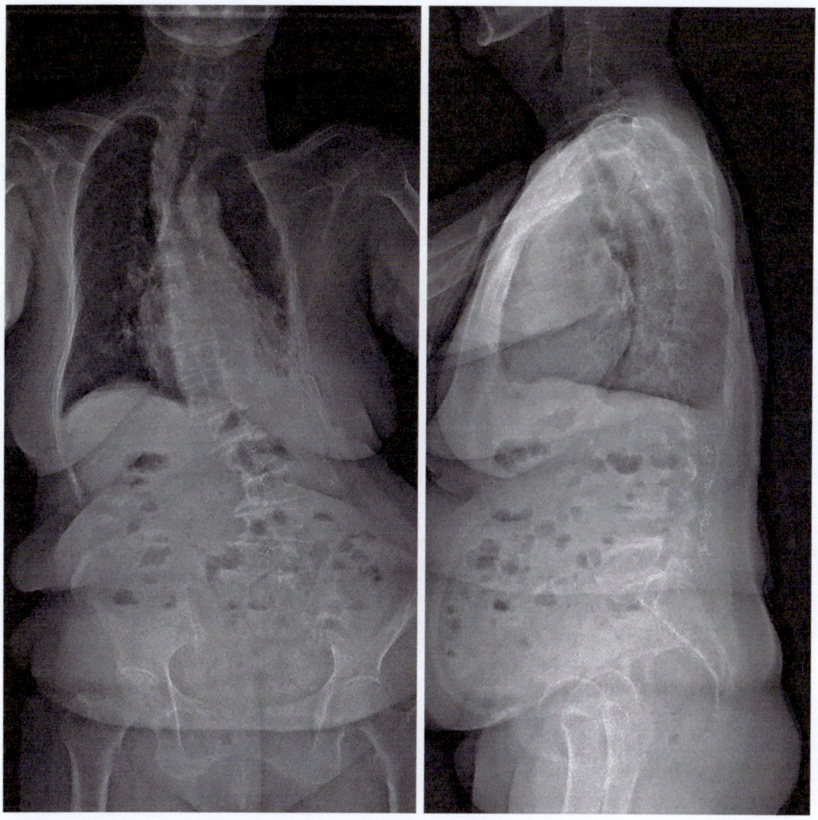

Fig. 23.2 The whole spine X-ray, compared to Fig. 23.1, shows no significant changes in coronal and sagittal imbalance

23.5 Commentary

Decompression and ligament reconstruction for soft stabilization can be presented as effective palliative surgical options for adult spinal deformity (ASD) patients who are not candidates for deformity correction surgeries due to advanced age, osteoporosis, or multiple comorbidities. Techniques like Open Midline Decompression and SH Lee Ligament Reconstruction, as performed at our institute, emphasize safety and efficacy, offering tailored solutions that improve quality of life and provide a sustainable alternative for high-risk patients.

References

1. Terran J, Schwab F, Shaffrey CI, Smith JS, Devos P, Ames CP, Fu K-MG, Burton D, Hostin R, Klineberg E, Gupta M, Deviren V, Mundis G, Hart R, Bess S, Lafage V. The SRS-Schwab adult spinal deformity classification: assessment and clinical correlations based on a prospective operative and nonoperative cohort. Neurosurgery. 2013;73(4):559–68. https://doi.org/10.1227/NEU.0000000000000012.
2. Hong KU, Hyun SJ, Lee JK, Kim KJ. Diagnosis and treatment of adult spinal deformity. J Korean Med Assoc. 2023;66(8):497–505. https://doi.org/10.5124/jkma.2023.66.8.497.
3. Kim HJ, Yang JH, Chang D-G, Suk S-I, Suh SW, Song K-S, Park J-B, Cho W. Adult spinal deformity: current concepts and decision-making strategies for management. Asian Spine J. 2020;14(6):886–97. https://doi.org/10.31616/asj.2020.0568.
4. Daubs MD, Lenke LG, Cheh G, Stobbs G, Bridwell KH. Adult spinal deformity surgery: complications and outcomes in patients over age 60. Spine. 2007;32(20):2238–44. https://doi.org/10.1097/BRS.0b013e31814cf24a.
5. Kim WJ, Cha YH. Complications and risk factors of surgery for adult spine deformity. J Korean Orthop Assoc. 2016;51(1):40–7. https://doi.org/10.4055/jkoa.2016.51.1.40.
6. Akıntürk N, Zileli M, Yaman O. Complications of adult spinal deformity surgery: a literature review. J Craniovertebral Junct Spine. 2022;13(1):17–26. https://doi.org/10.4103/jcvjs.jcvjs_159_21.
7. Di Silvestre M, Lolli F, Bakaloudis G, Parisini P. Dynamic stabilization for degenerative lumbar scoliosis in elderly patients. Spine. 2010;35(2):227–34. https://doi.org/10.1097/BRS.0b013e3181bd3be6.
8. Veresciagina K, Mehrkens A, Schären S, Jeanneret B. Minimum ten-year follow-up of spinal stenosis with degenerative spondylolisthesis treated with decompression and dynamic stabilization. J Spine Surg. 2018;4(1):93–101. https://doi.org/10.21037/jss.2018.03.20.
9. Lee SH, Enes M, Hoogland T. Soft stabilization with interspinous artificial ligament for mildly unstable lumbar spinal stenosis: a multicenter comparison. Arch Orthop Trauma Surg. 2009;130(8):967–73. https://doi.org/10.1007/s00402-009-1031-5.
10. Lee SH, Lee JH, Hong SW, Shim CS, Chung SE, Yoo SH, Lee HY. Clinical significance of achieving a flexion limitation with a tension band system in grade 1 degenerative spondylolisthesis: a minimum 5-year follow-up. Spine. 2015;40(6):E349–58. https://doi.org/10.1097/BRS.0000000000000766.
11. Lee DY, Lee SH, Shim CS, Lee HY. Decompression and interspinous dynamic stabilization using the locker for lumbar canal stenosis associated with low-grade degenerative spondylolisthesis. Minim Invasive Neurosurg. 2010;53(2):117–21. https://doi.org/10.1055/s-0030-1249704.
12. Lee SH, Lee JH, Hong SW, Chung SE, Yoo SH, Lee HY. Spinopelvic alignment after interspinous soft stabilization with a tension band system in grade 1 degenerative lumbar spondylolisthesis. Spine. 2010;35(15):E691–701. https://doi.org/10.1097/BRS.0b013e3181d2607e.

Ligamentoplasty for Proximal Soft Landing in Multi-Segment Fusion Surgery

24

Junseok Bae

Abstract

Proximal junctional kyphosis (PJK) remains one of the most challenging complications following long-segment spinal fusion in adult spinal deformity (ASD) surgery, with reported incidence rates of 20–40%. Ligamentoplasty, an emerging technique for creating a "soft landing" at the upper instrumented vertebra (UIV), offers a biomechanical transition zone to mitigate the abrupt rigidity change that predisposes patients to PJK. This chapter presents the rationale, surgical technique, and clinical outcomes of posterior ligamentoplasty using autologous fascia lata or synthetic substitutes. We describe a standardized approach for patient selection, preoperative planning, and step-by-step surgical implementation. Early clinical studies demonstrate promising reductions in PJK rates, with 2-year follow-up data showing decreased proximal junctional angle progression and lower revision surgery rates. Ligamentoplasty represents a valuable addition to the surgical armamentarium for addressing the challenging problem of junctional failure in ASD surgery.

Keywords

Proximal Junctional Kyphosis
Ligamentoplasty · Adult Spinal Deformity
Soft Landing · Biomechanical Transition

24.1 Introduction

Adult spinal deformity (ASD) represents a complex spectrum of conditions that often require long-segment spinal fusion for appropriate correction. While instrumented fusion effectively addresses deformity, the creation of abrupt transitions between highly rigid instrumented segments and more mobile unfused segments presents a significant clinical challenge. This transition zone, particularly at the proximal end of constructs, is vulnerable to accelerated degeneration and mechanical failure, manifesting as proximal junctional kyphosis (PJK) and, in more severe cases, proximal junctional failure (PJF).

PJK is radiographically defined as a proximal junctional angle increase of 10° or more between the lower endplate of the uppermost instrumented vertebra (UIV) and the upper endplate of the ver-

J. Bae (✉)
Department of Neurosurgery, Cheongdam Wooridul Spine Hospital, Seoul, Korea (Republic of)

S.-H. Lee et al. (eds.), *Ligament Reconstruction for Spine*,
https://doi.org/10.1007/978-981-95-3971-0_24

tebra two levels above (UIV+2) compared to preoperative measurements [1]. The reported incidence ranges from 20% to 40% following ASD surgery [2, 3]. Risk factors include older age, osteoporosis, greater preoperative sagittal imbalance, greater correction of sagittal deformity, and fusion to the sacrum [4, 5].

While not all cases of radiographic PJK are symptomatic, progression to PJF—characterized by vertebral fracture, implant failure, or neurological compromise—often necessitates revision surgery. The socioeconomic impact of these complications is substantial, with revision procedures increasing healthcare costs and patient morbidity.

Recent advances in understanding the biomechanical factors contributing to PJK have led to the development of "soft landing" techniques that aim to create a more gradual transition between fused and unfused segments. Ligamentoplasty represents one such approach, wherein synthetic or autologous ligamentous structures are used to augment the posterior tension band at the proximal junction, theoretically distributing mechanical stresses more evenly and reducing the risk of failure.

This chapter details the concept, technical considerations, and early clinical outcomes of ligamentoplasty for proximal soft landing in multi-segment fusion for ASD. By providing a comprehensive approach to implementation, we aim to standardize the technique and encourage further clinical investigation to establish its long-term efficacy.

24.2 Presentation of Patient

A 68-year-old female presented with progressive low back pain, left-sided radiculopathy, and increasing difficulty with ambulation over the past 2 years. Her symptoms were refractory to conservative management, including physical therapy, non-steroidal anti-inflammatory medications, and epidural steroid injections. The patient reported inability to stand upright for more than 15 minutes and had a walking tolerance limited to approximately 100 m before requiring rest due to pain and fatigue.

Physical examination revealed a significant sagittal plane deformity with forward stooping posture. The patient demonstrated a positive sagittal vertical axis (SVA) with compensatory knee flexion and hip extension. Neurological examination showed 4/5 weakness in left ankle dorsiflexion with otherwise preserved motor function. Sensory testing revealed decreased sensation in the left L5 distribution.

Radiographic evaluation included standing full-spine radiographs, which demonstrated thoracolumbar degenerative kyphosis with severe sagittal malalignment. Additional findings included multilevel disc degeneration and facet arthropathy from L2 to S1. Bone density scanning revealed moderate osteopenia (T-score: −2.1) (Fig. 24.1).

After thorough discussion of management options, including continued conservative care, limited decompression alone, or deformity correction with instrumented fusion, the patient elected to proceed with surgical intervention for comprehensive deformity correction. Given her age and bone quality, she was identified as having multiple risk factors for developing PJK, making her an appropriate candidate for proximal soft landing techniques, including ligamentoplasty.

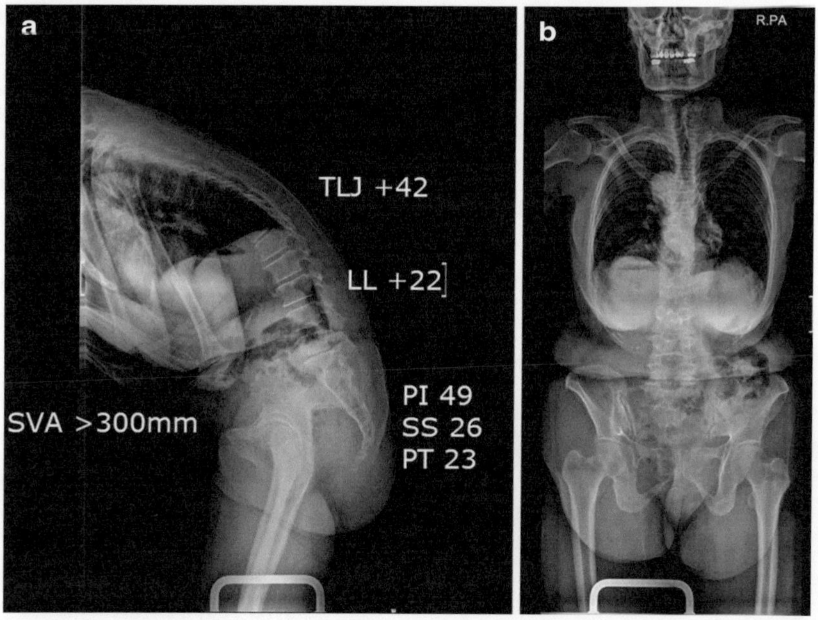

Fig. 24.1 Preoperative radiographic evaluation of a 68-year-old female with adult spinal deformity. The lateral standing radiograph (**a**) demonstrates severe sagittal imbalance with a sagittal vertical axis exceeding 300 mm, thoracolumbar junction kyphosis measuring +42°, reduced lumbar lordosis of +22°, and a pelvic incidence of 49° with elevated pelvic tilt of 23° and sacral slope of 26°. The anteroposterior standing radiograph (**b**) shows global coronal imbalance with pelvic obliquity and degenerative lumbar scoliosis

24.3 Preoperative Planning

24.3.1 Assessment of Deformity Parameters

Comprehensive radiographic analysis is essential for appropriate surgical planning. Standing full-spine radiographs should be obtained to assess the following parameters:

1. *Coronal plane deformity*: Cobb angles of major and minor curves.
2. *Sagittal plane parameters*:
   - Thoracic kyphosis (TK)
   - Lumbar lordosis (LL)
   - Pelvic incidence (PI)
   - Pelvic tilt (PT)
   - Sacral slope (SS)
   - Sagittal vertical axis (SVA)
   - T1 pelvic angle (TPA)
3. *Global alignment*:
   - Global coronal alignment
   - Global sagittal alignment
   - T1 spinopelvic inclination (T1-SPI)

Surgical planning should aim to achieve age-appropriate alignment targets as described by Schwab et al. [6], including SVA < 5 cm, PT < 25°, and LL = PI ± 9°.

24.3.2 UIV Selection and PJK Risk Assessment

Selection of the uppermost instrumented vertebra (UIV) is critical in mitigating PJK risk. Several factors guide this decision:

1. *Sagittal alignment of the thoracolumbar junction*: In patients with normal thoracic kyphosis, stopping at T10 or T11 may increase the risk of PJK due to the transition from the kyphotic thoracic spine to the lordotic lumbar spine.

2. *Extent of deformity*: For patients with significant thoracolumbar or thoracic deformity, UIV at T2-T4 may be necessary for adequate correction.
3. *Bone quality*: DEXA scanning helps identify patients with osteoporosis or osteopenia who may benefit from additional preventive measures.
4. *Age and comorbidities*: Older patients (>60 years) with comorbidities such as osteoporosis have increased PJK risk.

For our patient, given her age, osteopenia, and sagittal imbalance requiring substantial correction, we selected T10 as the UIV with plans to incorporate ligamentoplasty for proximal soft landing.

24.3.3 Material Selection for Ligamentoplasty

Options for ligamentoplasty include:

1. *Autologous tissue*:
   - Fascia lata graft: Harvested from the lateral thigh
   - Thoracolumbar fascia: Local tissue preservation and reinforcement
2. *Allograft options*:
   - Achilles tendon allograft
   - Fascia lata allograft
3. *Synthetic materials*:
   - Polyethylene tape (e.g., Mersilene tape)
   - Ultra-high molecular weight polyethylene (UHMWPE) sutures or tapes

For our patient, we selected autologous fascia lata graft to minimize risk of foreign body reaction while providing adequate tensile strength.

24.3.4 Additional PJK Prevention Strategies

Comprehensive PJK prevention involves multiple approaches:

1. *Vertebral body augmentation*: Prophylactic vertebroplasty or kyphoplasty at UIV and UIV+1 in osteoporotic patients
2. *Hook placement*: Use of transverse process hooks rather than pedicle screws at UIV
3. *Hybrid constructs*: Transition from rigid to semi-rigid fixation at proximal levels
4. *Appropriate correction targets*: Avoiding overcorrection of thoracic kyphosis

In our case, we planned ligamentoplasty in conjunction with prophylactic vertebroplasty at UIV and UIV+1, given the patient's osteopenia.

24.4 Surgical Technique

24.4.1 Patient Positioning and Approach

1. Position the patient prone on a Jackson table or similar frame that allows for appropriate intraoperative adjustment of spinal alignment.
2. Perform a standard posterior midline approach to expose the spine from T10 to S1, extending 2 levels above the planned UIV to allow adequate exposure for ligamentoplasty.
3. If using autologous fascia lata, prepare a separate surgical field on the lateral thigh for graft harvest.

24.4.2 Standard Deformity Correction and Instrumentation

1. Place pedicle screws at planned levels (in this case, T10 to S1 with iliac fixation).
2. Perform necessary decompression procedures at stenotic levels (L3-L4 and L4-L5 in our patient).
3. Execute planned osteotomies as needed for deformity correction.
4. Apply temporary rods and correct the deformity gradually using standard techniques.

5. Perform interbody fusion as planned stage surgery prior to posterior approach (in this case, OLIF at L2-3, L3-L4, L4-L5, and ALIF at L5-S1).
6. Secure final rods and confirm correction with intraoperative radiographs.

24.4.3 Ligamentoplasty Technique

1. *Preparation of Ligamentoplasty*:
   - Measure the distance between the spinous processes of UIV-2 and UIV+2 (in this case, from T8 to T12).
   - Prepare the graft to appropriate length, aiming for tension-free fixation in neutral alignment.
   - If using synthetic materials, cut to appropriate length according to manufacturer specifications.
2. *Fixation Technique*:
   - Expose the supraspinous and interspinous ligaments from UIV-2 to UIV+2.
   - Preserve these native ligamentous structures when possible.
   - Place the graft material in figure-of-eight configuration around the spinous processes of UIV-2, UIV-1, UIV, UIV+1, and UIV+2.
   - Secure the graft to each spinous process using heavy nonabsorbable sutures (e.g., #2 FiberWire).
   - Ensure appropriate tension of the construct, allowing for slight motion while providing support.

24.5 Postoperative Management

1. Mobilize the patient on postoperative day 1 with appropriate bracing.
2. Consider thoracolumbosacral orthosis (TLSO) for 24 weeks in high-risk patients.
3. Begin physical therapy focusing on proper body mechanics and core strengthening.
4. Implement osteoporosis treatment as indicated.
5. Obtain standing full-spine radiographs at 6 weeks, 3 months, 6 months, 1 year, and annually thereafter to monitor for development of PJK (Fig. 24.2).

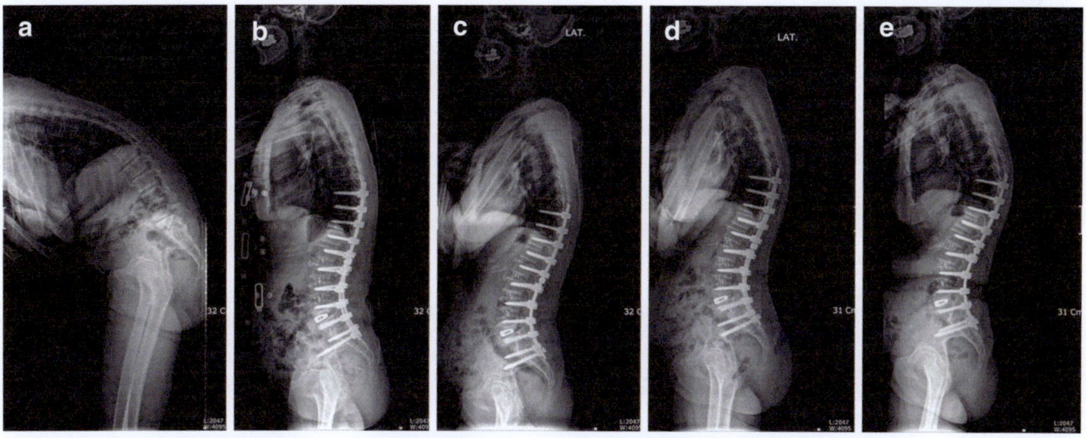

Fig. 24.2 Sequential lateral radiographs of a patient who underwent T10-S1 fusion with proximal ligamentoplasty for adult spinal deformity. The preoperative image (**a**) shows severe sagittal imbalance with insufficient lumbar lordosis. The three-month postoperative radiograph (**b**) demonstrates restored sagittal alignment following corrective surgery with ligamentoplasty at the proximal junction. At 1-year follow-up (**c**), the patient maintains good correction with no evidence of proximal junctional kyphosis. Three-year follow-up imaging (**d**) shows stable instrumentation and preserved sagittal alignment. The 6-year follow-up radiograph (**e**) confirms long-term durability of the construct with successful prevention of proximal junctional failure through the ligamentoplasty technique

24.6 Commentary

Ligamentoplasty for proximal soft landing represents a promising approach to addressing the persistent challenge of PJK in ASD surgery. The technique aims to create a biomechanical transition zone at the proximal end of long constructs, potentially mitigating the abrupt change in stiffness implicated in junctional failure.

24.7 Evidence from Clinical Studies

Several recent studies have evaluated the efficacy of various soft landing techniques, including ligamentoplasty:

Pehlivanoglu et al. [7] reported on 58 ASD patients who underwent posterior ligamentoplasty using autologous fascia lata with a minimum 2-year follow-up. The PJK rate was 12.1% in the ligamentoplasty group compared to 34.5% in a matched control group without ligamentoplasty ($p < 0.01$).

Safaee et al. [8] described a technique using Mersilene tape for posterior tension band ligamentoplasty in 42 patients with ASD. At mean follow-up of 18 months, the PJK rate was 14.3%, lower than historical controls from the same institution (28.7%).

Viswanathan et al. [9] evaluated a combined approach using prophylactic vertebroplasty at UIV and UIV+1 along with ligamentoplasty in 45 patients with osteoporosis undergoing ASD surgery. The PJK incidence was 11.1% at 2-year follow-up, suggesting a synergistic benefit of combining these techniques.

These preliminary results are encouraging, though longer-term follow-up and prospective randomized trials are needed to definitively establish the efficacy of ligamentoplasty.

24.8 Technical Considerations and Pitfalls

Several technical considerations warrant attention:

1. *Material selection*: While autologous fascia provides excellent biocompatibility, synthetic materials may offer more consistent mechanical properties. The ideal material should balance durability, biocompatibility, and ease of handling.
2. *Tensioning*: Appropriate tensioning of the ligamentoplasty construct is critical. Too tight may limit motion and transfer stress to adjacent levels, while too loose may not provide adequate support.
3. *Fixation method*: Secure fixation to each spinous process is essential for long-term function. Bone quality must be considered when selecting fixation techniques.
4. *Learning curve*: The technique requires additional operative time and technical expertise, particularly when harvesting autologous fascia lata.

24.9 Conclusion

Ligamentoplasty represents a promising addition to the surgical armamentarium for preventing PJK in ASD surgery. The technique is particularly valuable for high-risk patients, including older individuals with osteoporosis undergoing substantial sagittal correction. By creating a more gradual transition between fused and mobile segments, ligamentoplasty addresses the fundamental biomechanical issue underlying junctional failure.

As with any evolving technique, standardization of the approach and prospective evaluation are essential to establish best practices. The current clinical experience suggests that ligamentoplasty, especially when combined with other preventive strategies, may substantially reduce the burden of PJK. Future refinements in technique and materials will likely further enhance outcomes for patients with adult spinal deformity.

References

1. Glattes RC, Bridwell KH, Lenke LG, Kim YJ, Rinella A, Edwards C 2nd. Proximal junctional kyphosis in adult spinal deformity following long instrumented posterior spinal fusion: incidence, outcomes, and risk factor analysis. Spine (Phila Pa 1976). 2005;30(14):1643–9.
2. Yagi M, Rahm M, Gaines R, et al. Characterization and surgical outcomes of proximal junctional failure in surgically treated patients with adult spinal deformity. Spine (Phila Pa 1976). 2014;39(10):E607–14.
3. Kim HJ, Iyer S. Proximal junctional kyphosis. J Am Acad Orthop Surg. 2016;24(5):318–26.
4. Lau D, Clark AJ, Scheer JK, et al. Proximal junctional kyphosis and failure after spinal deformity surgery: a systematic review of the literature as a background to classification development. Spine (Phila Pa 1976). 2014;39(25):2093–102.
5. Park SJ, Lee CS, Chung SS, Lee JY, Kang SS, Park SH. Different risk factors of proximal junctional kyphosis and proximal junctional failure following long instrumented fusion to the sacrum for adult spinal deformity: survivorship analysis of 160 patients. Neurosurgery. 2017;80(2):279–86.
6. Schwab F, Ungar B, Blondel B, et al. Scoliosis Research Society-Schwab adult spinal deformity classification: a validation study. Spine (Phila Pa 1976). 2012;37(12):1077–82.
7. Pehlivanoglu T, Akgul T, Bayram S, Meric E, Ozdemir M, Yazicioglu O. Effect of posterior ligamentoplasty on adjacent segment pathology after long segment fusion in adult spinal deformity: a retrospective comparative study. Spine J. 2020;20(10):1620–8.
8. Safaee MM, Deviren V, Dalle Ore C, Scheer JK, Lau D, Osorio JA, Nicholls F, Ames CP. Ligament augmentation for prevention of proximal junctional kyphosis and proximal junctional failure in adult spinal deformity. J Neurosurg Spine. 2018;28(5):512–9.
9. Viswanathan VK, Kukreja S, Minnema AJ, Farhadi HF. Proximal junctional kyphosis prevention strategies: a review of current literature. Global Spine J. 2022;12(4):684–95.

Part IV

Complication and Its Management of Ligament Reconstruction

Postoperative Infection

25

Shin-Jae Kim

Abstract

Material innovations are reshaping infection management in artificial ligament reconstruction, offering new strategies to combat bacterial adhesion and biofilm formation. Recent advances include antimicrobial coatings, biofilm-resistant surfaces, and hybrid materials engineered to disrupt microbial colonization. Techniques such as vancomycin-coated grafts, hydrophobic surface treatments, and controlled-release drug delivery systems enhance infection prevention and postoperative care. These innovations can be integrated with orthopedic principles, optimizing implant design, and improving tissue integration. By reducing microbial load, minimizing biofilm development, and maintaining effective antimicrobial concentrations at the surgical site, these approaches help curb persistent infections, lower revision rates, and enhance patient comfort. Ultimately, combining cutting-edge material science with clinical expertise provides a robust framework for safer spinal surgeries, improved healing, and superior long-term outcomes.

Keywords

Postoperative infection · Ligament reconstruction · Polyethylene terephthalate · Poly propylene

25.1 Introduction

Infections in spinal surgeries involving artificial ligaments pose significant challenges, jeopardizing both surgical outcomes and patient safety [1]. Synthetic materials like the SHLee ligament are integral to structural repair but can act as scaffolds for bacterial colonization and biofilm formation [2]. These infections are particularly difficult to treat due to the inherent resistance of biofilms to antibiotics and immune defenses [3].

Material science has emerged as a critical tool in addressing these challenges, drawing inspiration from advancements in orthopedic surgeries, such as anterior cruciate ligament (ACL) and shoulder ligament reconstructions. Techniques like antimicrobial coatings, surface modifications, and controlled drug delivery systems have demonstrated remarkable efficacy in reducing infection risks [4, 5]. For instance, vancomycin-coated ligaments have shown significant success in minimizing postoperative infections in orthopedic applications, suggesting similar potential for spinal surgery [6]. Additionally, biofilm-

S.-J. Kim (✉)
Department of Neurosurgery, Cheongdam Wooridul Spine Hospital, Seoul, Korea (Republic of)

S.-H. Lee et al. (eds.), *Ligament Reconstruction for Spine*,
https://doi.org/10.1007/978-981-95-3971-0_25

resistant surface treatments and hybrid materials are being developed to further inhibit bacterial adhesion and prevent biofilm formation [7].

In this chapter, we explore how these material innovations and lessons from orthopedics are reshaping infection prevention and management in spinal ligament reconstruction. By integrating these advancements, surgeons can enhance surgical outcomes, reduce complications, and improve the long-term success of artificial ligament implantation. The incorporation of antimicrobial strategies not only mitigates infection risks but also supports the longevity and functionality of artificial ligaments in the demanding environment of the spinal column.

Ultimately, the convergence of material science and surgical expertise offers a robust framework for combating infections in spinal surgeries, ensuring safer procedures and better patient prognoses. This comprehensive approach underscores the importance of interdisciplinary collaboration in advancing spinal surgery techniques and improving patient care.

25.2 Incidence and Pathophysiology of Infection

Surgical site infections (SSIs) in spinal surgeries involving synthetic materials occur at rates ranging from 0.7% to 12% [8–10]. The SHLee ligament, while offering significant biomechanical advantages, shares a common challenge with anterior cruciate ligament (ACL) grafts: the propensity for biofilm formation [11]. Biofilms—dense microbial colonies on artificial surfaces—substantially reduce antibiotic efficacy and complicate treatment, often necessitating surgical intervention [12]. Literature from orthopedic studies on ACL reconstruction reports infection rates of 0.5–2%, providing an analogous context to spinal cases [13]. Key pathogens, including *Staphylococcus aureus* and coagulase-negative staphylococci, are notorious for their ability to rapidly colonize synthetic surfaces, forming resilient biofilms that resist both antibiotic therapy and immune responses [12].

25.3 Diagnostic Protocols

Early diagnosis of infections is critical to preserving the integrity of artificial ligaments [14]. Biomarkers such as C-reactive protein (CRP) and erythrocyte sedimentation rate (ESR) remain standard for detecting inflammatory responses indicative of infection [15]. Advanced imaging modalities, particularly contrast-enhanced MRI (Fig. 25.1), excel in identifying deep infections and differentiating them from noninfectious inflammatory changes [13]. Insights from orthopedic ACL reconstruction emphasize the importance of routine postoperative surveillance, especially in high-risk patients, a practice that may significantly improve outcomes in spinal surgeries [12]. Regular monitoring enables the

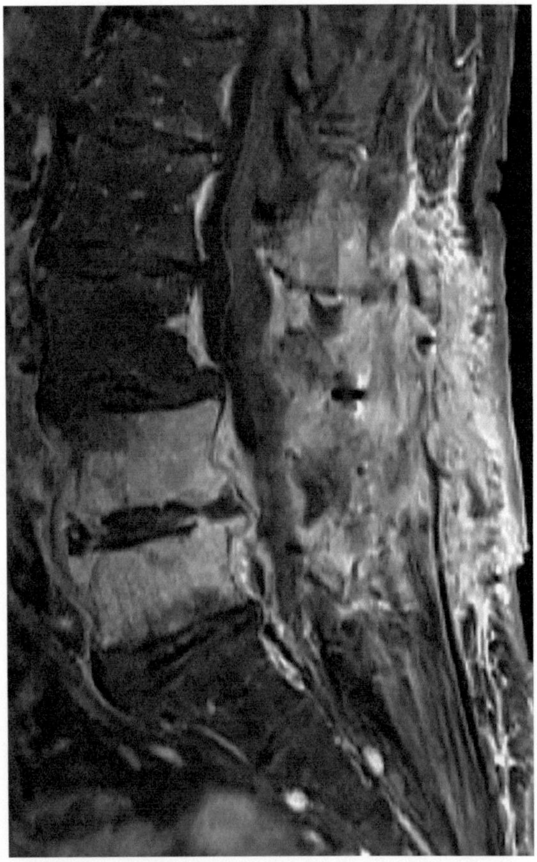

Fig. 25.1 Contrast-enhanced MRI shows the infectious spondylodiscitis at L4–5 level with posterior ligament, muscle infection image 2 weeks after artificial ligament insertion surgery

timely detection of infections, facilitating prompt intervention and reducing the likelihood of severe complications [15].

25.4 Treatment Strategies

Orthopedic management principles for infected ACL grafts provide a foundational framework for spinal ligamentoplasty [16]. Effective management begins with early debridement and irrigation to reduce microbial load and delay biofilm maturation [17].

25.4.1 Antibiotic Therapy

Antibiotic therapy is paramount in managing SSIs, particularly in cases involving artificial ligaments [18]. The primary goal is to control the infection, prevent further complications, and preserve the artificial ligament when possible. The process begins with empirical antibiotic treatment, which evolves to targeted therapy based on culture results, and may include local delivery systems for enhanced efficacy [19]. Empirical antibiotics are chosen based on the most common pathogens associated with SSIs, typically *Staphylococcus aureus* (including methicillin-resistant strains) and coagulase-negative staphylococci [20]. For instance, vancomycin or daptomycin (targeting gram-positive bacteria) combined with ceftriaxone or cefepime (addressing gram-negative organisms) are commonly used [21]. As culture results become available, antibiotic regimens are refined to target specific pathogens, reducing unnecessary broad-spectrum antibiotic exposure and minimizing resistance risks [22].

Localized antibiotic delivery systems, such as antibiotic-impregnated beads, sponges, or hydrogels, provide high drug concentrations directly at the infection site, enhancing antimicrobial efficacy while minimizing systemic toxicity [23]. These methods are particularly effective against biofilm-associated infections on synthetic ligaments. However, biofilms present significant challenges, as they protect bacteria from antibiotics and immune responses, often necessitating surgical removal of the infected graft [1]. Lessons from orthopedic ACL reconstruction, such as the use of vancomycin-soaked grafts and aggressive debridement, demonstrate high success rates in managing localized infections and preserving graft integrity [2]. Emerging therapies, including quorum-sensing inhibitors and nanoparticle-based antibiotic carriers, offer promising avenues for more effective biofilm disruption and infection control [3].

25.4.2 Early Debridement and Irrigation

Managing SSIs effectively begins with early debridement and irrigation. These techniques are vital in procedures involving artificial ligaments, as they help control bacterial colonization, reduce biofilm formation, and create a healthier environment for healing [4]. Debridement involves the removal of infected or necrotic tissue to minimize bacterial load and disrupt early-stage biofilm formation [5]. High-volume lavage with sterile saline or antiseptic solutions, often utilizing pulsatile lavage systems, effectively cleanses irregular surfaces and synthetic materials like artificial ligaments [24]. Incorporating antibiotics such as vancomycin or gentamicin into irrigation fluids enhances local antimicrobial activity, directly targeting the infection site [6]. Early intervention, ideally within 48–72 hours of symptom onset, is crucial for successful infection control and graft preservation [7]. Orthopedic case studies demonstrate that aggressive debridement and antibiotic irrigation can salvage up to 80% of infected grafts, underscoring the potential application of these techniques in spinal ligament reconstruction.

25.5 Material Innovations to Reduce Infection Risk

Advancements in material science are significantly improving infection management in artificial ligament reconstruction. These innovations are particularly valuable in spinal surgeries, where synthetic materials like the SHLee ligament are integral but can also serve as substrates for bacterial colonization. Key material innovations include antimicrobial coatings, biofilm-resistant surfaces, and hybrid materials designed to disrupt microbial colonization.

25.5.1 Antimicrobial Coatings

Antimicrobial coatings provide a protective barrier on the surface of artificial ligaments, actively preventing bacterial adhesion. Vancomycin-coated ligaments have shown remarkable success in reducing postoperative infections in orthopedic applications, suggesting similar potential for spinal surgery. Additionally, coatings using metals like silver, copper, and titanium offer broad-spectrum antimicrobial properties, disrupting bacterial membranes and preventing biofilm formation.

25.5.2 Biofilm-Resistant Surfaces

Biofilm-resistant surface treatments, such as smooth-surface materials and hydrophobic coatings, minimize bacterial adhesion and inhibit biofilm formation [3]. Polypropylene (PP) and hydrophobic materials inspired by natural surfaces like lotus leaves effectively repel water and bacteria, reducing infection risks. Although polypropylene (PP) has slightly lower tensile strength compared to PET, it demonstrates significantly lower infection rates, higher resilience, and faster tissue integration. These properties make PP-based artificial ligaments a promising alternative material that can address several limitations of PET.

25.5.3 Hybrid and Composite Materials

Hybrid materials combine synthetic fibers with biologically derived components like collagen, promoting cell growth while resisting bacterial adhesion [25]. Nanocomposites incorporating nanoparticles such as zinc oxide or graphene oxide provide sustained antimicrobial activity, enhancing the resistance of artificial ligaments to infections. Controlled drug release systems embedded within ligaments allow for the gradual release of antibiotics, ensuring continuous antimicrobial action at the implant site.

25.6 Lessons from Orthopedic Surgery

Orthopedic surgery, particularly ACL and shoulder ligament reconstructions, offers significant insights into managing infections in artificial ligament surgeries. These insights are invaluable for spinal surgeries, where synthetic materials present similar infection challenges.

25.6.1 Infection Prevention

Preoperative antibiotic prophylaxis is a cornerstone in orthopedic ligament reconstructions [26]. Administering antibiotics like cefazolin or vancomycin within an hour before surgery has been shown to significantly reduce infection rates. Additionally, soaking grafts in vancomycin before implantation minimizes postoperative infections, a practice adaptable to spinal surgeries.

25.6.2 Antibiotic Therapy and Biofilm Management

Early, aggressive antibiotic therapy and biofilm-disrupting techniques from orthopedics are applicable to spinal ligamentoplasty. Empirical antibiotic treatment followed by targeted therapy based on culture results ensures effective infection control. The use of localized antibiotic delivery systems in orthopedics, such as antibiotic-laden hydrogels, can be translated to spinal surgeries to enhance antimicrobial efficacy.

25.6.3 Graft Retention Versus Removal

Orthopedic practices emphasize the importance of timely decision-making in graft retention versus removal [27]. In ACL reconstructions, localized infections responsive to early treatment can often be managed without graft removal, whereas advanced infections necessitate graft removal to fully eradicate the infection. This staged approach, balancing infection control with structural preservation, is equally relevant in spinal surgeries.

25.6.4 Fusion Surgery

Even after the removal of the artificial ligament, if the infection is not well-controlled with antibiotic therapy or progresses to infectious spondylodiscitis with destruction of the bony structure, fusion surgery may be required to stabilize the affected level. In cases where the posterior structure is severely affected by infection leading to significant adhesion, an anterior approach such as ALIF (anterior lumbar interbody fusion) can be a viable alternative [28].

25.7 Conclusion

By integrating material science innovations and lessons from orthopedic surgery, spinal ligament reconstruction can achieve enhanced infection prevention and management. These strategies not only reduce infection risks but also support the longevity and functionality of artificial ligaments, ultimately improving patient outcomes in spinal surgeries.

25.8 Summary

Infection management in spinal surgeries involving artificial ligaments has reached a new frontier with the integration of material innovations and orthopedic insights. Antimicrobial coatings, such as those infused with vancomycin or silver nanoparticles, have proven highly effective in preventing bacterial colonization. Biofilm-resistant surfaces, including smooth-surfaced polypropylene and superhydrophobic materials, further reduce the risk of infections by minimizing bacterial adhesion. Additionally, hybrid materials and nanocomposites provide both antimicrobial properties and enhanced biocompatibility. Controlled drug release systems represent another breakthrough, enabling targeted delivery of antibiotics to the site of infection. These systems reduce systemic side effects while maintaining high local drug concentrations, effectively preventing early infections. Smart drug delivery technologies that respond to environmental triggers, such as pH or temperature changes, add a new layer of precision to infection management. Orthopedic practices, particularly those from ACL reconstruction, offer invaluable guidance for spinal surgeons. Strategies like graft preparation with vancomycin and staged surgical management for infected implants have set a precedent for success. Adopting these approaches in spinal surgeries can significantly enhance infection control and improve patient outcomes. As material science continues to evolve, emerging technologies such as quorum-sensing inhibitors and biodegradable ligaments hold promise for the future. These innovations aim to further reduce infection risks, enhance the longevity of artificial ligaments, and make spinal ligament reconstruction safer and more effective. By integrating these advancements, spinal surgeons can not only address the challenges of infection management but also set new standards for success in artificial ligament reconstruction. This synergy of material innovation and surgical expertise represents a paradigm shift in the field, paving the way for better outcomes and improved patient care.

References

1. Atesok K, Papavassiliou E, Heffernan MJ, Tunmire D, Sitnikov I, Tanaka N, et al. Current strategies in prevention of postoperative infections in spine surgery. Glob Spine J. 2020;10(2):183–94.
2. Numazaki H, Kobayashi H, Yoshida K, Hakozaki M, Konno S. Prolonged infection at the tibial bone tun-

nel after anterior cruciate ligament reconstruction. Fukushima J Med Sci. 2017;63(2):121–5.
3. Veerachamy S, Yarlagadda T, Manivasagam G, Yarlagadda PKDV. Bacterial adherence and biofilm formation on medical implants: a review. Proc Inst Mech Eng H. 2014;228(10):1083–99.
4. Jägersberg M, Feihl S, Ringel F. Future directions of postoperative spinal implant infections. J Spine Surg. 2020;6(4):814–9.
5. Garcia DR, Deckey DG, Zega A, Mayfield C, Spake CSL, Emanuel T, et al. Analysis of growth and biofilm formation of bacterial pathogens on frequently used spinal implant materials. Spine Deform. 2020;8(4):389–96.
6. Li H, Chen S. Biomedical coatings on polyethylene terephthalate (PET) artificial ligaments. J Biomed Mater Res A. 2015;103(12):839.
7. Nishizawa M, Hu D, Serhan H, Saleh B, Marcucio RS, Morioka K. A novel approach to reducing spinal implant-associated infections. bioRxiv. 2024.
8. Deyo RA, Mirza SK, Martin BI. Back pain prevalence and visit rates: estimates from U.S. national surveys, 2002. Spine (Phila Pa 1976). 2006;31(23):2724–7.
9. Kalichman L, Cole R, Kim DH, et al. Spinal stenosis prevalence and association with symptoms: the Framingham study. Spine J. 2009;9(7):545–50.
10. Genevay S, Atlas SJ. Lumbar spinal stenosis. Best Pract Res Clin Rheumatol. 2010;24(2):253–65.
11. Deyo RA, Cherkin DC, Loeser JD, et al. Morbidity and mortality in association with operations on the lumbar spine: the influence of age, diagnosis, and procedure. J Bone Joint Surg Am. 1992;74(4):536–43.
12. Yang JC, Kim SG, Kim TW, Park KH. Analysis of factors contributing to postoperative spinal instability after lumbar decompression for spinal stenosis. Korean J Spine. 2013;10(3):149–54.
13. Kim HJ, Chun HJ, Kang KT, et al. The biomechanical influence of the facet joint orientation and tropism in the lumbar spine. Spine J. 2013;13(10):1301–8.
14. Panjabi MM. The stabilizing system of the spine. Part II. Neutral zone and instability hypothesis. J Spinal Disord. 1992;5(4):390–6.
15. Adams MA, Roughley PJ. What is intervertebral disc degeneration, and what causes it? Spine (Phila Pa 1976). 2006;31(18):2151–61.
16. Stoll TM, Dubois G, Schwarzenbach O. The dynamic neutralization system for the spine: a multi-center study of a novel non-fusion system. Eur Spine J. 2002;11(Suppl 2):S170–8.
17. Gao K, Chen S, Wang L, et al. Anterior cruciate ligament reconstruction with LARS artificial ligament: a multicenter study with 3- to 5-year follow-up. Arthroscopy. 2010;26(4):515–23.
18. Cakir B, Richter M. Dynamic stabilization of the lumbar spine. Curr Orthop. 2007;21(4):270–7.
19. Schnake KJ, Schaeren S, Jeanneret B. Dynamic stabilization in addition to decompression for lumbar spinal stenosis with degenerative spondylolisthesis. Spine. 2006;31(7):442–9.
20. Fay LY, Wu JC, Tsai TY, et al. Dynamic stabilization for degenerative spondylolisthesis: evaluation of radiographic and clinical outcomes. Clin Neurol Neurosurg. 2016;144:60–7.
21. Dhammi IK, Haq RU, Kumar S. Graft choices for anterior cruciate ligament reconstruction. Indian J Orthop. 2015;49(2):127–8.
22. Ibrahim AMS, Vargas CR, Colakoglu S, Nguyen JT, Lin SJ, Lee BT. Properties of meshes used in hernia repair: a comprehensive review of synthetic and biologic meshes. J Reconstr Microsurg. 2015;31(2):83.
23. Schöttle PB, Fucentese SF, Romero J. Clinical and radiological outcome of medial patellofemoral ligament reconstruction with a semitendinosus autograft for patella instability. Knee Surg Sports Traumatol Arthrosc. 2005;13(7):516–21.
24. Anwar FN, Roca AM, Khosla I, Medakkar SS, Loya AC, Federico VP, et al. Antibiotic use in spine surgery: a narrative review based on principles of antibiotic stewardship. NASSJ. 2023;16:100278.
25. Li S, Wang S, Liu W, Zhang C, Song J. Current strategies for enhancement of the bioactivity of artificial ligaments: a mini-review. J Orthop Translat. 2022;36:205–15.
26. Queiroz R, Grinbaum RS, Galvão LL, Tavares FG, Bergsten-Mendes G. Antibiotic prophylaxis in orthopedic surgeries: the results of an implemented protocol. Braz J Infect Dis. 2005;9(3):283–7.
27. Sinagra ZP, Kop A, Pabbruwe M, Parry J, Clark G. Foreign body reaction associated with artificial LARS ligaments: a retrieval study. Orthop J Sports Med. 2018;6(12):2325967118811604.
28. Kim SH, Kang MS, Chin DK, Kim KS, Cho YE, Kuh SU. Anterior lumbar interbody fusion for the treatment of postoperative spondylodiscitis. J Korean Neurosurg Soc. 2014;56(4):310–4.

Postoperative Hematoma

26

Ju Hyung Lee

Keywords

Ligament reconstruction · Postoperative hematoma · Surgical complication · Symptomatic epidural hematoma · Open midline decompression

26.1 Introduction

Open midline decompression and soft stabilization with artificial ligament has been a successful spinal procedure to treat spinal stenosis and instability. This procedure offers several advantages over conventional laminectomy. This procedure can preserve the facet joint so as to provide stability to the spinal structures. But it has several complications like other spinal procedures, which includes postoperative dysesthesia associated with dorsal root ganglion, incidental durotomy, surgical site infection, and hematoma [1].

Postoperative hematoma is the most important complication of spinal surgery. Risk factors are old age, multilevel surgery, anemia, preoperative coagulopathy, long operation time, and large amount of blood loss [2]. Most cases are asymptomatic, but in rare conditions, it becomes symptomatic. Once neurological change occurs, emergency evacuation is required as soon as possible [3].

26.2 Blood Supply of the Lumbar Spine (Anatomical Focuses of Postoperative Hematoma)

26.2.1 Blood Supply of Vertebrae

The lumbar segmental arteries provide blood supply to the segments of the lumbar spine. The unbranched arteries that connect to the anterior spinal artery (ASA) or the posterior spinal arteries (PSAs) are referred to as "segmental medullary arteries" to distinguish them from the radicular arteries, which primarily supply the nerve roots. These segmental medullary arteries are also known as "radiculomedullary arteries" or "radicular feeders." [4].

Spinal branches enter the vertebral canal through the intervertebral foramen, where they supply the vertebral body, ligaments, and meninges. These spinal branches then divide into radicular arteries and segmental medullary arteries, which supply the spinal nerve roots and the spinal cord (Fig. 26.1).

J. H. Lee (✉)
Department of Neurosurgery, Cheongdam Wooridul Spine Hospital, Seoul, Korea (Republic of)
e-mail: leejh55@wooridul.co.kr

S.-H. Lee et al. (eds.), *Ligament Reconstruction for Spine*,
https://doi.org/10.1007/978-981-95-3971-0_26

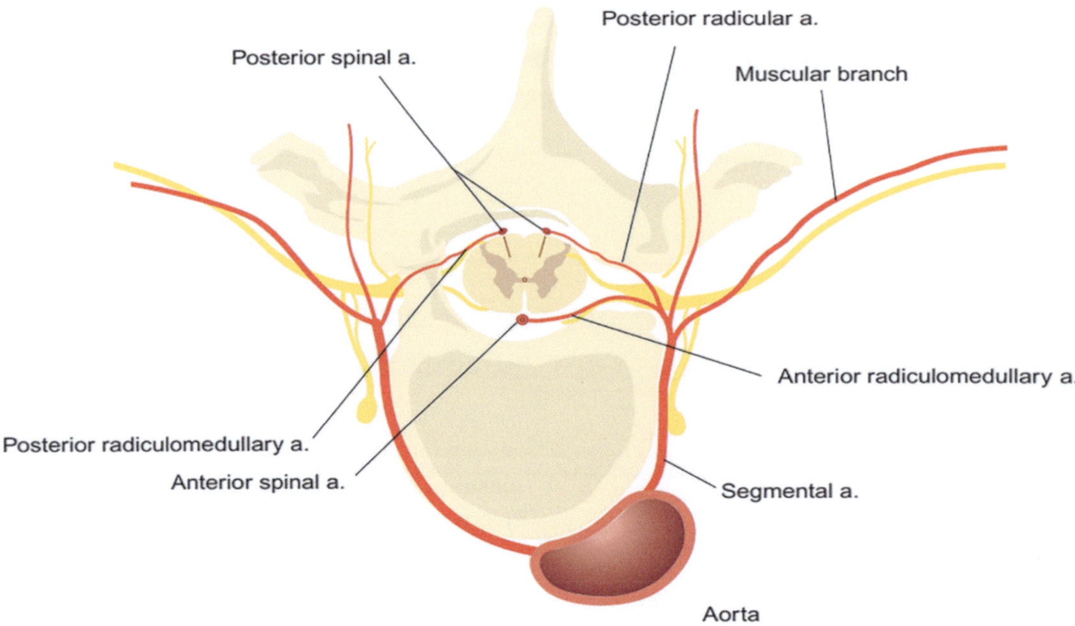

Fig. 26.1 Arterial blood supply of vertebrae

26.2.2 Vasculature of the Spinal Cord and Spinal Nerve Roots

The spinal cord receives its blood supply from the anterior spinal artery (ASA) and the posterior spinal arteries (PSAs). These arteries give rise to multiple branches that form anastomotic connections at the level of the conus medullaris. The ASA originates from the distal V4 segment of the vertebral arteries and supplies the anterior two-thirds of the spinal cord. In contrast, the PSAs arise from either the distal vertebral arteries or the posterior inferior cerebellar arteries (PICAs) and are responsible for supplying the posterior one-third of the spinal cord.

Anastomoses between the ASA and PSAs, known as the arterial vasocorona, provide vascular supply to the peripheral lateral aspects of the spinal cord. The lumbar spinal nerve roots receive their blood supply through branches arising from the conus medullaris vasculature, as well as the dorsal and ventral proximal radicular arteries. The proximal radicular arteries run along the nerve roots distally and contribute to the collateral circulation of the ASA and PSAs medially. The proximal regions of the nerve roots are already vascularized by collateral branches between the radiculomedullary arteries and the ASA or PSAs. These smaller arterial branches tend to run parallel to the nerve root fascicles.

At the intervertebral foramen, the spinal branch can divide into an anterior radicular branch and a posterior radicular branch, both of which supply their respective nerve roots before disappearing within the structures. The posterior radicular artery gives off a ganglionic branch near its origin. From this point, it extends both proximally and distally along the nerve root to supply its vascular needs. As the distal radicular artery travels proximally, it establishes numerous arterio-venous anastomoses with adjacent veins.

The venous drainage of the lumbar nerve roots is divided into two systems: the proximal and distal radicular venous systems. The distal radicular veins empty into the lumbar veins at the level of the intervertebral foramen, while the proximal radicular veins drain into the spinal cord venous plexuses. These veins have been observed to return via the arterial vasocorona before passing proximally into the anterior and posterior longitudinal veins of the spinal cord [5] (Fig. 26.2.)

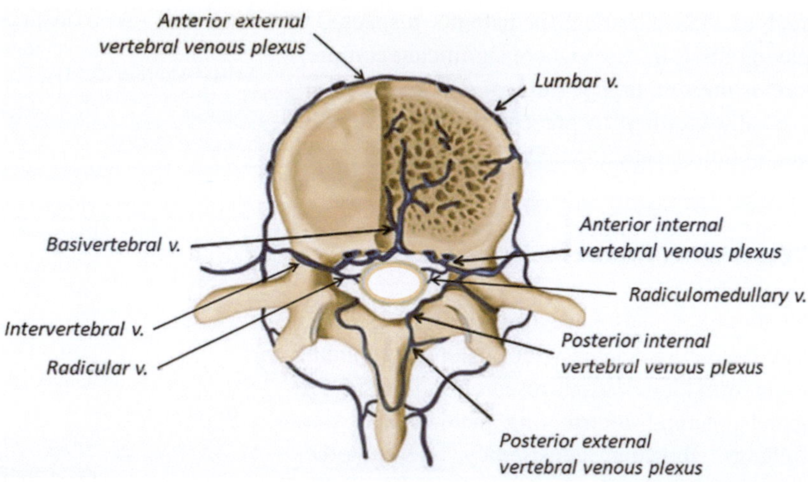

Fig. 26.2 Venous drainage of vertebrae

26.3 General Features of Postoperative Hematoma

26.3.1 Incidence

Most cases of the spinal epidural hematoma have no clinical symptoms. In a few patients, the postoperative hematoma compresses the dural sac, nerve roots or caudal equine, leading to the deterioration of nerve function, with sensory and motor dysfunction in the innervated area, which is called symptomatic spinal epidural hematoma [6]. The reported incidence of symptomatic postoperative hematoma requiring surgical evacuation varies significantly from 0.1% up to 1% [7, 8]. Interestingly, over 70% of spinal surgeons consider the risk of SEH after a major spinal surgery to be over 1% [9]. In addition, a recent systematic review found an overall calculated incidence of 0.2% [10].

Spinal epidural hematoma (SEH) is a relatively uncommon condition, and in most cases, it remains asymptomatic. However, in certain patients, particularly after spinal surgery, a postoperative hematoma may develop and exert pressure on critical structures such as the dural sac, nerve roots, or the cauda equina. When this compression leads to neurological deterioration, including sensory and motor dysfunction in the affected innervated areas, the condition is referred to as symptomatic spinal epidural hematoma [6].

The clinical presentation of symptomatic SEH can vary widely, depending on the location and extent of the hematoma. Patients may experience progressive limb weakness, sensory deficits, radicular pain, or even bowel and bladder dysfunction in severe cases. Early recognition of these symptoms is crucial, as delayed diagnosis and intervention can lead to permanent neurological impairment. The reported incidence of symptomatic postoperative SEH requiring surgical evacuation varies significantly across studies, with estimates ranging from 0.1% to 1% [7, 8]. Interestingly, surveys of spinal surgeons indicate that over 70% of them perceive the risk of SEH after major spinal surgery to be greater than 1% [9]. This discrepancy between actual incidence rates and clinical perception highlights the concern among surgeons regarding this potential complication.

Additionally, a recent systematic review analyzing multiple studies found the overall calculated incidence of symptomatic postoperative SEH to be approximately 0.2% [10]. While the condition is rare, its potentially severe consequences emphasize the importance of careful perioperative management, including meticulous hemostasis during surgery, appropriate use of anticoagulation therapy, and close postoperative monitoring for early signs of hematoma formation.

Given the potential for neurological deterioration, timely diagnosis through imaging studies such as MRI is critical for patients suspected of having SEH. In cases where significant compression is present, urgent surgical decompression is typically required to prevent permanent deficits and optimize patient outcomes.

26.3.2 Risk Factors

Numerous studies have been published on the risk factors associated with postoperative hematoma formation. Various researchers have investigated potential contributing factors, with some findings showing consistency, while others remain debated.

Kou et al. suggested that multilevel surgical procedures increase the risk of venous plexus rupture, thereby raising the likelihood of developing a compressive hematoma. Additionally, they identified preoperative coagulopathy as a significant risk factor. However, other variables such as age, body mass index (BMI), perioperative durotomy, and the use of surgical drains did not appear to increase the risk when compared to matched controls [7].

In a meta-analysis conducted by Awad et al., the researchers also recognized multilevel procedures as a significant risk factor. However, in contrast to Kou et al., they found that patients older than 60 years had an increased risk of developing postoperative hematomas. Interestingly, their analysis did not identify coagulopathy as a significant risk factor when age and the number of surgical levels were taken into account [11] (Table 26.1).

Sokolowski et al. further examined the determinants of hematoma volume and found several significant risk factors. These included advanced age (greater than 60 years), elevated preoperative international normalized ratio (INR), multilevel procedures, and increased estimated blood loss (EBL) during surgery. Their findings reinforce the notion that both patient-related and surgical factors contribute to the development of postoperative hematoma [12].

While some studies emphasize the role of coagulopathy, others prioritize the influence of age and procedural factors. Despite some variations in findings, the consensus indicates that multilevel procedures and advanced age are among the most consistently reported risk factors for postoperative hematoma formation.

Table 26.1 Summary of previously identified significant risk factors for developing symptomatic postoperative SEH. (Amiri et al. [2])

Author	Risk factors
Awad et al. [11]	
	Age > 60 years
	Preoperative NSAIDs
	Rh-positive blood type
	Involvement of >5 operating levels
	Hb <10 g/dL
	Blood loss >1 L
	INR >2 within first 48 postoperative hours
Kou et al. [7]	
	Multilevel procedure
	Preoperative coagulopathy

SEH spinal epidural hematoma, *NSAIDs* nonsteroidal anti-inflammatory drugs, *Hb* hemoglobin, *INR* international normalized ratio

26.3.3 Hematoma Formation Following Ligament Reconstruction Surgery: Comparison with General Spinal Surgery and Considerations for Management

Hematoma formation after ligament reconstruction surgery is not fundamentally different from hematoma development following general spinal surgery. In most cases, postoperative hematoma results from surgical trauma, leading to blood accumulation within the operative site. However, certain factors specific to ligament reconstruction procedures may influence the extent and characteristics of hematoma formation.

In particular, open midline decompression surgery is designed to achieve wide decompression while preserving the facet joints as much as possible. This approach helps maintain spinal stability while effectively relieving neural compression. However, due to the nature of this procedure, the postoperative hematoma may occupy a relatively larger space compared to other spinal surgeries where facet joints are more extensively resected. The larger decompression area creates a broader potential space for hematoma formation, which can sometimes lead to increased hematoma volume on postoperative imaging.

Additionally, the use of artificial ligaments introduces another potential factor in fluid accumulation. Some patients may experience an allergic reaction to artificial ligament materials, leading to fluid collection at the surgical site. This fluid accumulation can manifest as seroma formation, which itself may not cause significant compression. However, if blood mixes with the serous fluid, it may appear as a large hematoma on imaging studies, potentially leading to misinterpretation of the findings. Differentiating between a true hematoma and a mixed seroma-hematoma is crucial in postoperative management, as their clinical significance and treatment approaches may differ.

From a clinical and radiological perspective, it is essential to assess the degree of dural sac compression and determine whether there are neurological symptoms caused by neural compression. While small hematomas may resolve spontaneously without intervention, larger hematomas or those causing significant neurological deficits may require careful management,

26.4 Management of the Hemorrhages

26.4.1 Preoperative Management

Preoperative management is a fundamental aspect of reducing the risk of postoperative hematoma and ensuring optimal patient recovery following surgery. A thorough patient assessment is the first step in this process, which includes a detailed review of medical history, identification of pre-existing conditions such as bleeding disorders, and an evaluation of any prior episodes of abnormal bleeding or hematoma formation. A physical examination is also essential, focusing on vital signs, signs of coagulopathy, or conditions that may contribute to increased bleeding risk. Additionally, laboratory tests such as coagulation profiles (PT, aPTT, INR) and platelet counts are performed to assess the patient's clotting ability and determine if any corrective measures are needed before surgery.

Medication management is another crucial component of preoperative care. Many patients undergoing surgery are on anticoagulants or antiplatelet agents such as warfarin, aspirin, or clopidogrel, which can significantly increase the risk of postoperative hematoma. These medications must be carefully managed, with temporary discontinuation or dose adjustment based on the patient's condition, the urgency of the procedure, and the expected bleeding risk. The timing of discontinuation and reinitiation should be guided by clinical protocols to balance the risks of excessive bleeding and thromboembolic complications. In some cases, bridging therapy with short-acting anticoagulants, such as low-molecular-weight heparin (LMWH), may be considered to minimize both risks [13].

Patient education is another essential aspect of preoperative management, ensuring that patients are well informed about steps they can take to optimize surgical outcomes. Smoking cessation is strongly encouraged, as smoking negatively impacts blood circulation and wound healing, increasing the likelihood of postoperative complications, including hematoma formation. Similarly, alcohol restriction is recommended, as excessive alcohol consumption can interfere with normal coagulation and immune function. Patients should also receive clear preoperative instructions, including fasting guidelines, hydration recommendations, and information about which medications should or should not be taken before surgery.

26.4.2 Intra-, Postoperative Management

Effective intraoperative bleeding control is paramount in preventing postoperative hematoma, which can lead to serious complications. One of the most crucial strategies in reducing intraoperative bleeding is subperiosteal dissection, particularly when working with muscle tissue. This technique minimizes muscle damage and reduces the risk of excessive bleeding. In surgeries aimed at evacuating a hematoma, the most common sources of bleeding include muscular arterial bleeding or diffuse muscle bleeding. Thus, careful muscle coagulation and precise subperiosteal dissection during the initial surgery are essential for minimizing the risk of postoperative hematoma formation.

As previously mentioned, the radiculomedullary artery, vasocorona, and Batson's venous plexus are among the most significant sources of postoperative hematoma. Because these vascular structures play a crucial role in spinal cord circulation, failure to adequately control their bleeding can lead to severe complications. Therefore, meticulous attention must be given to vascular bleeding control during surgery.

A bipolar coagulator is an effective tool for achieving precise hemostasis. However, when operating near the nerve roots or the dural sac, additional protective measures are required to prevent unintended neural damage. In these cases, placing a protective cotton pad around the nerve structures can serve as a safeguard against thermal or mechanical injury.

In situations where direct coagulation of bleeding vessels proves to be challenging—especially in the case of venous bleeding, where coagulation can be more difficult than arterial bleeding—hemostatic agents are often required. A variety of hemostatic agents are available, each suited for different types of bleeding and surgical needs [14].

Commonly Used Hemostatic Agents

- Vegetal-origin hemostatic agents such as Surgicel®, Tabotamp®, and Hemostase® are widely utilized for promoting clot formation in surgical fields.
- Fibrin sealants, including Tachosil® and Tisseel®, function by mimicking the body's natural coagulation process to enhance hemostasis.
- Gelatin-based sponge products such as Gelfoam®, which consist solely of gelatin, provide an additional means of controlling bleeding.
- Polyvinyl alcohol sponges, such as Merocel®, offer specialized applications for hemostasis.

Among these, gelatin-thrombin matrix sealants are frequently used in intraoperative settings due to their ability to act at the final stage of the coagulation cascade, facilitating fibrin formation and promoting clot stabilization. These agents are composed of a flowable gelatin matrix (derived from either bovine or porcine sources) combined with a human-derived thrombin component. For example:

Floseal® (Baxter Healthcare Corporation, Fremont, CA, USA) consists of a bovine gelatin matrix and thrombin, making it highly effective for immediate hemostasis.

Surgiflo® (Ethicon Endo-Surgery, a Johnson & Johnson company, New Jersey, USA) utilizes a porcine gelatin matrix and thrombin, offering similar efficacy in controlling surgical bleeding.

Both of these products are typically prepared immediately before use and directly injected into the bleeding site to achieve rapid and localized coagulation.

To further reduce the risk of postoperative hematoma, the placement of a drainage tube is a standard preventive measure. However, the positioning of the drainage tube is critical—if placed too close to the dural sac, there is a risk of injury to the decompressed and expanded dura mater due to negative pressure effects. This could lead to cerebrospinal fluid (CSF) leakage, neural damage, or delayed healing [15].

The drainage tube should be closely monitored, and its function must be regularly assessed to ensure proper evacuation of excess fluids. The tube can be safely removed once the drainage volume decreases to an acceptable level, indicating reduced risk of hematoma formation. However, particular attention should be given to potential obstruction of the drainage tube, as blockage can lead to fluid accumulation and increased intracranial or intraspinal pressure, which are primary causes of hematoma development [13].

26.5 Summary

Open midline decompression and ligament reconstruction is an effective treatment for spinal stenosis and instability, preserving spinal structure stability while avoiding excessive facet joint resection. However, complications such as postoperative hematoma, dysesthesia, incidental durotomy, and infection can occur, with hematoma being particularly critical due to its potential to compress neural structures and cause neurological deficits, sometimes requiring emergency evacuation. Major risk factors include multilevel surgery, advanced age, coagulation disorders, prolonged operation time, and significant blood loss. Effective management requires meticulous intraoperative hemostasis, with the use of advanced hemostatic agents such as gelatin-thrombin matrix sealants (e.g., Floseal®, Surgiflo®), fibrin sealants (e.g., Tachosil®, Tisseel®), and cellulose-based agents (e.g., Surgicel®) playing a crucial role in controlling surgical bleeding. Proper placement and monitoring of drainage tubes are essential to prevent cerebrospinal fluid leakage and neural injury. Additionally, careful preoperative assessment, anticoagulation management, and postoperative neurological monitoring are necessary to minimize the risk of hematoma formation and ensure optimal patient outcomes.

References

1. Lho HW, Shin SH. Hematoma. In: Transforaminal endoscopy for lumbar spine. Singapore: Springer Nature Singapore; 2023. p. 285–92.
2. Amiri AR, Fouyas IP, Cro S, Casey AT. Postoperative spinal epidural hematoma (SEH): incidence, risk factors, onset, and management. Spine J. 2013;13(2):134–40.
3. Aono H, Ohwada T, Hosono N, Tobimatsu H, Ariga K, Fuji T, Iwasaki M. Incidence of postoperative symptomatic epidural hematoma in spinal decompression surgery. J Neurosurg Spine. 2011;15(2):202–5.
4. Bosmia AN, Hogan E, Loukas M, Tubbs RS, Cohen-Gadol AA. Blood supply to the human spinal cord: part I. Anatomy and hemodynamics. Clin Anat. 2015;28(1):52–64.
5. Griessenauer CJ, Raborn J, Foreman P, Shoja MM, Loukas M, Tubbs RS. Venous drainage of the spine and spinal cord: a comprehensive review of its history, embryology, anatomy, physiology, and pathology. Clin Anat. 2015;28(1):75–87.
6. Chen Q, Zhong X, Liu W, Wong C, He Q, Chen Y. Incidence of postoperative symptomatic spinal epidural hematoma requiring surgical evacuation: a systematic review and meta-analysis. Eur Spine J. 2022;31(12):3274–85.
7. Kou J, Fischgrund J, Biddinger A, Herkowitz H. Risk factors for spinal epidural hematoma after spinal surgery. Spine (Phila Pa 1976). 2002;27:1670–3.
8. Cabana F, Pointillart V, Vital J, Senegas J. Postoperative compressive spinal epidural hematomas. 15 cases and a review of the literature. [Article in French]. Rev Chir Orthop Reparatrice Appar Mot. 2000;86:335–45.
9. Glotzbecker MP, Bono CM, Harris MB, et al. Surgeon practices regarding postoperative thromboembolic prophylaxis after high-risk spinal surgery. Spine (Phila Pa 1976). 2008;33:2915–21.
10. Glotzbecker MP, Bono CM, Wood KB, Harris MB. Postoperative spi nal epidural hematoma: a systematic review. Spine. 2010;Phila Pa 1976(35):E413–20.
11. Awad JN, Kebaish KM, Donigan J, Cohen DB, Kostuik JP. Analysis of the risk factors for the development of post-operative spinal epidural haematoma. J Bone Joint Surg Br. 2005;87(9):1248–52.
12. Sokolowski MJ, Garvey TA, John Perl II, Sokolowski MS, Cho W, Mehbod AA, et al. Prospective study of postoperative lumbar epidural hematoma: incidence and risk factors. Spine. 2008;33(1):108–13.
13. Zeng XJ, Wang W, Zhao Z, Li M. Causes and preventive measures of symptomatic spinal epidural haematoma after spinal surgery. Int Orthop. 2017;41:1395–403.
14. Szpalski M, Gunzburg R, Sztern B. An overview of blood-sparing techniques used in spine surgery during the perioperative period. Eur Spine J. 2004;13(Suppl 1):S18–27.
15. Echave M, Oyagüez I, Casado MA. Use of Floseal®, a human gelatine-thrombin matrix sealant, in surgery: a systematic review. BMC Surg. 2014;14:1–13.

Spinous Process Fracture in Ligament Reconstruction: Mechanisms, Prevention, and Management

27

Ju-Wan Seuk

Abstract

Spinous process fractures are a relatively rare but significant complication associated with lumbar ligament reconstruction. They often result from excessive mechanical stress during artificial ligament placement, ligament tension imbalance, or patient-related factors such as osteoporosis. These fractures can cause postoperative localized pain, reduced mobility, and mechanical instability, potentially delaying recovery or necessitating revision surgery. Key risk factors include over-distraction during ligament placement, over-resection during decompression, and inadequate preoperative bone health optimization. Symptoms typically present as focal tenderness, mechanical back pain, and restricted range of motion, with imaging techniques such as CT and MRI playing a critical role in diagnosis.

Effective prevention strategies emphasize meticulous surgical techniques, including preserving spinous process integrity, gentle ligament handling, and balanced ligament tensioning. Preoperative optimization of bone density through medications such as bisphosphonates or teriparatide is particularly crucial for osteoporotic patients. Postoperative care should include gradual rehabilitation and activity modifications to minimize stress on the spinous processes.

Management of fractures varies depending on severity and symptoms, ranging from conservative measures such as pain control, bracing, and restricted activity to surgical interventions like extension of ligament reconstruction. Future advancements in surgical techniques and patient-specific care are essential to further reduce the risk of spinous process fractures and improve clinical outcomes.

Keywords

Spinal stabilization · Artificial ligament Ligament reconstruction · Spinous process fracture · H-ligament augmentation

J.-W. Seuk (✉)
Department of Neurosurgery, Cheongdam Wooridul Spine Hospital, Seoul, Korea (Republic of)
e-mail: imaxpert@wooridul.co.kr

27.1 Introduction

Ligament reconstruction is a specialized surgical intervention aimed at restoring spinal stability and maintaining the integrity of the posterior ligamentous complex while alleviating symptoms of spinal disorders such as lumbar spinal stenosis. This technique is increasingly utilized as an adjunct to traditional decompression procedures, particularly in cases where maintaining spinal stability is essential, but fusion is either not

S.-H. Lee et al. (eds.), *Ligament Reconstruction for Spine*,
https://doi.org/10.1007/978-981-95-3971-0_27

desired or deemed unnecessary [1, 2]. By reconstructing or augmenting the ligamentous structures, surgeons aim to preserve segmental mobility, reduce the risk of adjacent segment disease, and provide durable symptom relief [3, 4].

Despite its advantages, lumbar ligament reconstruction carries a risk of complications, among which spinous process fracture is of particular concern [5, 6]. The spinous processes, located posteriorly along the vertebrae, play a crucial role in the structural and functional dynamics of the spine. They serve as attachment points for the interspinous ligament, supraspinous ligament, and surrounding musculature, all of which contribute to spinal stability [7, 8]. When these structures are manipulated or augmented during ligament reconstruction, the spinous processes are subjected to mechanical stress, which can lead to fractures under certain conditions [9, 10].

Spinous process fractures, though uncommon, have been increasingly reported in association with procedures involving interspinous devices or posterior ligament reconstruction [1, 4, 11]. These fractures can result in significant postoperative pain, delay recovery, and, in severe cases, necessitate additional surgical intervention [5, 12]. Various factors, including surgical technique, device design, and patient-related variables such as osteoporosis or preexisting spinal deformities, contribute to the risk of fracture [2, 9]. Understanding these risk factors and their interplay is crucial for minimizing complications and optimizing surgical outcomes [3, 6, 10].

Moreover, spinous process fractures are not merely mechanical failures; they can disrupt the delicate balance of spinal biomechanics, leading to altered load distribution, instability, or even adjacent segment degeneration over time [4, 7]. Therefore, the management of such fractures requires a nuanced approach that considers the biomechanical and clinical implications of the injury [5, 11].

This chapter delves into the complexities of spinous process fractures in the context of ligament reconstruction. It examines the mechanisms underlying their occurrence, identifies key risk factors, and outlines evidence-based strategies for prevention and management. By synthesizing current research and clinical insights, this chapter aims to provide a comprehensive understanding of this complication, enabling surgeons to make informed decisions and improve patient outcomes in ligament reconstruction procedures [1, 8, 9].

27.2 Mechanisms of Spinous Process Fracture

Spinous process fractures are rare but significant complications associated with lumbar ligament reconstruction. They result from various mechanical and biomechanical factors, which are detailed below.

27.2.1 Structural Damage During Surgery

Intraoperative errors or excessive manipulation can weaken the structural integrity of the spinous processes, making them more susceptible to fractures.

1. *Over-resection During Decompression*

During decompression procedures, excessive resection of the parts of the spinous process can weaken its structural stability (Fig. 27.1). Particularly, over-resection at the base of the spinous process can compromise its load-bearing capacity, increasing the likelihood of fractures.

2. *Direct Instrumentation-Related Trauma*

Spinous processes may sustain direct mechanical damage during the placement of surgical instruments or devices. For example, improper alignment or excessive force during the insertion of interspinous devices can cause microcracks or outright fractures.

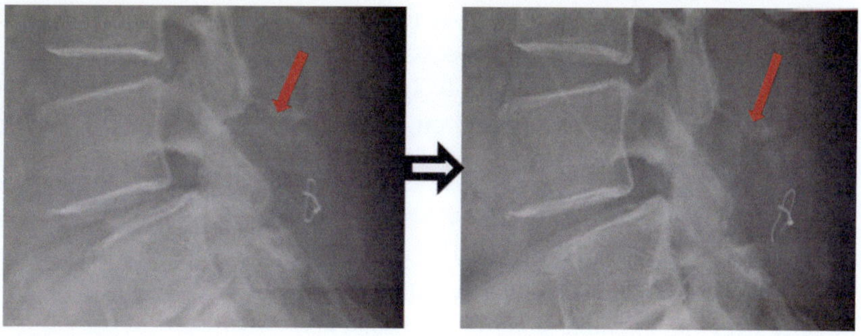

Fig. 27.1 Excessive resection of the spinous process can lead to spinous process fractures

27.2.2 Repetitive Stress-Related Damage

Postoperative repetitive stress on the spinous processes can result in stress fractures over time.

1. *Excessive Rehabilitation or Physical Activity*

Patients engaging in overly aggressive physical therapy or rehabilitation exercises immediately after surgery may subject the spinous processes to repetitive stress before they have fully healed. Activities involving excessive lumbar flexion or extension are particularly harmful and can predispose the spinous processes to fatigue fractures.

2. *Micro-movements of Implanted Devices*

Micro-movements of the implanted device against the spinous process may cause chronic stress and eventual fatigue fractures. This often occurs when the fixation of the device is incomplete or when spinal motion is excessive postoperatively.

27.2.3 Patient-Related Factors

Patient-specific factors also play a critical role in the occurrence of spinous process fractures.

1. *Osteoporosis*

Elderly or osteoporotic patients are particularly susceptible to spinous process fractures due to reduced bone density and structural weakness. The decreased bone mass and quality in these patients cannot withstand the repetitive or concentrated mechanical loads applied during and after surgery.

2. *Preexisting Spinal Deformities*

Conditions like scoliosis or kyphosis may alter the mechanical load distribution across the spinous processes, increasing fracture risk. The abnormal curvature can lead to asymmetric loading and heightened stress on specific spinous processes, making them more prone to fractures.

27.3 Clinical Features of Spinous Process Fracture

The clinical presentation of spinous process fractures following lumbar ligament reconstruction can vary in severity, ranging from mild discomfort to significant functional impairment. Understanding these features is crucial for timely diagnosis and management.

27.3.1 Symptoms

1. *Localized Pain*

Patients commonly report sharp or dull pain localized to the surgical site. This pain may intensify during movement or changes in posture, such as bending or twisting. Pain typically arises within the first few days to weeks after surgery but can sometimes appear later, especially in cases of stress fractures.

2. *Mechanical Pain*

Patients may experience mechanical back pain, characterized by worsening symptoms during physical activity or weight-bearing and improvement with rest. Spinous process fractures alter the biomechanics of the posterior spinal column, leading to increased stress on adjacent segments.

3. *Palpable Tenderness*

Physical examination often reveals tenderness directly over the affected spinous process. This finding is particularly noticeable when manual pressure is applied to the surgical area.

4. *Reduced Range of Motion*

Fractures can cause stiffness and limit the patient's ability to perform daily activities, such as bending, twisting, or lifting objects. Severe fractures may result in gross instability, causing significant impairment.

27.3.2 Associated Signs

1. *Visible Swelling or Deformity*

In cases where the fracture is severe or associated with soft tissue injury, localized swelling or visible deformity over the surgical site may be noted.

2. *Adjacent Segment Dysfunction*

Altered load distribution from the fracture may lead to compensatory stress and symptoms in adjacent segments, such as muscle spasms or disc-related issues.

27.3.3 Diagnostic Modalities

1. *Plain Radiography (X-Ray)*

X-rays are often the initial imaging modality but may not always reveal minor fractures. Stress fractures or early microfractures are particularly difficult to detect.

2. *Computed Tomography (CT)*

CT is the gold standard for evaluating spinous process fractures. It provides detailed information about fracture location, pattern, and severity.

3. *Magnetic Resonance Imaging (MRI)*

MRI is helpful in assessing soft tissue involvement, including the posterior ligamentous complex, and identifying adjacent segment complications. MRI also helps differentiate fractures from other postoperative complications, such as infection or hematoma.

4. *Bone Scan or Dual-Energy X-ray Absorptiometry (DXA)*

A bone scan can detect metabolic activity at the fracture site, while DXA evaluates the patient's bone density, particularly in osteoporotic individuals.

27.4 Strategies for Prevention

Preventing spinous process fractures requires a multifaceted approach that includes careful surgical planning, patient-specific considerations, and appropriate postoperative care.

27.4.1 Optimizing Surgical Techniques

1. *Preservation of Spinous Process Integrity*

Avoid excessive resection of bone or surrounding soft tissues during decompression. Minimize direct mechanical stress on the spinous process during instrumentation or device placement.

2. *Balanced Ligament Tension*

Ensure that reconstructed ligaments are tensioned appropriately to avoid overloading the spinous process. Adjustments should consider the patient's specific spinal dynamics and bone quality.

3. *Gentle Instrument Handling*

Employ meticulous surgical techniques to prevent iatrogenic damage to the spinous process. Avoid applying excessive force during device placement or fixation.

27.4.2 Addressing Patient-Specific Factors

1. *Preoperative Bone Health Optimization*

Perform preoperative assessment of bone density using DXA, especially in elderly or osteoporotic patients. Prescribe medications such as bisphosphonates or teriparatide to improve bone quality in at-risk individuals. Encourage adequate calcium and vitamin D intake before surgery.

2. *Risk Stratification*

Evaluate patients for conditions like scoliosis, kyphosis, or other spinal deformities that may predispose them to uneven load distribution and fracture risk.

27.4.3 Postoperative Care

1. *Rehabilitation Protocols*

Develop a structured and gradual physical therapy plan to avoid premature loading of the spinous process. Educate patients on safe movements and restrictions to prevent stress on the reconstructed spine.

2. *Use of Braces*

In high-risk patients, consider postoperative lumbar bracing to reduce motion and support the spinous process during healing.

27.5 Management and Treatment

Managing spinous process fractures depends on the severity of the fracture, the presence of instability, and the patient's symptoms.

27.5.1 Nonsurgical Management

1. *Pain Management*

Prescribe NSAIDs or acetaminophen for pain relief. Avoid long-term use of opioids unless absolutely necessary. Consider localized injections (e.g., corticosteroids) for refractory pain.

2. *Activity Modification*

Restrict activities that place undue stress on the spine, such as heavy lifting, bending, or prolonged standing. Encourage low-impact exercises such as walking or swimming as tolerated.

3. *Bracing*

Apply a lumbar brace to stabilize the spine and prevent further stress on the fracture site during healing.

4. *Bone Health Improvement*

For osteoporotic patients, continue or initiate pharmacologic treatment to enhance bone density and promote fracture healing.

27.5.2 Surgical Management

27.5.2.1 Ligament Reconstruction Extension (H-Ligament Augmentation)

Spinous process fractures can be effectively managed by extending ligament reconstruction to adjacent segments, redistributing mechanical stress, and enhancing stability while preserving spinal mobility. This approach involves removing the fractured spinous process, then extending the artificial ligament to adjacent segments to redis-

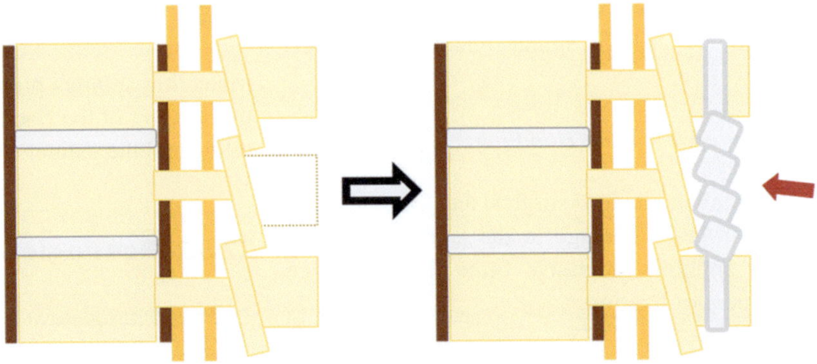

Fig. 27.2 The space left by the fractured spinous process is filled with an H-ligament (H-ligament augmentation) to restore structural continuity and provide additional support

tribute mechanical stress and enhance stability. Following this, the space left by the removed spinous process is filled with an H-ligament to restore structural continuity and provide additional support (Fig. 27.2). This approach creates a balanced load-sharing mechanism while preserving spinal mobility, aligning with the principles of non-fusion stabilization.

27.6 Conclusion

Spinous process fractures are rare but significant complications of lumbar ligament reconstruction. They arise from complex interactions between mechanical forces, surgical techniques, and patient-specific factors such as bone quality [2, 7, 8]. Early diagnosis through advanced imaging and a thorough understanding of risk factors are crucial for effective prevention and management [4–6]. Adopting meticulous surgical techniques, optimizing preoperative bone health, and ensuring structured postoperative rehabilitation can significantly reduce the incidence of spinous process fractures [1, 3, 9]. In cases of spinous process fractures, treatment can involve extending the artificial ligament to adjacent segments for stability, and filling the resulting space with an H-ligament to restore structural continuity while preserving spinal mobility.

References

1. Kazarian GS, Jordan YJ, Johnson M, Bhargava S, Cecere R, Hirase T, Qureshi S, Dowdell J, Sheha E, Lovecchio F, Iyer S. Analysis of 1027 adverse events reports for interspinous process devices from the US FDA MAUDE database. Int J Spine Surg. 2024;18(3):452–9.
2. Epstein NE. A review of interspinous fusion devices: high complication, reoperation rates, and costs with poor outcomes. Surg Neurol Int. 2020;11:102.
3. Skoblar M, Hedman T, Rogers AJ, Jasper GP, Beall DP. Instrumented posterior arthrodesis of the lumbar spine: prospective study of a minimally invasive interspinous fixation device. J Pain Res. 2021;14:1231–40.
4. Aggarwal N, Chow R. Real-world adverse events of interspinous spacers using manufacturer and user facility device experience (MAUDE) data. Anesth Pain Med. 2020;10(2):93–8.
5. Florence TJ, Say I, Patel KS, Unterberger A, Laiwalla A, Vivas AC, Lu DC. Neurosurgical management of interspinous device complications: a case series. Front Surg. 2022;9:812.
6. Hao-Ju Lo H.-J, Chen H.-M, Yi-Jie Kuo Y.-J, Yang S.-W. Effect of different designs of interspinous process devices on the instrumented and adjacent levels after double-level lumbar decompression surgery: a finite element analysis. PLoS One. 2020;15(12):e0244571.
7. Li K.-Y, Li H.-L, Chen L.-J, Xiang J.-W, Li C.-C, Weng J.-J, Tian N.-F. Complications and radiographic changes after implantation of interspinous process devices: a five-year follow-up. BMC Musculoskelet Disord. 2023;24:119.
8. Gazzeri R, Galarza M, Neroni M, Fiore C, Faiola A, Puzzilli F, Callovini G, Alfieri A. Failure rates and complications of interspinous process decompres-

sion devices: a clinical study. J Neurosurg Spine. 2015;23(4):356–64.
9. Park WM, Choi DK, Kim YH, Kim K. Pre-tension effects from tightening the ligature on spinous process fracture risk in interspinous process devices implantation. Int J Precis Eng Man uf. 2014;15(10):2109–14.
10. Kim DH, Shanti N, Tantorski ME, Shaw JD, Li L, Martha JF, Thomas AJ, Parazin SJ, Rencus TC, Kwon B. Association between degenerative spondylolisthesis and spinous process fracture after interspinous process spacer surgery. S pine J. 2012;12(4):322–9.
11. Bowers C, Amini A, Dailey AT, Schmidt MH. Dynamic interspinous process stabilization: review of complications associated with the X-STOP device. Neurosurg Focus. 2010;28(6):E8.
12. Xu C, Ni W.-F, Tian N.-F, Hu X.-Q, Li F, Xu H.-Z. Complications in degenerative lumbar disease treated with a dynamic interspinous spacer (Coflex): is it a safe implant? Int Orthop. 2013;37(5):1001–6.

Foreign Body Reaction and Allergic Reaction Associated with Artificial Ligaments in Degenerative Lumbar Spinal Stenosis

28

Hyoung-Woo Lho

Abstract

Degenerative lumbar spinal stenosis (DLSS) is a common spinal disease in elderly patients. For elderly patients, midline decompression surgery for DLSS is a more suitable approach, as it preserves the disc, lamina, and facet joints while reconstructing the posterior tension bands. In this context, we discuss ligament reconstruction using interspinous artificial ligaments for soft stabilization after microsurgical fenestration to prevent post-decompression segmental instability.

Foreign body reaction is a very rare postoperative complication following artificial ligament reconstruction surgery. However, if such a reaction occurs, it can be managed with antihistamines or steroids to control the allergic response. Artificial ligaments are typically made of polyethylene terephthalate, a material with a minimal risk of foreign body reaction; thus, its occurrence is extremely rare. In most cases, removal is unnecessary, as favorable outcomes are observed even in the presence of a foreign body reaction.

Keywords

Polyethylene terephthalate · Foreign body reaction · Foreign body response · Allergic reaction · Artificial ligament

28.1 Introduction

Degenerative lumbar spinal stenosis (DLSS) is a common condition among elderly patients. With an aging population and increasing life expectancy, a growing number of geriatric patients present with DLSS alongside complex medical conditions such as frailty, sarcopenia, osteoporosis, and cardiovascular diseases. Given the high surgical risks associated with multilevel fusion surgery in this population, alternative treatments such as midline decompression surgery combined with soft stabilization using artificial ligaments have been introduced.

Artificial ligaments, such as the SHLee ligament made from polyethylene terephthalate (PET), provide mechanical stabilization while preserving spinal structures like the disc, lamina, and facet joints. However, despite PET's proven biocompatibility, complications such as foreign body reaction (FBR) and, rarely, allergic reactions may occur postoperatively. This chapter reviews the incidence, mechanisms, and manage-

H.-W. Lho (✉)
Department of Neurosurgery, Cheongdam Wooridul Spine Hospital, Seoul, Korea (Republic of)
e-mail: nhw724@wooridul.co.kr

S.-H. Lee et al. (eds.), *Ligament Reconstruction for Spine*,
https://doi.org/10.1007/978-981-95-3971-0_28

ment strategies for these reactions in the context of artificial ligament reconstruction in elderly DLSS patients [1–3].

28.2 Biocompatibility of Polyethylene Terephthalate (PET)

Polyethylene terephthalate (PET) is widely used in medical implants due to its high tensile strength, durability, and biocompatibility. It has been employed in various applications, including vascular grafts, sutures, and artificial ligaments like the SHLee ligament. PET's key advantages include:

Mechanical Stability: Resistance to wear and degradation under stress [4, 5].

Hydrophobicity: Minimal water absorption, preserving mechanical integrity [1, 6].

Surface Chemistry: Facilitates protein adsorption and cellular interactions without inducing significant toxicity [2, 7].

While PET is generally well tolerated, it is not completely inert. Protein adsorption on its surface can initiate mild inflammatory responses, which, in rare cases, progress to complications such as foreign body reactions or hypersensitivity [8–10].

28.3 Foreign Body Reaction to Artificial Ligaments

28.3.1 Incidence

Foreign body reactions (FBRs) associated with PET-based artificial ligaments are rare, with reported rates ranging from 1% to 3% for mild to moderate reactions. Severe cases, including granuloma formation or fibrosis, occur in less than 1% of patients [2, 5, 6, 7, 9].

28.3.2 Mechanisms

FBR occurs when the immune system identifies PET as a foreign material. Upon implantation, the following sequence occurs:

Protein Adsorption: Host proteins coat the PET surface, forming a conditioning layer [1, 9, 11].

Macrophage Activation: Immune cells recognize the coated surface and release inflammatory cytokines such as IL-1 and TNF-α [6, 8, 11].

Foreign Body Giant Cell (FBGC) Formation: Persistent macrophage activity may lead to the development of FBGCs, which promote fibrosis or encapsulation of the ligament [2, 9, 11, 12].

28.3.3 Risk Factors

Several factors can increase the likelihood of FBR:

Surface Irregularities: Rough or irregular PET surfaces enhance protein adsorption and immune activation [2, 6, 10].

Mechanical Stress: Repeated stress on the ligament can cause microabrasions, exposing new surfaces for immune recognition [9, 12].

Patient-Specific Factors: Comorbidities such as diabetes, smoking, or autoimmune diseases may amplify the immune response [8, 10].

28.3.4 Management

Foreign body reactions are often manageable with conservative therapies:

Medication: Antihistamines or steroids can control inflammation and allergic responses [5, 7, 9].

Monitoring: Most cases resolve without requiring surgical intervention. If necessary, long-term follow-up should be done [2, 6, 12].

Despite these rare complications, favorable clinical outcomes are commonly observed, even when mild FBR occurs [8–10].

28.4 Allergic Reactions to Artificial Ligaments

28.4.1 Incidence

Allergic reactions to PET are exceedingly rare, as PET itself is nonimmunogenic. However, residual chemicals from manufacturing, such as stabilizers or catalysts, may provoke hypersensitivity in predisposed individuals [1, 2, 5].

28.4.2 Mechanisms

Type I Hypersensitivity: Immediate allergic reactions mediated by IgE antibodies, resulting in swelling, rash, or localized inflammation [6, 8, 10].

Type IV Hypersensitivity: Delayed-type reactions involving T-cells, which may cause localized dermatitis or chronic inflammation [7, 9, 13].

These reactions may arise from the following:

Contaminants or Degradation Products: Chemicals like terephthalic acid can bind to host proteins, forming neoantigens that trigger immune responses [1, 2, 8].

Patient Predisposition: Individuals with a history of allergies or atopy are at increased risk [5, 6, 8].

28.4.3 Risk Factors and Prevention

Manufacturing Quality: Ensuring the removal of processing residues can minimize allergenic potential [5, 10, 12].

Patient Screening: Preoperative assessment of allergy history can help identify at-risk individuals [1, 5, 10].

28.5 Clinical Applications and Advantages of Artificial Ligaments

Artificial ligament reconstruction, combined with microsurgical midline decompression surgery, provides a viable alternative to multilevel fusion surgery in elderly patients with DLSS. Key advantages include:

Preservation of Spinal Structures: Unlike fusion surgeries, artificial ligaments preserve the disc, lamina, and facet joints.

Soft Stabilization: Artificial ligaments offer sufficient stabilization to prevent post-decompression segmental instability.

Shorter Surgical Time: Soft stabilization simplifies the procedure, reducing operative time and associated risks, which is particularly beneficial for patients with significant comorbidities.

28.6 Case Presentation

28.6.1 Introduction

The incidence of allergic or foreign body reactions following ligament reconstruction has not been clearly established, primarily due to the exceptional rarity of such events. When these reactions do occur, they are typically characterized by localized radiating pain, often in the absence of systemic symptoms such as malaise or fever. Diagnostic imaging, particularly magnetic resonance imaging (MRI) and computed tomography (CT), can play a critical role in identifying these adverse responses.

This report documents a single case of allergic reaction identified among more than 80,000 ligament reconstruction procedures performed at a single specialized spine center over a 24-year period (2000–2024), highlighting the exceptional rarity of this complication.

28.6.2 Case

A 59-year-old male patient presented with lateral calf pain, tingling sensations, and an antalgic gait secondary to pain. Neurological examination revealed motor weakness in dorsiflexion of both great toes, along with difficulty performing heel walking. Lumbar spine magnetic resonance imaging (MRI) demonstrated hypertrophic ligamentum flavum resulting in significant canal compression at the L3–4 and L4–5 levels (Fig. 28.1). In addition, MRI myelography showed signal blockage at the L3–4 and L4–5 levels, consistent with the areas of stenosis (Fig. 28.1).

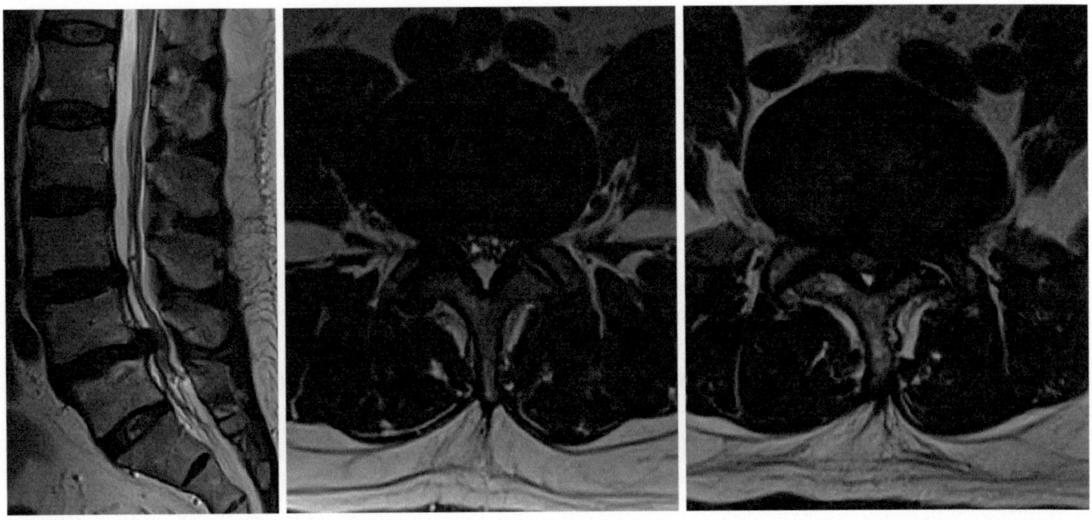

Fig. 28.1 Preoperative MRI demonstrated spinal stenosis at the L3/4, L4/5

The patient underwent open midline decompression at the L3–4 and L4–5 levels, including flavectomy, to achieve neural decompression. Subsequently, ligament reconstruction was performed to provide soft stabilization. Postoperative magnetic resonance imaging (MRI) confirmed complete neural decompression at L3–4 and L4–5 (Fig. 28.2). The patient's symptoms showed significant improvement, and he was discharged on postoperative day 6.

Three weeks after discharge, the patient presented to the outpatient clinic with complaints of low back pain and right buttock pain. Follow-up magnetic resonance imaging (MRI) revealed epidural fluid accumulation causing compression of the thecal sac at the L3–4 and L4–5 levels (Fig. 28.3).

The patient was treated with a single intramuscular steroid injection and initiated on pheniramine therapy. Following this treatment, his low back pain and right buttock pain gradually improved. Serial follow-up MRI demonstrated progressive resolution of the epidural fluid accumulation (Fig. 28.4).

If an allergic reaction or foreign body reaction is suspected, the first-line treatment typically involves anti-inflammatory medications, such as corticosteroids or antihistamines. The patient's symptoms generally improve rapidly, and the epidural fluid collection is expected to resolve gradually over time. In such cases, there is no necessity for the removal of the artificial ligament, as the allergic or foreign body reaction does not typically warrant surgical intervention.

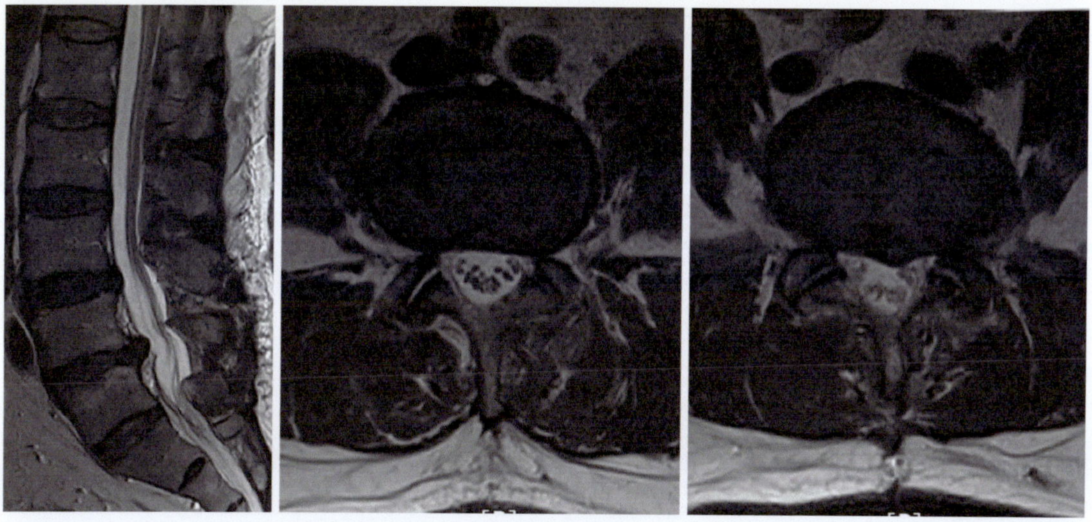

Fig. 28.2 Postoperative MRI showed fully neural decompression at the L3–4, L4–5

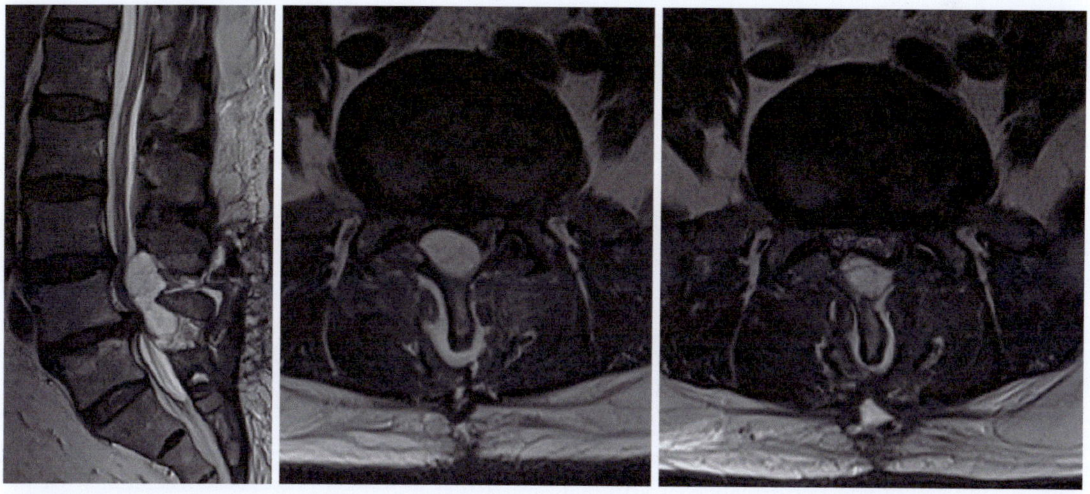

Fig. 28.3 Fluid accumulation on the epidural space of the previous surgical site on the follow-up MRI. It is presumed to be an allergic reaction of the artificial ligament

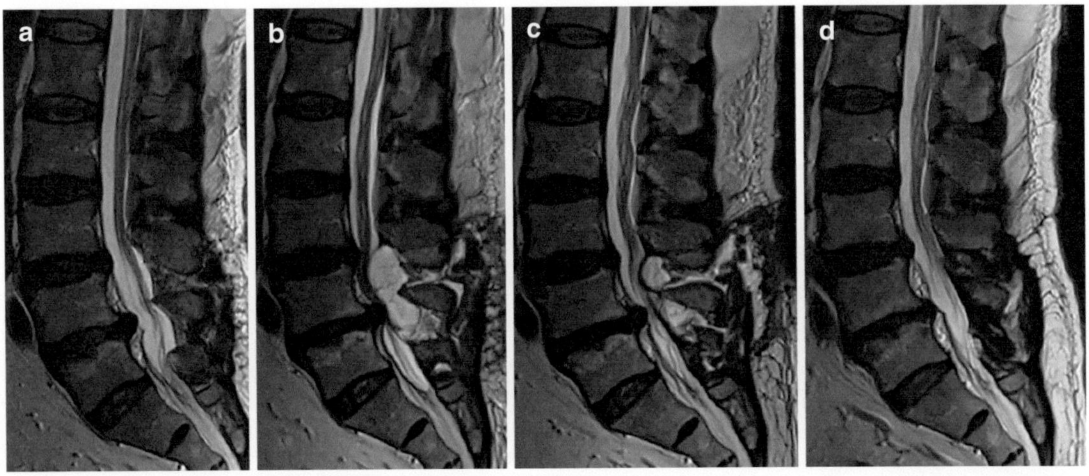

Fig. 28.4 Immediate postoperative MRI showed fully neural decompression at the L3–4, L4–5 on the postoperative day one (**a**), 3 weeks after surgery, first follow-up MRI demonstrated fluid accumulation on the epidural space of the previous surgical site (**b**), 7 weeks after surgery, the epidural fluid gradually disappeared (**c**), 3 months after surgery, the epidural fluid totally disappeared (**d**)

28.7 Conclusion

The use of PET-based artificial ligaments, such as the SHLee ligament, demonstrates excellent biocompatibility and durability, making it an effective solution for soft stabilization in elderly DLSS patients. While rare, foreign body reactions and allergic responses can occur and should be managed through appropriate medical interventions and patient monitoring. Advances in material engineering, such as surface modifications and improved manufacturing processes, continue to enhance the safety and performance of artificial ligaments. Soft stabilization with artificial ligaments represents a promising option for patients who are elderly or have comorbidities that preclude traditional fusion surgery.

References

1. Ratner BD, Bryant SJ. Biomaterials: where we have been and where we are going. Annu Rev Biomed Eng. 2004;6:41–75.
2. Williams DF. On the mechanisms of biocompatibility. Biomaterials. 2008;29(20):2941–53.
3. Teo AJT, Mishra A, Park I, Kim YJ, Park WT, Yoon YJ. Polymeric biomaterials for medical implants and devices. ACS Biomater Sci Eng. 2016;2:454–72.
4. Katti KS. Biomaterials in total joint replacement. Colloids Surf B Biointerfaces. 2004;39(3):133–42.
5. Paxton NC, Allenby MC, Lewis PM, Woodruff MA. Biomedical applications of polyethylene. Eur Polym J (Elsevier Ltd). 2019;118:412–28.
6. Fishman JM, Wiles K, Wood KJ. The acquired immune system response to biomaterials, including both naturally occurring and synthetic biomaterials. In: Host response to biomaterials: the impact of host response on biomaterial selection. Elsevier Inc; 2015. p. 151–87.
7. Wang CH, Guo ZS, Pang F, Zhang LY, Yan M, Yan JH, et al. Effects of graphene modification on the bioactivation of polyethylene-terephthalate-based artificial ligaments. ACS Appl Mater Interfaces. 2015;7(28):15263–76.
8. Anderson JM, Jiang S. Implications of the acute and chronic inflammatory response and the foreign body reaction to the immune response of implanted biomaterials. In: The immune response to implanted materials and devices: the impact of the immune system on the success of an implant. Springer International Publishing; 2016. p. 15–36.
9. Anderson JM, Rodriguez A, Chang DT. Foreign body reaction to biomaterials. Semin Immunol. 2008;20:86–100.
10. Meyers SR, Grinstaff MW. Biocompatible and bioactive surface modifications for prolonged in vivo efficacy. Chem Rev. 2012;112:1615–32.

11. Klopfleisch R, Jung F. The pathology of the foreign body reaction against biomaterials. J Biomed Mater Res A (John Wiley and Sons Inc.). 2017;105:927–40.
12. Swar S, Zajícová V, Rysová M, Lovětinská-Šlamborová I, Voleský L, Stibor I. Biocompatible surface modification of poly(ethylene terephthalate) focused on pathogenic bacteria: promising prospects in biomedical applications. J Appl Polym Sci. 2017;134(26).
13. Saito T, Takemoto M, Fukuda A, Kuroda Y, Fujibayashi S, Neo M, et al. Effect of titania-based surface modification of polyethylene terephthalate on bone-implant bonding and peri-implant tissue reaction. Acta Biomater. 2011;7(4):1558–69.

29 Dural Tear

Pratyush Shahi and Sang-Ha Shin

Abstract

Like other lumbar spine surgeries, dural tear is a known complication of open midline decompression (OMD) and ligament reconstruction. It is mostly identified and repaired intraoperatively. Repair can be direct (suture repair) (preferred method) or indirect (fat/muscle graft, artificial dura, collagen matrix, gelatin sponge, fibrin, fibrin glue, polyethylene glycol). In case of large dural defect where suture repair alone is insufficient for closure, we prefer using artificial dura as inlay graft and securing it to the dura with sutures leading to a watertight closure. Revision surgery may be required in cases with symptomatic delayed presentation due to CSF leak or pseudomeningocele formation. Scar tissue formation is less after ligament reconstruction compared to conventional decompression enabling an easier dissection in revision surgery. Horizontal ligament is removed, which gives access to the spinal canal. Dural defect is identified and repaired. After dural repair, horizontal ligament is reattached to maintain ligament reconstruction.

Keywords

Dural tear · Durotomy · Ligament reconstruction · Soft stabilization · Dura repair · Artificial dura

29.1 Introduction

Dural tear is a common complication seen in lumbar spine surgery. Although it is mostly identified and addressed intraoperatively, patients can also have a delayed presentation with symptoms resulting from cerebrospinal fluid (CSF) leak and pseudomeningocele formation [1, 2]. Similar to other types of lumbar spine surgery, open midline decompression (OMD) and ligament reconstruction surgery can also be associated with dural tear and its associated complications. In this chapter, we describe the surgical management of dural tear occurring in OMD and ligament reconstruction surgery.

P. Shahi
Department of Orthopedics, Cheongdam Wooridul Spine Hospital, Seoul, Korea (Republic of)

S.-H. Shin (✉)
Department of Neurosurgery, Cheongdam Wooridul Spine Hospital, Seoul, Korea (Republic of)
e-mail: burrhoer@wooridul.co.kr

S.-H. Lee et al. (eds.), *Ligament Reconstruction for Spine*,
https://doi.org/10.1007/978-981-95-3971-0_29

29.2 Dural Tear in Lumbar Spine Surgery

Dural tear with CSF leak is reported to be seen in 6–10% of lumbar spine surgeries [3]. It can be classified as acute or chronic (delayed), primary (pathological) or secondary (procedural), and intentional or accidental. Pathologies known to cause dural defect are ossified posterior longitudinal ligament (OPLL), ossified ligamentum flavum (OLF), hard/calcified disc, tumor, and trauma. Procedures associated with a higher risk of dural tear are revision surgery (adhesions), minimally invasive surgery (less visualization), and deformity surgery. Complications of dural tear include pseudomeningocele, nerve root entrapment (radiculopathy, cauda equina syndrome), intracranial hypotension (postural headache, photophobia, intracranial hemorrhage), delayed wound healing, and infection (meningitis, arachnoiditis) [4].

29.3 Dural Repair After OMD and Ligament Reconstruction

29.3.1 Primary Closure

Dural tear is identified and repaired intraoperatively in most cases. A primary closure of dural tear is performed as it is easy to secure adequate working space in OMD and ligament reconstruction surgery. Direct suture repair is preferred and can be performed with simple interrupted or continuous sutures (Fig. 29.1). 5–0/6–0 reverse cutting /round silk/prolene is utilized. Microsurgical instruments include micro-Bayonet forceps, micro-needle holder, micro-scissors, micro-dissector, and atraumatic suction tip. Indirect closure using fat/muscle graft, artificial dura (Neuropatch, Lyoplant, Duragen), collagen matrix (Durafoam), gelatin sponge (Gelfoam), fibrin (Tachocomb, Tachosil), fibrin glue (Tisseel), and polyethylene glycol (Duraseal) can also be performed [5]. In case of large dural defect where suture repair alone is insufficient for closure, we prefer using artificial dura as inlay graft and securing it to the dura with sutures leading to a watertight closure.

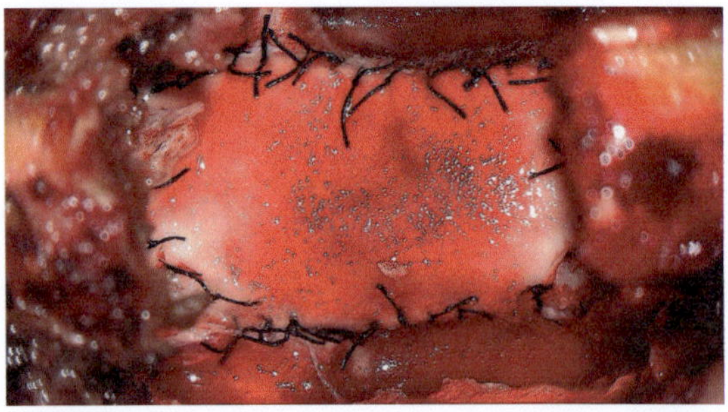

Fig. 29.1 Direct suture repair

29.3.2 Delayed Presentation

The same surgical incision is utilized for exposure. Postoperative fibrotic scar tissue formation is less after OMD and ligament reconstruction surgery compared to conventional decompression. Scar tissue is hence easier to dissect. The horizontal ligament is then removed and the spinal canal is exposed. Dural tear is identified and repaired. After this, the horizontal ligament is reattached and watertight closure is done. Unlike other artificial ligaments, the SH ligament incudes sagittal and horizontal ligaments. The operative field can be secured by removing only the horizontal ligament without cutting the ligament. After surgery, the horizontal ligament can be reattached to maintain ligament reconstruction. The conventional 8-shaped and 11-shaped ligaments require the removal of ligament.

29.4 Postoperative Protocol

Suction drain is kept for 2 days. It is maintained at half pressure until postoperative day 2. Drainage amount is monitored every 8 hours. If the drainage amount is >100 mL, suction pressure is removed. Patients are adviced bed rest for 2 days after which they are ambulated.

29.5 Illustrative Case

A 62-year-old female presented with low back pain, bilateral lower limb radiculopathy, and claudication for 3 years. She also complained of paresthesia in both lower limbs. There was no motor deficit. Magnetic Resonance Imaging (MRI) and myelogram showed L1-S1 spinal stenosis (Fig. 29.2a–f). Upon failure of conservative treatment, L1-S1 OMD and ligament reconstruction was performed. Postoperative MRI and myelogram showed adequate decompression (Fig. 29.2g–l). Patient reported significant improvement in symptoms after surgery. However, she presented with low back pain, radiculopathy, and urinary incontinence after 3 months. There was no postural headache or photophobia. MRI showed a large subcutaneous fluid collection due to CSF leak at L4–5 (Figs. 29.3 and 29.4). Revision surgery with dura repair was performed. The L4–5 horizontal ligament was removed and dural defect site was identified (Fig. 29.5a). The defect was too large for suture repair alone and hence was closed with the help of artificial dura (Lyodura). The artificial dura was used as an inlay graft and secured to the dura with sutures providing a watertight closure (Fig. 29.5b–h). Following watertight closure of the dural defect, CSF leakage was not seen. Tachosil was placed over the repair site (Fig. 29.5i). L4–5 horizontal ligament was reattached (Fig. 29.5j). Adequate irrigation was performed and wound closure was done in layers. Postoperative MRI was satisfactory and showed no CSF leakage (Fig. 29.6). Patient reported significant improvement in symptoms after surgery.

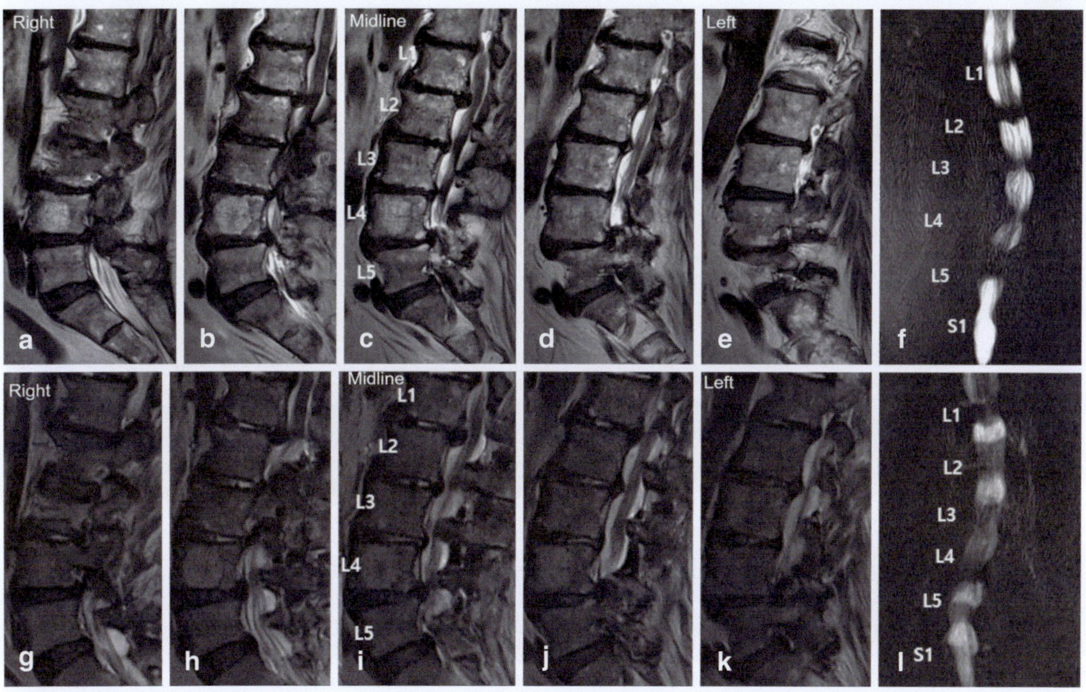

Fig. 29.2 (**a–f**) Preoperative MRI and myelogram showed L1-S1 spinal stenosis (**g–l**) Postoperative MRI and myelogram showed adequate decompression. MRI Magnetic Resonance Imaging

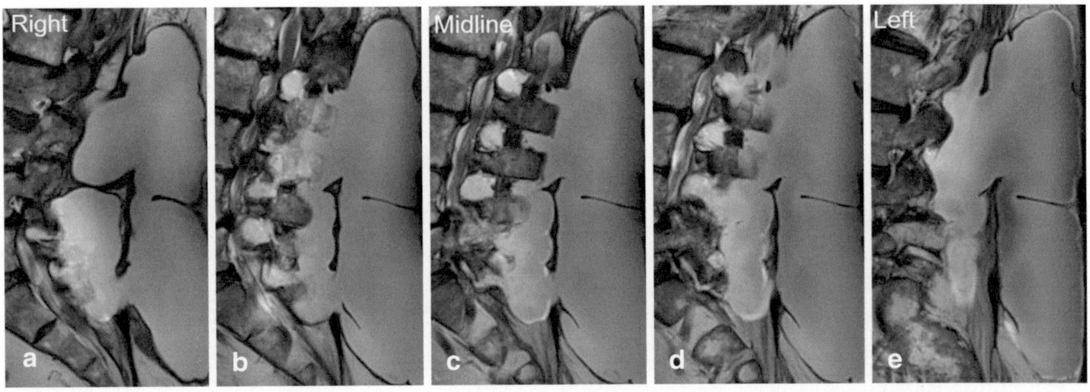

Fig. 29.3 Sagittal MRI showed large subcutaneous fluid collection. MRI Magnetic Resonance Imaging

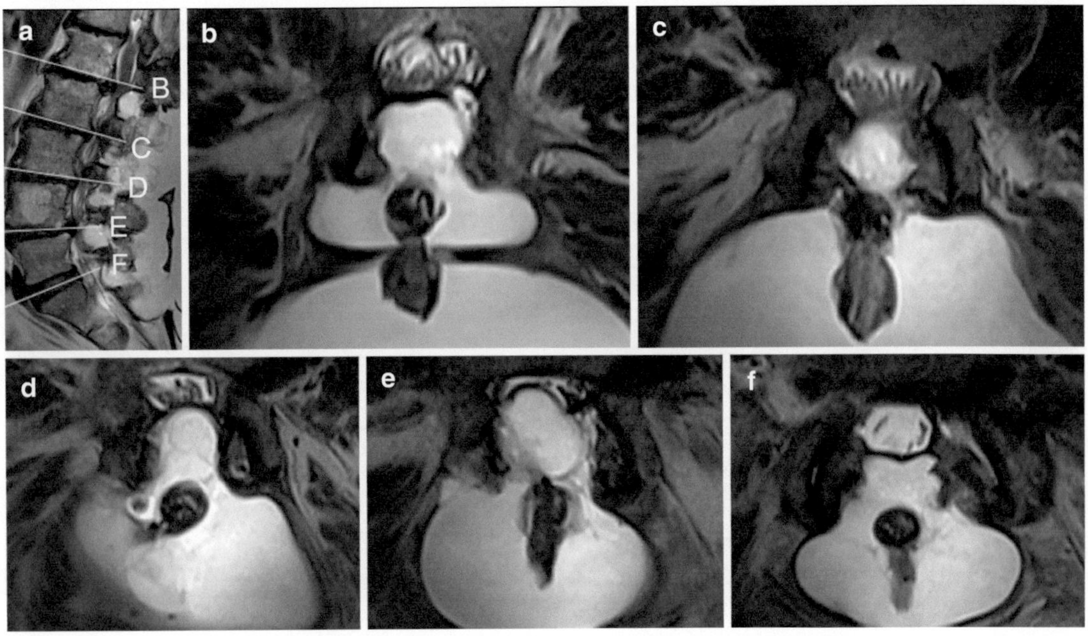

Fig. 29.4 Axial MRI showed CSF leak at L4–5. MRI Magnetic Resonance Imaging, CSF cerebrospinal fluid

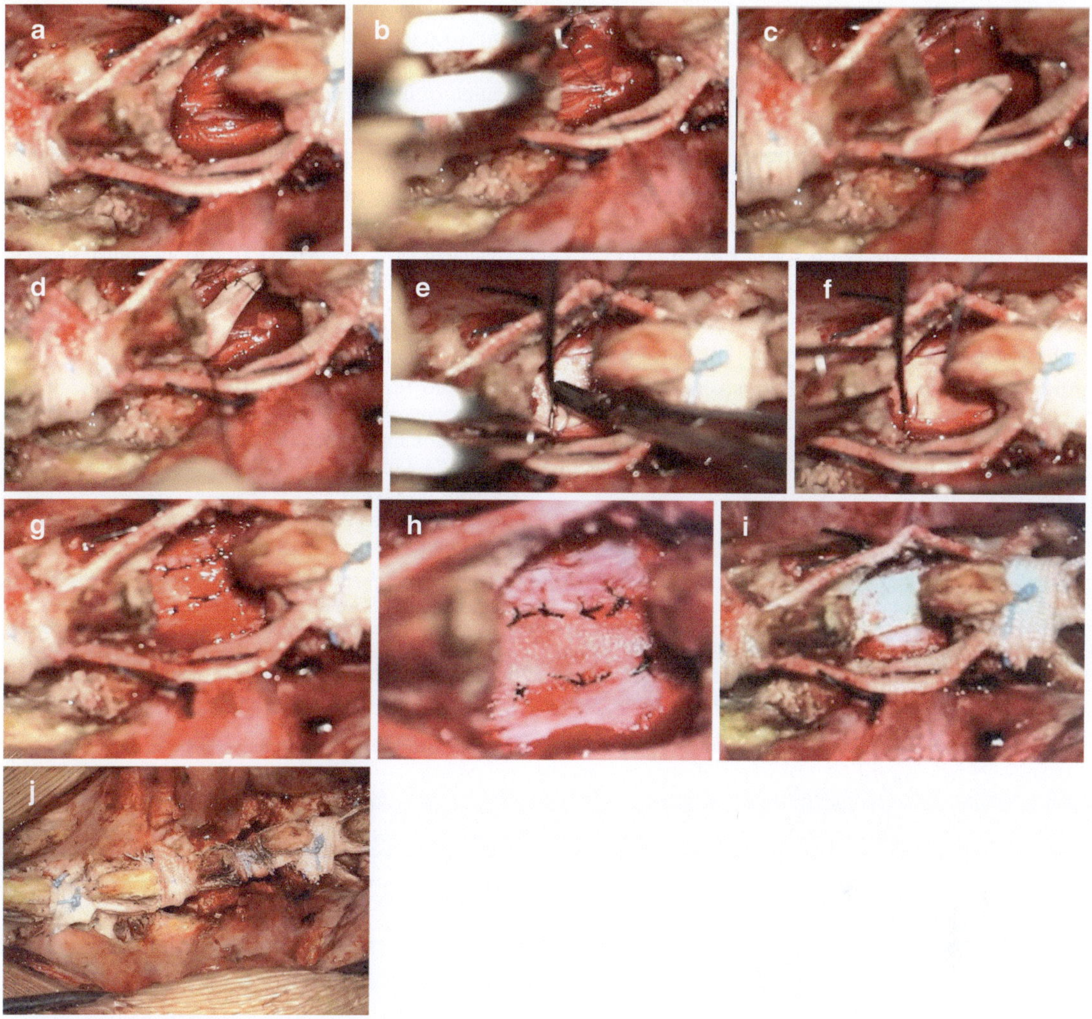

Fig. 29.5 Revision surgery for dural defect closure. (**a**) L4–5 horizontal ligament was removed and dural defect site was identified. (**b–h**) Artificial dura was used as an inlay graft and secured to the dura with sutures providing a watertight closure. (**i**) Tachosil was placed over the repair site. (**j**) L4–5 horizontal ligament was reattached to maintain ligament reconstruction

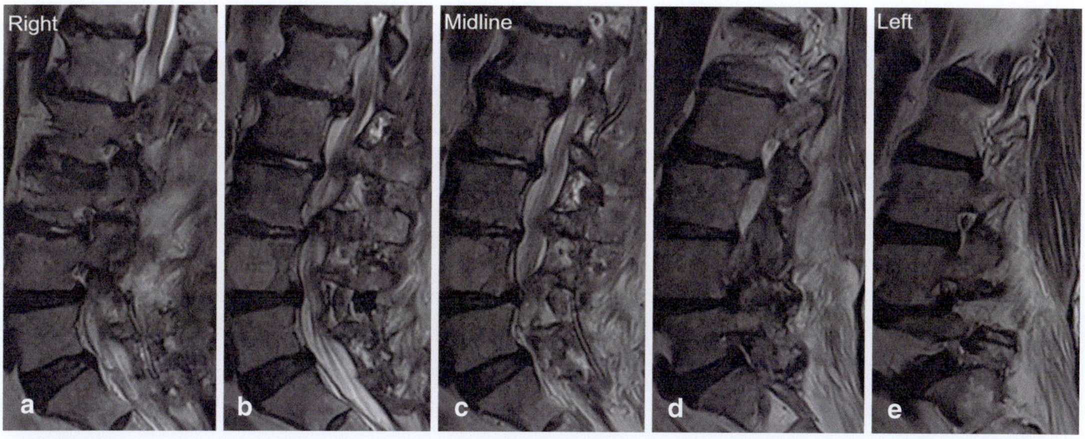

Fig. 29.6 Postoperative MRI showed no CSF leakage. MRI Magnetic Resonance Imaging, CSF cerebrospinal fluid

29.6 Summary

Dural tear can occur during OMD and ligament reconstruction surgery. It is mostly identified and repaired intraoperatively. Patients can also have a delayed presentation due to symptoms caused by CSF leakage and pseudomeningocele formation. Direct suture repair is the preferred method. In cases of large dural defect, suture repair alone is insufficient and artificial dura is used for a watertight closure. Revision surgery for dura repair after OMD and ligament reconstruction can be performed by removing the horizontal ligament and reattaching it after repair to maintain ligament reconstruction.

References

1. Espiritu MT, Rhyne A, Darden BV 2nd. Dural tears in spine surgery. J Am Acad Orthop Surg. 2010;18(9):537–45. https://doi.org/10.5435/00124635-201009000-00005. PMID: 20810935.
2. Xu C, Dong RP, Cheng XL, Zhao JW. Late presentation of dural tears: two case reports and review of literature. World J Clin Cases. 2023;11(11):2464–73. https://doi.org/10.12998/wjcc.v11.i11.2464. PMID: 37123324; PMCID: PMC10130997.
3. Alshameeri ZAF, El-Mubarak A, Kim E, Jasani V. A systematic review and meta-analysis on the management of accidental dural tears in spinal surgery: drowning in information but thirsty for a clear message. Eur Spine J. 2020;29(7):1671–85. https://doi.org/10.1007/s00586-020-06401-y. Epub 2020 Apr 15. PMID: 32296949.
4. Bosacco SJ, Gardner MJ, Guille JT. Evaluation and treatment of dural tears in lumbar spine surgery: a review. Clin Orthop Relat Res. 2001;389:238–47. https://doi.org/10.1097/00003086-200108000-00033. PMID: 11501817.
5. Choi EH, Chan AY, Brown NJ, Lien BV, Sahyouni R, Chan AK, Roufail J, Oh MY. Effectiveness of repair techniques for spinal dural tears: a systematic review. World Neurosurg. 2021;149:140–7. https://doi.org/10.1016/j.wneu.2021.02.079. Epub 2021 Feb 25. PMID: 33640528; PMCID: PMC8102333.

Facet Synovial Cyst

30

Pratyush Shahi and Sang-Ha Shin

Abstract

Facet cyst results from increased degeneration and fluid collection in the facet joint and can cause radiculopathy secondary to nerve compression. It can be seen after open midline decompression (OMD) and ligament reconstruction surgery. Surgical treatment is required upon failure of conservative measures. Scar tissue formation is less after ligament reconstruction compared to conventional decompression. Revision surgery can be performed by removing the horizontal ligament and reattaching it after resection of the facet cyst. Further extended laminectomy and facetectomy necessitating fusion are usually not required.

Keywords

Facet cyst · Resection · Revision surgery · Complication · Ligament reconstruction

P. Shahi
Department of Orthopedics, Cheongdam Wooridul Spine Hospital, Seoul, Korea (Republic of)

S.-H. Shin (✉)
Department of Neurosurgery, Cheongdam Wooridul Spine Hospital, Seoul, Korea (Republic of)
e-mail: burrhoer@wooridul.co.kr

S.-H. Lee et al. (eds.), *Ligament Reconstruction for Spine*,
https://doi.org/10.1007/978-981-95-3971-0_30

30.1 Introduction

Facet cyst arises from the anteromedial portion of the facet and can cause symptoms because of compression of the nerve roots and thecal sac. Surgical treatment is indicated upon failure of conservative measures. Although facet cyst mostly presents as a primary lesion, it has also been reported to develop after lumbar decompression surgery [1–3]. In this chapter, we discuss the occurrence of facet cyst after open midline decompression (OMD) and ligament reconstruction and describe its management.

30.2 Pathophysiology of Facet Cyst

Facet joints are lined by synovial membrane and lubricated by synovial fluid. These joints allow for smooth movements of the spine. With disc degeneration and loss of disc height, more load is transmitted through the facet joints causing facetal arthrosis. Degeneration of the facet joints and associated micromotion cause an increase in the production of synovial fluid. The accumulated fluid can cause outpouching of the synovial membrane and facet capsule, leading to the formation of a facet cyst [4].

This pathological process can be aggravated after lumbar decompression surgery because of two reasons [1–3]. Firstly, the medial portion of the facet joint becomes weaker after removal of ligamentum flavum. This enables an easy outpouching of the synovial membrane and facet capsule. The requirement of partial medial facetectomy for complete decompression may further weaken the medial portion and facilitate outpouching. Secondly, laminectomy can cause iatrogenic segmental instability. This causes micromotion in the facet joint and can lead to the formation of a facet cyst secondary to increased production of facetal fluid. OMD and soft stabilization require less removal of lamina and facet compared to conventional decompression and provide stability to the spine because of ligament reconstruction. Although the risk of facet cyst formation after OMD and soft stabilization is theoretically less compared to conventional decompression, it can still be seen postoperatively and needs to be adequately managed.

30.3 Surgical Treatment of Facet Cyst Occuring After Ligament Reconstruction

Patients with occurrence of facet cyst after OMD and ligament reconstruction surgery usually present with radiculopathy. A trial of conservative treatment including medications and physical therapy is first given. Upon failure of conservative measures, revision surgery is indicated.

30.3.1 Surgical Technique

The same surgical incision is utilized for exposure (Fig. 30.1a). Postoperative fibrotic scar tissue formation is less after OMD and ligament reconstruction surgery compared to conventional decompression. Scar tissue is hence easier to dis-

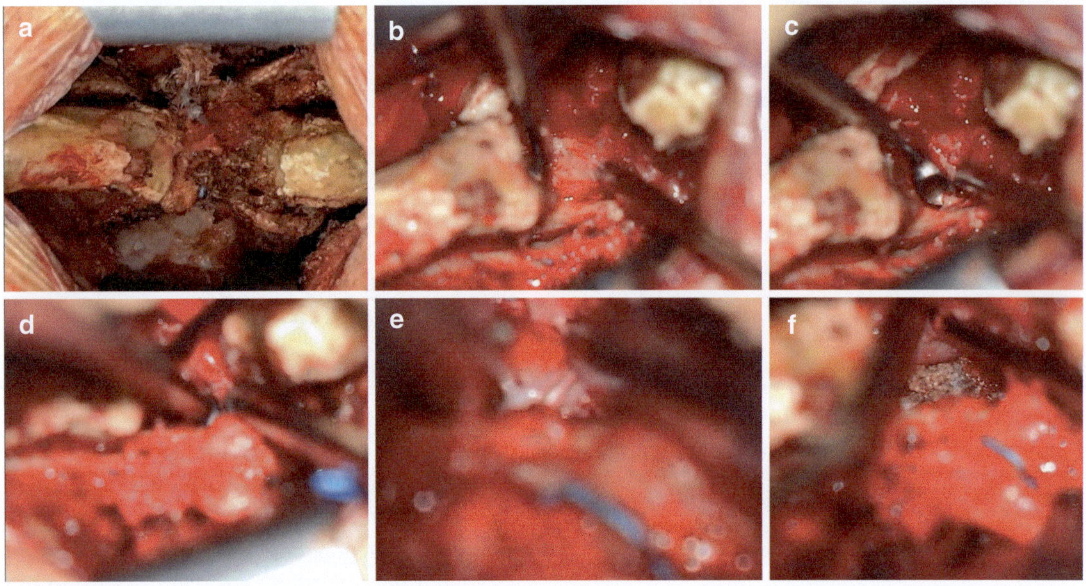

Fig. 30.1 (**a**) Artificial ligaments are seen after exposure; (**b**) Facet cyst is visualized; (**c**) Cyst is detached from the facet with a curette; (**d**) Some amount of medial facetectomy may be needed; (**e**) Facet cyst usually has fibrotic adhesions with the dura; (**f**) Complete removal of the facet cyst

sect, and bypassing it using further extended laminectomy and facetectomy is not required. The horizontal ligament is then removed and the spinal canal is exposed. Some amount of laminectomy may be required. The facet cyst is identified (Fig. 30.1b) and internally decompressed by opening its lining and evacuating its gel-like content. This relieves the nerve compression. The cyst is detached from the facet with the help of a curette (Fig. 30.1c). Some amount of medial facetectomy may be needed (Fig. 30.1d) to completely resect the lateral wall of the cyst for adequate decompression and prevention of recurrence. Facet cyst is usually found adhered to the dura (Fig. 30.1e). These fibrous adhesions are removed with a dissector. After separation from the dura, the cyst can be completely removed with the pituitary rongeur or Kerrison punch. After removal of facet cyst and adequate decompression (Fig. 30.1f), the horizontal ligament is reattached and closure is done. The conventional 8-shaped and 11-shaped ligaments require the removal of ligament, hence necessitating fusion.

30.4 Illustrative Cases

A 73-year-old woman presented with low back pain, radiating leg pain, and claudication for 3 years. Magnetic Resonance Imaging (MRI) and myelogram revealed significant spinal stenosis at L2–3, L3–4, and L4–5 (Fig. 30.2a–f). Multilevel OMD and ligament reconstruction were performed. Postoperative MRI and myelogram showed adequate decompression (Fig. 30.2g–l). Patient reported significant improvement in symptoms postoperatively. Three years after surgery, she presented again with radiating leg pain.

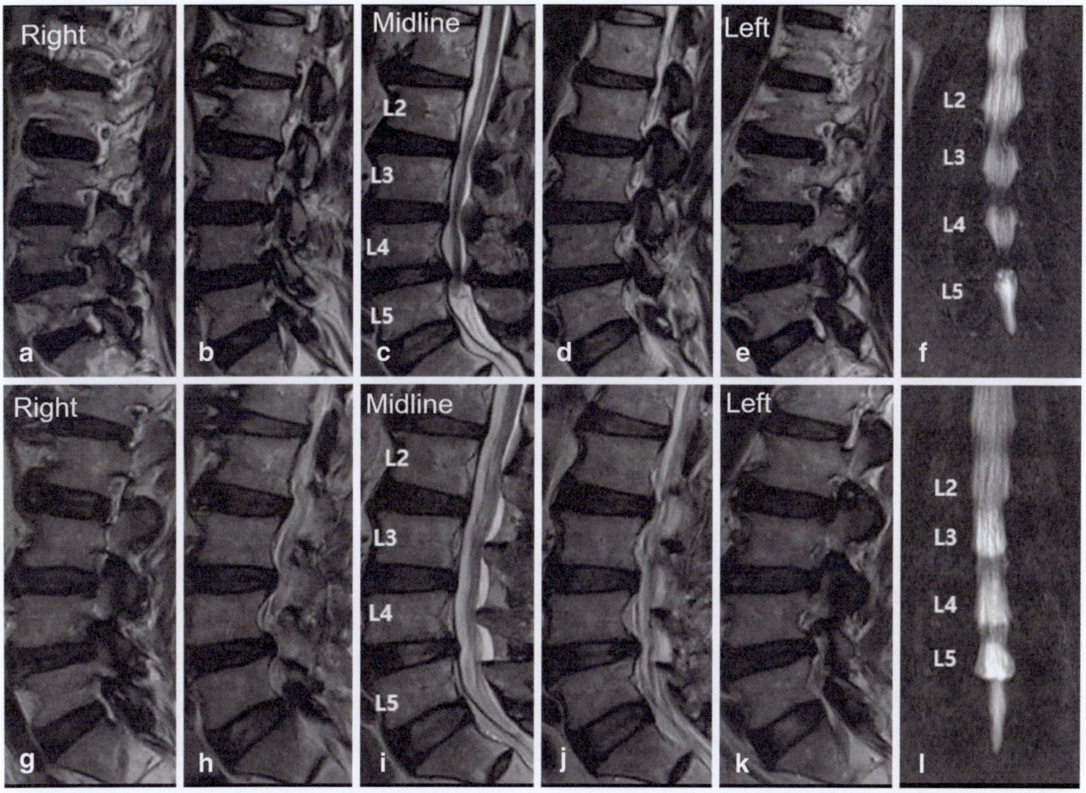

Fig. 30.2 (**a–f**) Preoperative MRI and myelogram showed spinal stenosis at L2–3, L3–4, and L4–5; (**g–l**) Postoperative MRI and myelogram after multilevel OMD and ligament reconstruction showed adequate decompression. MRI Magnetic Resonance Imaging, OMD open midline decompression

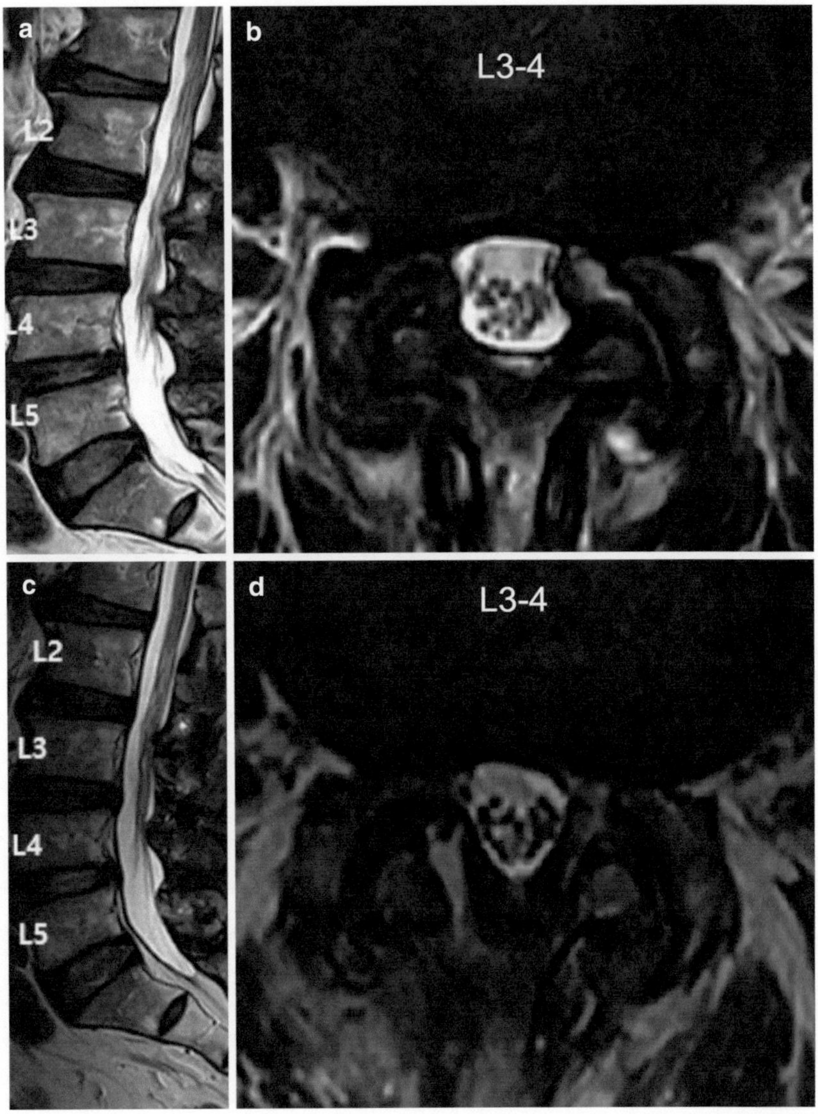

Fig. 30.3 (**a**, **b**) Preoperative MRI showed left-sided facet cyst at L3–4 after ligament reconstruction surgery; (**c**, **d**) Postoperative MRI showed complete removal of facet cyst and adequate decompression after revision surgery. MRI Magnetic Resonance Imaging

MRI showed left-sided facet cyst at L3–4 (Fig. 30.3a, b). Upon failure of conservative treatment, resection of the facet cyst was performed as describe above. Postoperative MRI showed complete removal of the cyst and adequate decompression (Fig. 30.3c, d). Surgery led to resolution of the patient's symptoms.

Preoperative and postoperative MRI of three other cases where resection of facet cyst occurring after ligament reconstruction surgery was performed with the same surgical technique have been demonstrated in Figs. 30.4, 30.5, and 30.6.

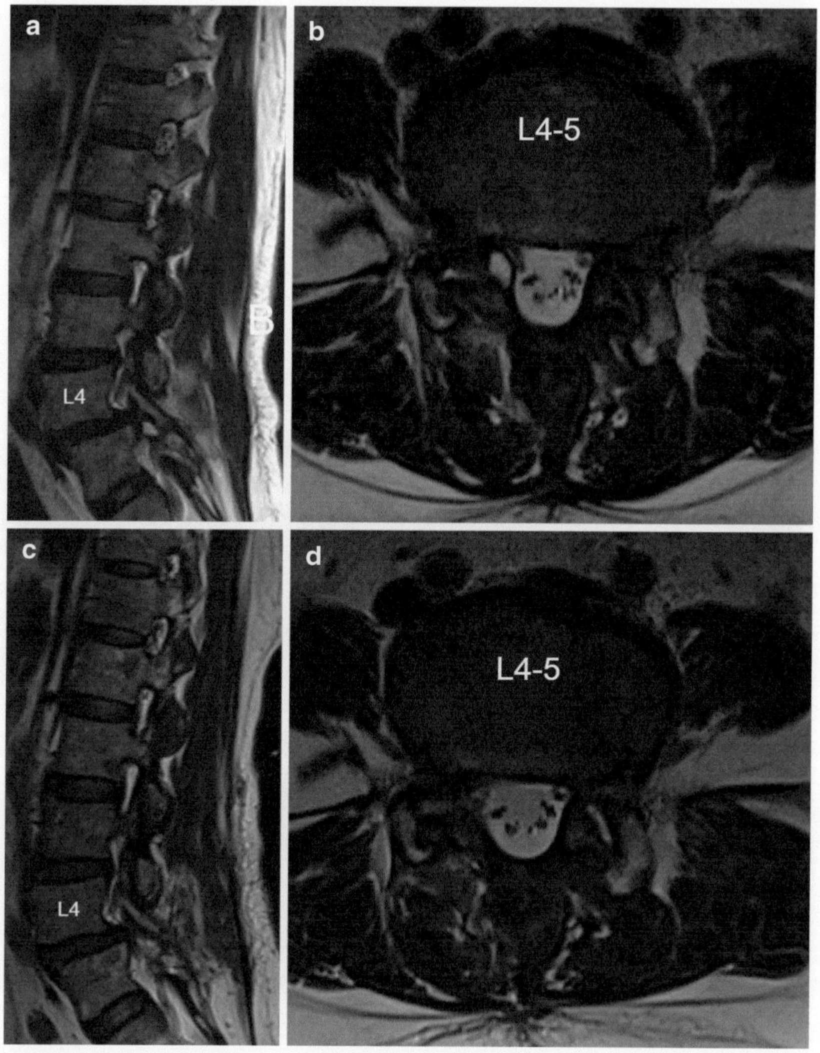

Fig. 30.4 (**a, b**) Preoperative MRI showed right-sided facet cyst at L4–5 after ligament reconstruction surgery; (**c, d**) Postoperative MRI showed complete removal of facet cyst and adequate decompression after revision surgery. MRI Magnetic Resonance Imaging

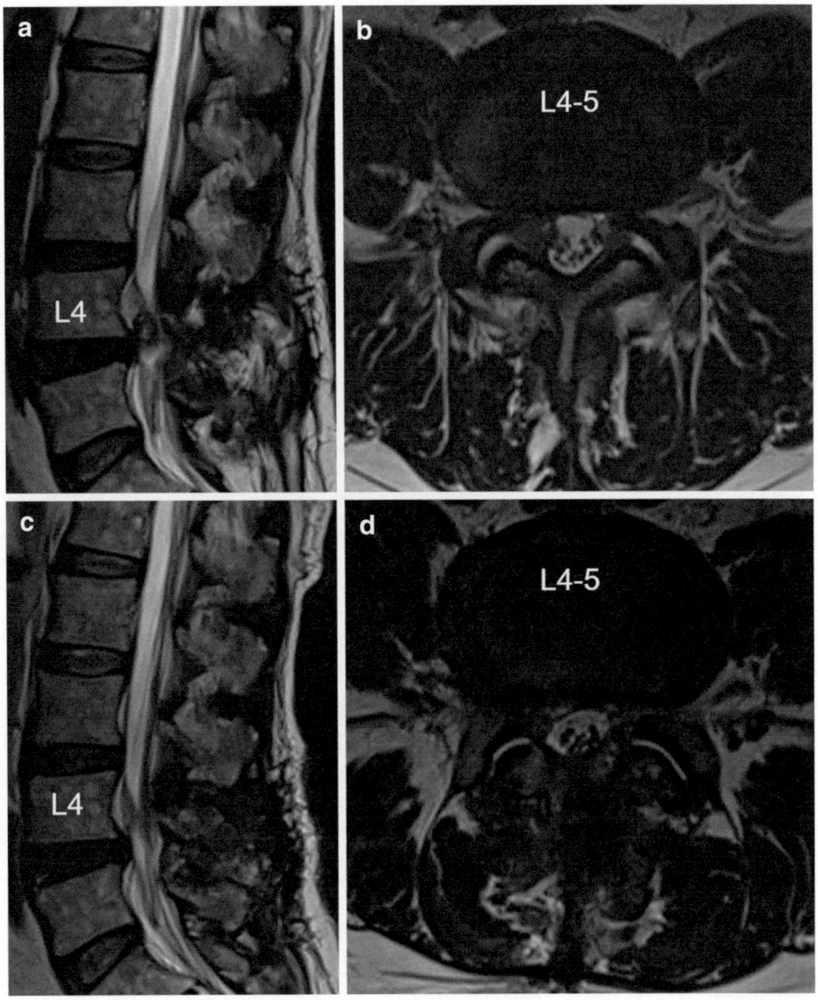

Fig. 30.5 (**a**, **b**) Preoperative MRI showed right-sided facet cyst at L4–5 after ligament reconstruction surgery; (**c**, **d**) Postoperative MRI showed complete removal of facet cyst and adequate decompression after revision surgery. MRI Magnetic Resonance Imaging

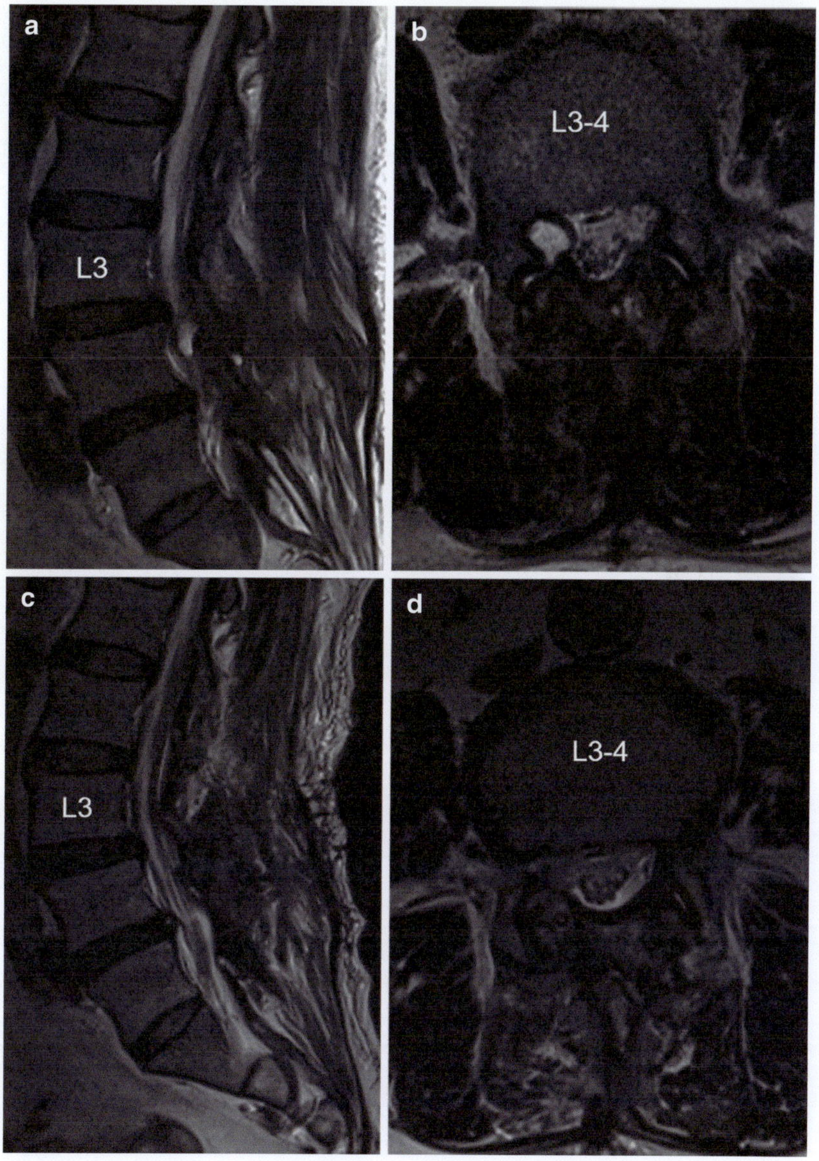

Fig. 30.6 (**a**, **b**) Preoperative MRI showed right-sided facet cyst at L3–4 after ligament reconstruction surgery; (**c**, **d**) Postoperative MRI showed complete removal of facet cyst and adequate decompression after revision surgery. MRI Magnetic Resonance Imaging

30.5 Summary

Formation of facet cyst can occur after OMD and ligament reconstruction surgery. Revision surgery is indicated if conservative treatment fails. Removal of facet cyst after ligament reconstruction does not require further extended laminectomy and facetectomy. Scar tissue formation is less compared to conventional decompression. Resection of the facet cyst can be performed by removing the horizontal ligament, which can be reattached after surgery.

References

1. Morishita Y, Taniguchi R, Kawano O, Maeda T. Synovial facet joint cysts after lumbar posterior decompression surgery. J Neurosurg Spine. 2021;35(6):704–9. https://doi.org/10.3171/2021.2.SPINE201671. PMID: 34416717.

2. Ikuta K, Tono O, Oga M. Prevalence and clinical features of intraspinal facet cysts after decompression surgery for lumbar spinal stenosis. J Neurosurg Spine. 2009;10(6):617–22. https://doi.org/10.3171/2009.2.SPINE08769. PMID: 19558297.
3. Seo JH, Park G, Ju CI, Kim SW, Lee SM. Radiological analysis of symptomatic complications after bilateral laminotomy for lumbar spinal stenosis. Korean J Spine. 2012;9(1):18–23. https://doi.org/10.14245/kjs.2012.9.1.18. Epub 2012 Mar 31. PMID: 25983783; PMCID: PMC4432379.
4. Boody BS, Savage JW. Evaluation and treatment of lumbar facet cysts. J Am Acad Orthop Surg. 2016;24(12):829–42. https://doi.org/10.5435/JAAOS-D-14-00461. PMID: 27792054.

MIX
Papier aus verantwortungsvollen Quellen
Paper from responsible sources
FSC® C105338

If you have any concerns about our products,
you can contact us on
ProductSafety@springernature.com

In case Publisher is established outside the EU,
the EU authorized representative is:
Springer Nature Customer Service Center GmbH
Europaplatz 3, 69115 Heidelberg, Germany

Printed by Libri Plureos GmbH
in Hamburg, Germany